Commissioning Editor: *Ellen Green/Pauline Graham*
Development Editor: *Ailsa Laing*
Project Manager: *Joannah Duncan*
Designer: *Stewart Larking*
Illustrations Manager: *Gillian Murray*

MUNRO KERR'S OPERATIVE OBSTETRICS

CENTENARY EDITION (ELEVENTH)

THOMAS F. BASKETT

MB BCh BAO(The Queen's University of Belfast)
FRCS(C) FRCS(Ed) FRCOG FACOG DHMSA

Professor, Department of Obstetrics and Gynaecology,
Dalhousie University, Halifax,
Nova Scotia, Canada

ANDREW A. CALDER

MB ChB, MD(University of Glasgow)
FRCS(Ed) FRCP(Glas) FRCP(Ed) FRCOG HonFCOG(SA)

Professor and Head, Department of Obstetrics and Gynaecology,
University of Edinburgh, UK

SABARATNAM ARULKUMARAN

MB BS(University of Ceylon) MD PhD FRCS(Ed)
FRCOG FACOG HonFCOG(SA)

Professor and Head, Department of Obstetrics and Gynaecology,
St. George's University Medical School,
London, UK

Illustrated by IAN RAMSDEN

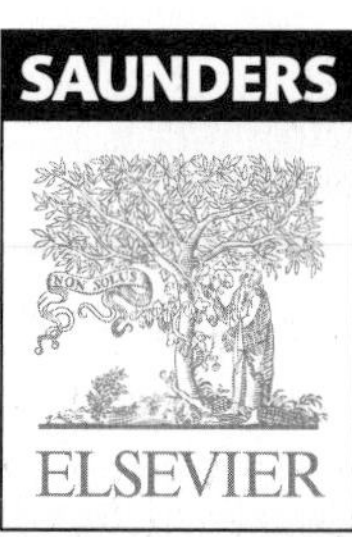

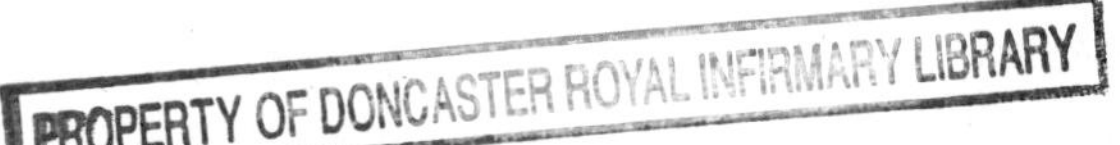

Edinburgh London New York Oxford Philadelphia St Louis Sydney Toronto 2007

SAUNDERS
ELSEVIER

First published 1908 as *Operative Midwifery* by J. Munro Kerr
Second edition 1911
Third edition 1916
Fourth edition 1937 as *Operative Obstetrics* by J. Munro Kerr, D. McIntyre and D. Fyfe Anderson
Fifth edition 1949 by J. Munro Kerr and J. Chassar Moir
Sixth edition 1956 and Seventh edition 1964 as *Munro Kerr's Operative Obstetrics* by J. Chassar Moir
Eighth edition 1971 by J. Chassar Moir and P. R. Myerscough
Ninth edition 1977 and Tenth edition 1982 by P. R. Myerscough
Eleventh (Centenary) edition 2007 by T. F. Baskett, A.A. Calder and S. Arulkumaran

ISBN 978-0-7020-2746-8

British Library Cataloguing in Publication Data
A catalogue record for this book is available from the British Library

Library of Congress Cataloging in Publication Data
A catalog record for this book is available from the Library of Congress

Note
Medical knowledge is constantly changing. Standard safety precautions must be followed, but as new research and clinical experience broaden our knowledge, changes in treatment and drug therapy may become necessary or appropriate. Readers are advised to check the most current product information provided by the manufacturer of each drug to be administered to verify the recommended dose, the method and duration of administration, and contraindications. It is the responsibility of the practitioner, relying on experience and knowledge of the patient, to determine dosages and the best treatment for each individual patient. Neither the Publisher nor the authors assume any liability for any injury and/or damage to persons or property arising from this publication.

The Publisher

Printed in China

Contents

It must be acknowledged that all errors of practice do not proceed from ignorance of the art. Some of them may justly be imputed to our entertaining too much confidence in our own dexterity, or too little dependence on the natural efforts and resources of the constitution... The abuse of art produces more and greater evils than are occasioned by the imperfections of Nature.

Thomas Denman, 1795

Preface

After a lapse of a quarter century since the tenth edition, we are pleased to produce the centenary edition of *Munro Kerr's Operative Obstetrics*. When Munro Kerr took up his pen to write the first edition in 1908, the maternal mortality in Britain was about 4 per thousand and the perinatal mortality was approximately 80 per thousand. At the time of writing this centenary edition those figures are about 0.1 and 10 respectively, which illustrates the enormous social and medical advances of the past century. However, in a number of developing countries the maternal and perinatal figures remain similar to or worse than when Munro Kerr wrote the first edition of his book. Many of the poor outcomes associated with intrapartum care are not due to a lack of elaborate technical equipment, but the misapplication of sound clinical and surgical principles.

In the first edition there were 37 chapters and 705 pages. The first 20 chapters (322 pages) dealt with dystocia involving the three Ps: the powers, the passenger and the passages – emphasizing the focus of intrapartum care in an era of contracted pelvis and high maternal mortality rates associated with caesarean section. Such has been the enormous decline in both maternal and perinatal mortality in the past century that obstetric practice has changed beyond recognition. As maternal mortality rates have fallen, the emphasis during intrapartum care has changed from the mother to the fetus. Within the era of the current authors' clinical practice, fetal viability has gone from 30–32 weeks to 24–25 weeks gestation, while caesarean section has gone from an operation of last resort to, in many hands, the operation of first resort. Nevertheless, the imperative of ensuring a safe outcome for both the mother and her baby continues to be based on tried and tested principles of high quality clinical care.

As with previous editions, a background knowledge in obstetrics is assumed and this book is directed at the postgraduate student and practising obstetrician. Midwives working independently may also find much of relevance in these pages. The book is aimed at an international audience and some of the procedures outlined here will only have application in regions with few technical and hospital facilities. Thus, the advice and management outlined herein should be relevant for those working with limited resources, as well as those working in fully equipped tertiary care hospitals.

We have retained Munro Kerr's and his successors' rather pragmatic style without references to back every statement. We have therefore supplied a limited number of references and additional bibliography. Although we are in the evidence-based era of medicine, much of operative obstetrics remains *secundum artem*. However, we advise the reader to make use of the *Pregnancy and Childbirth Module of the Cochrane Database of Systematic Reviews*, particularly for areas where management is clearly unfolding.

We have included a number of historical quotes, as Munro Kerr himself was wont to do, to provide both historical and educational context.

We are grateful to Elsevier for allowing us to bring *Munro Kerr* back into the postgraduate obstetric educational fold.

T.F. Baskett
A.A. Calder
S. Arulkumaran

Introduction

'Munro Kerr', for almost a century a cornerstone of guidance and instruction on intrapartum care to generations of obstetricians, first made its appearance in 1908 entitled *Operative Midwifery*. Its author, John Martin Munro Kerr, described on the title page as President of the Glasgow Obstetrical and Gynaecological Society and formerly Assistant to the Regius Professor of Midwifery at Glasgow University, was at that time Obstetric Physician at Glasgow Maternity Hospital and Gynaecologist at the Western Infirmary, Glasgow, Scotland.

The first edition, published as were the first ten by Ballière, Tindall and Cox of London, ran to 705 pages and contained 294 illustrations. The second edition published a mere three years later in 1911 had seven fewer pages and five more illustrations. Several years later a third edition was published, followed in 1937 by the fourth, which saw a change in title to *Operative Obstetrics*. This ran to 847 pages and contained 338 illustrations. For this edition Kerr enlisted the assistance of Donald McIntyre and David Fyfe Anderson, two young Glasgow colleagues. The fifth edition, in 1949, was a joint production with John Chassar Moir, to whom he handed the baton for sole authorship of *Munro Kerr's Operative Obstetrics*, the title it has since retained. After the sixth (1956) and the seventh (1964) editions, Moir teamed up with Philip Roger Myerscough for the eighth edition in 1971 and in turn Myerscough was principal author of the ninth (1977) and tenth (1982) editions.

Following this, Myerscough invited Andrew Calder, then Senior Lecturer in Obstetrics and Gynaecology in the University of Glasgow, to work with him on an eleventh edition. The need to find a new publisher and other difficulties occasioned substantial delays and by the end of the century Philip Myerscough, who had retired from clinical practice in 1992, felt that he should withdraw from the project. Prospective publishers also felt that a more international dimension might be served by a wider geographical spread of the authors. The triumvurate who have produced this eleventh edition will, we hope, fulfil this objective.

John Martin Munro Kerr was born in Glasgow in 1868 – the year after Lister had

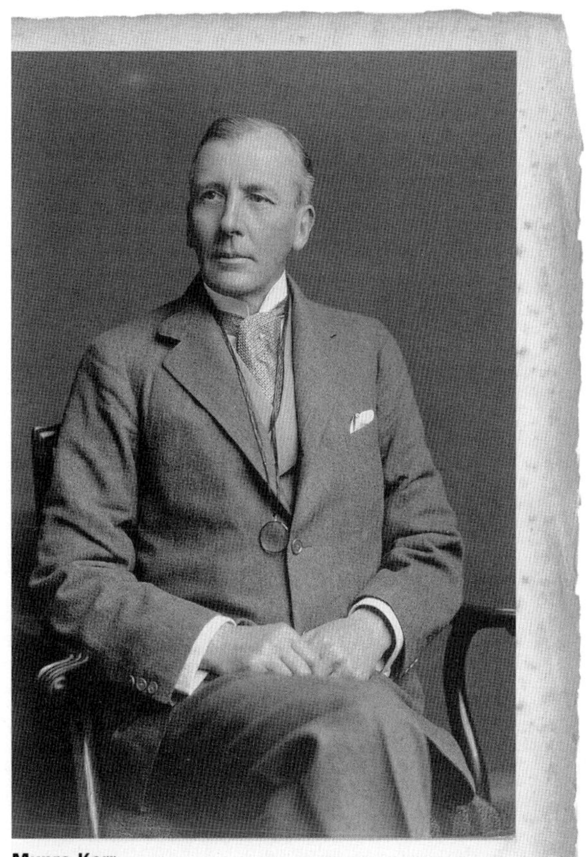

Munro Kerr

introduced his principles of antiseptic surgery in that city. Educated at Glasgow Academy and Glasgow University he occupied three different Chairs of 'Midwifery' in Glasgow: first and briefly in 1910 in Anderson's College of Medicine, then from 1911 till 1927 as the first occupant of the Muirhead Chair in Glasgow University, which was endowed to enhance the medical education of women, and finally, from 1927 until his retirement in 1934, he was Regius Professor of Midwifery. Foundation Vice-President of the (later Royal) College of Obstetricians and Gynaecologists in 1927, his other major publications were a classic monograph *Maternal Mortality and Morbidity* (1933) and his *Combined Textbook of Obstetrics and Gynaecology*, first published in 1923.

His most notable clinical innovations were his introduction and popularisation of the lower segment caesarean section in preference to the classical operation – for many years this was known in many parts of Europe as 'Kerr's operation' – and his development of the principles of 'trial of labour' in the management of cases of suspect cephalo-pelvic disproportion – the subject of an almost obsessive focus among the stunted, malnourished and rachitic gravidae in late 19th and early 20th century Glasgow.

Among his students and trainees Kerr could number many distinguished clinicians and academics, most notably Dugald Baird of Aberdeen.

Munro Kerr (Figure 1) received many honours and much international recognition. At the age of 87 he delivered the first William Hunter Memorial Lecture to the Glasgow Obstetrical and Gynaecological Society. He retired to Canterbury and in 1960 he died at the age of 92.

John Chassar Moir was born in Montrose, Scotland in 1900. A medical graduate of Edinburgh University he was the foundation Nuffield Professor of Obstetrics and Gynaecology when the Chair was established at the University of Oxford in 1937. Moir (Figure 2) is best remembered for his work with Sir Henry Dale and Harold Dudley on the isolation and clinical application of ergometrine in the prevention and management of postpartum haemorrhage. He was a brilliant gynaecological surgeon, notably in the treatment of vesico-vaginal fistulae, upon which subject he wrote a classic monograph. He died in 1977.

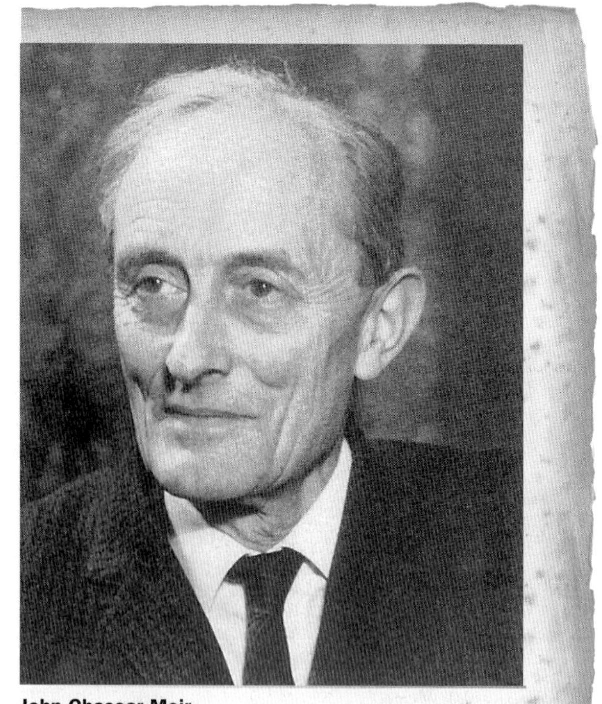

John Chassar Moir

Philip Roger Myerscough was born in Lancashire in 1924 and studied medicine in Edinburgh, where he spent his entire clinical career apart from a spell as WHO Visiting Professor at the University of Baroda in India. The consummate clinician and a highly prized teacher he was latterly Senior Obstetrician at the Simpson Memorial Maternity Pavilion at Edinburgh Royal Infirmary, until his retirement from the National Health Service in 1988. Myerscough (Figure 3) then spent a further 3 years in Muscat, Sultanate of Oman, teaching and directing the development of clinical services.

Thomas Firth Baskett was born in Belfast, Northern Ireland where he attended Belfast Royal Academy and the Queen's University of Belfast Medical School. Since completing his specialist training in the Belfast Teaching Hospitals he has lived and worked in Canada. He spent 10 years in Winnipeg, during which time he acted as a Consultant in Obstetrics

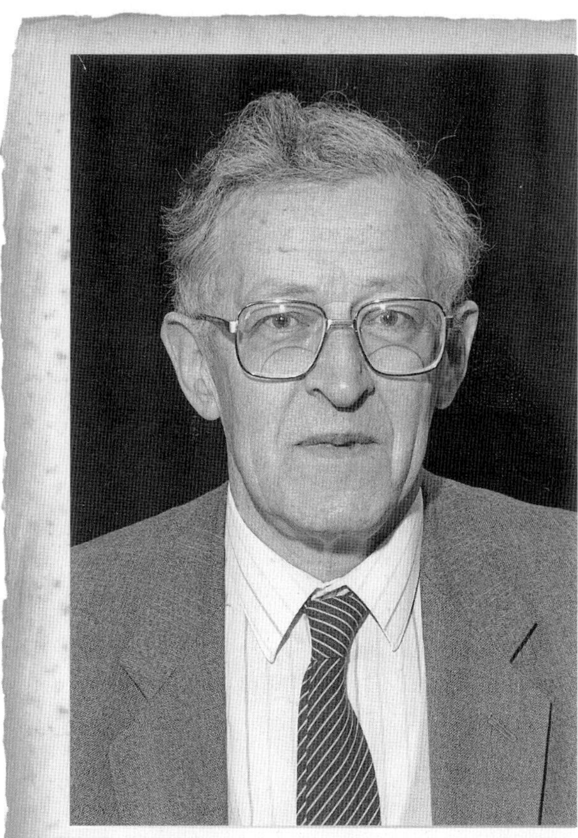

Philip Roger Myerscough

and Gynaecology to the Central Canadian Arctic, which he visited regularly. In 1980 he moved to Dalhousie University in Halifax, Nova Scotia where he is currently a Professor of Obstetrics and Gynaecology. He is a former President of the Society of Obstetricians and Gynaecologists of Canada and has written widely on clinical obstetrics and the history of medicine.

Andrew Alexander Calder was born in Aberdeen, Scotland and, like Munro Kerr, was educated at Glasgow Academy and the Glasgow University Medical School. After completing his basic specialist training in Glasgow Teaching Hospitals he was for 3 years Clinical Research Fellow in the Nuffield Department of Obstetrics and Gynaecology at Oxford with Sir Alexander Turnbull and Mostyn Embrey. After clinical academic posts at Glasgow Royal Maternity Hospital he was appointed in 1986 to the Chair of Obstetrics and Gynaecology in the University of Edinburgh. Formerly Chairman of The Academy of Royal Colleges and Faculties in Scotland and Vice Dean of the Edinburgh Medical School, he is currently Head of the Division of Reproductive and Developmental Sciences based at the Queen's Medical Research Institute and the Royal Infirmary of Edinbugh.

Sabaratnam Arulkumaran was born in Jaffa, Sri Lanka and undertook his medical training at the University of Ceylon. He took his clinical specialist training in Sri Lanka, the United Kingdom and Singapore. He became Professor and Head of the Department of Obstetrics and Gynaecology at the National University of Singapore from 1995 to 1997, Professor of Obstetrics and Gynaecology at the University of Nottingham in the UK from 1997 to 2001, and is currently Professor and Head of Obstetrics and Gynaecology at St. George's University of London. He was Secretary General of the International Federation of Gynecology and Obstetrics (FIGO) and is currently Vice President of Education at the Royal College of Obstetricians and Gynaecologists. He has wide international experience in teaching and publishing in the field of obstetrics.

1

Human birth

The safe and effective management of labour and delivery requires a clear understanding on the part of the birth attendant of the anatomy, physiology and biochemistry of human parturition and of its central participants – the mother and infant.

The 20th century, across most of which 'Munro Kerr' has stretched, witnessed the most spectacular growth and advance of medical science and with it a steady improvement in our understanding of the birth process. A hundred years ago the obstetrician's art depended mainly on the insights brought by the giants of 18th century obstetrics, notably William Smellie (1697–1763) and William Hunter (1718–1783), both incidentally born within 20 miles of Munro Kerr's birthplace. Smellie, who became acknowledged as 'The Master of British Midwifery', was the consummate man-midwife and teacher. His monumental *Treatise on the Theory and Practice of Midwifery* (1752), based on his extensive clinical experience, described and defined the birth process as never before and formed the basis for the clinical conduct of labour. His definition of the mechanisms of labour shed light on the convoluted journey through the birth canal which the fetus is required to follow. His *Sett of Anatomical Tables with Explanations and an Abridgement of the Practice of Midwifery* (1754) amplified these fundamental principles. This atlas, for which Smellie employed the Dutch artist Jan van Rymsdyk, was only surpassed 20 years later when Hunter, employing the same artist, published his spectacular *Anatomy of the Human Gravid Uterus* (1774).

A century ago when Munro Kerr was preparing *Operative Midwifery* there had been little additional progress. The relevant anatomy was fairly well understood but the physiology of the myometrium and cervix, and the biochemistry, endocrinology and pharmacology of human labour were almost entirely unknown. At the start of the new millennium the young obstetrician may consider that those mysteries have almost all been solved following a century of discoveries which saw the emergence of oxytocin, oestrogen, progesterone, prostaglandins and many other hitherto unknown substances. But it would be surprising indeed if the close of the 21st century does not reveal an even more complex picture.

Current understanding

As a starting point for the wide range of clinical issues addressed within this textbook, a brief review follows of some of the key elements of basic medical science pertaining to human labour and delivery as currently understood. This, by necessity, will be superficial and selective. For more detailed and comprehensive accounts the reader is referred to current textbooks of reproductive physiology, anatomy, biochemistry and endocrinology.

Myometrial function

The myometrium is the engine which drives human labour, during which it displays a highly sophisticated and co-ordinated set of forces. The simple objective of these is to efface and dilate the cervix and drive the fetus through the birth canal. In contrast to other smooth muscle systems, the myometrium displays three unique properties which are crucial for its function:

1. It must remain quiescent for the greater part of human pregnancy, suppressing its natural instinct to contract until called upon to do so at the appointed time.
2. During labour it must display a pattern which affords adequate periods of relaxation between contractions without which placental blood flow and fetal oxygenation would be compromised.
3. It possesses the capacity for *retraction*, vital to prevent exsanguination after delivery but also essential during labour. Retraction is a unique property of uterine muscle whereby a shorter length of the muscle fibre is maintained, without the consumption of energy, even after the contraction that produced the decrease in length has passed. As the cervix is effaced and pulled around the fetal presenting part, an inability of the myometrial fibres in the uterine corpus to retract, in essence to steadily reduce their relaxed lengths, would mean that the tension on the cervix could not be maintained.

At its most basic, human labour may be regarded as an interaction between the corpus and the cervix (Fig 1.1). For the maintenance of pregnancy the corpus must be quiescent and the cervix closed and uneffaced. In labour the corpus contracts and the cervix yields. A useful analogy may be to compare this process to the experience of putting on, for the first time, a roll-neck pullover. Just as with the fetus, the head must be flexed to present its smallest

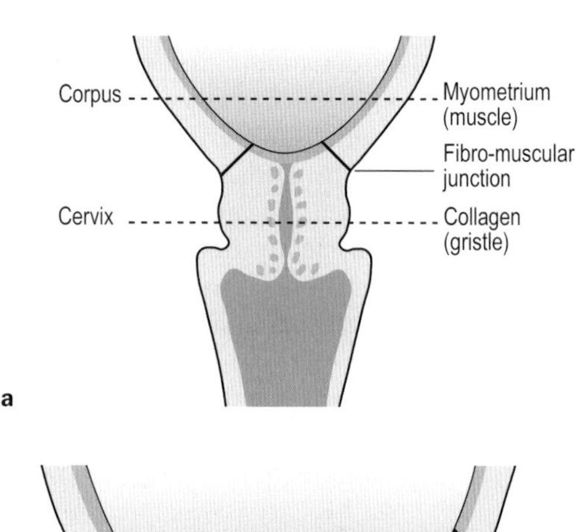

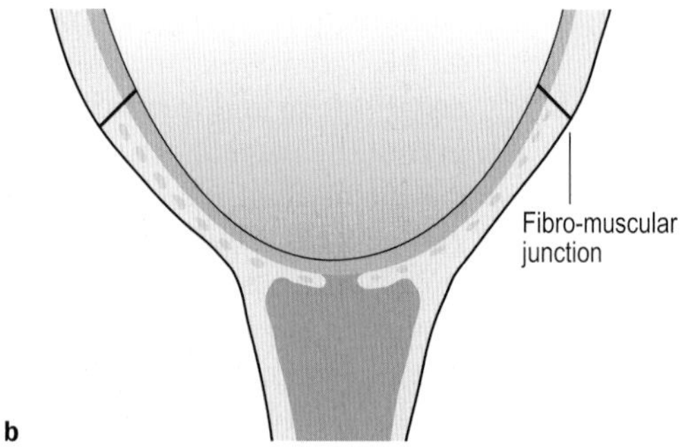

Figure 1.1 (a) Diagrammatic representation of the relationship of the uterine corpus and cervix in mid pregnancy. The interface between them is usefully described as the fibro-muscular junction (FMJ). (b) Cervix fully effaced at start of labour, in the primigravida

diameters to the cervix, or neck of the pullover, which is effaced round the presenting part and ultimately dilated as a result of traction applied by the arms, which are in this connection analogous to the myometrial fibres.

Although it has been conventional to acknowledge a 'lower uterine segment' arising from the uterine isthmus (between the nonpregnant corpus and cervix), in practice it may be more helpful simply to see the boundary between corpus and cervix as the 'fibromuscular junction' which marks the change from a mostly muscular corpus to a predominantly fibrous cervix. Obstetric purists may argue that the concept of a 'lower segment' is helpful in the definition of placenta praevia and in directing the site of contemporary caesarean sections but, those issues apart, it is of little relevance and it is a difficult concept to define either anatomically or physiologically.

At its simplest, contraction of the myometrial cell requires actin and myosin to combine in the contractile filament actomyosin (Fig 1.2). This reaction is catalyzed by the enzyme myosin-light-chain-kinase which is heavily calcium dependent. Calcium in turn relies for its availability on oxytocin and prostaglandin $F_{2\alpha}$ which transport it into the cell and also free it from intracellular stores. On the other hand this reaction is inhibited by progesterone, cyclic AMP and β-adrenergic agents. A particular insight into how the myometrial effort is co-ordinated into a concerted function came from the recognition of the essential requirement for gap junctions (biochemically characterized as Connexin-43) to be formed between individual myometrial cells, allowing cell-to-cell transmission of electrical impulses and ions. Thus, the corpus can display a wave of contractility propagated across its cell population which becomes a functional syncytium rather than a disorganized rabble of individual muscle fibres.

The cervix

The recognition, little more than 50 years ago, that the cervix possesses a distinct structure based on collagen-rich connective tissue rather than smooth muscle has been fundamental to a better understanding of its function. It is thus not a 'sphincter' of the uterus but rather a tough, rigid obstacle to delivery which has to undergo a profound change in consistency

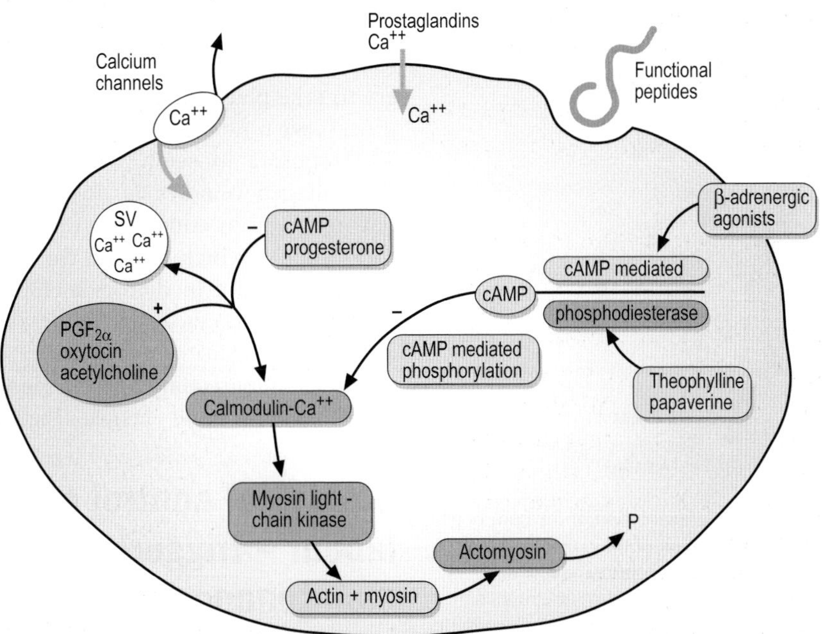

Figure 1.2 Schematic representation of the contractile process of the myometrial cell. Those components shown in dark boxes represent contraction, those in light boxes represent relaxation.

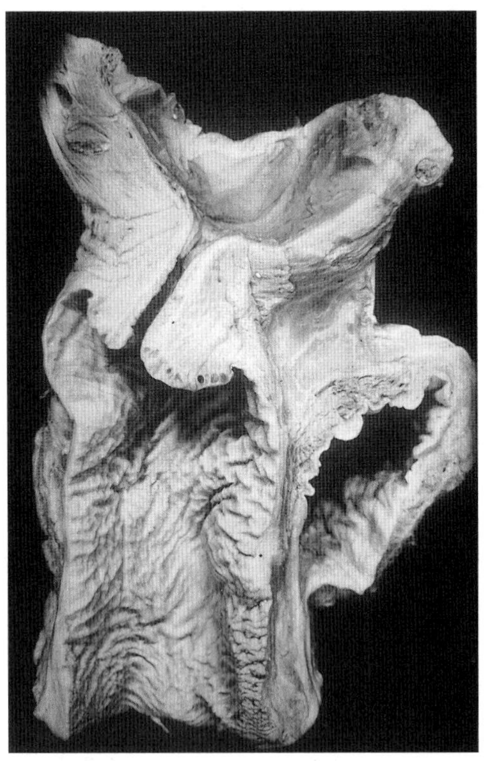

a

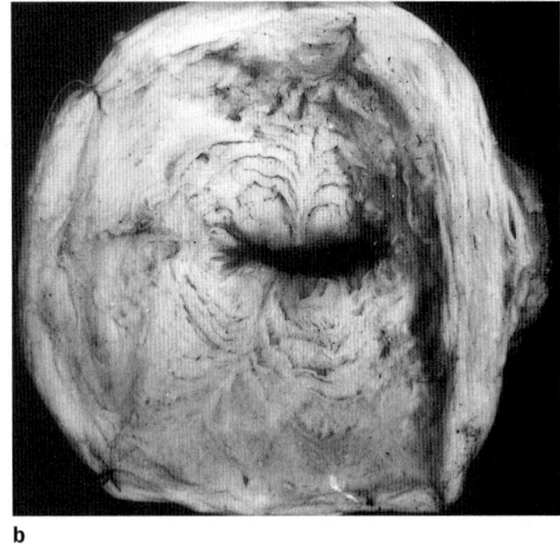

b

Figure 1.3 Original dissections prepared by William Hunter in the 18th century. That on the left (a) shows the lower part of the uterus, cervix, vagina, bladder and urethra in sagittal section in the last few weeks of pregnancy. That on the right (b) shows the cervix from the intrauterine aspect as it undergoes effacement in the last month of pregnancy (the fibromuscular junction is now at the periphery of this specimen).

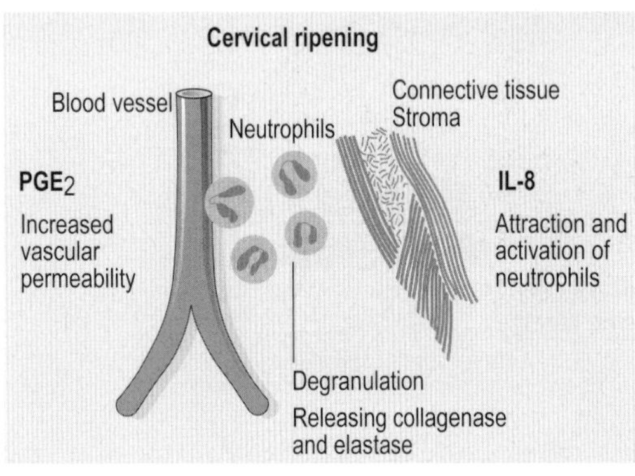

Figure 1.4 Schematic representation of the control of cervical ripening. The collagen of the cervical stroma is broken down by matrix metalloproteinases, such as collagenase and elastase derived from neutrophils in an inflammatory-like process which requires them to be drawn into the tissue under the influence of interleukin-8 (IL8) from capillaries which have been dilated and made more permeable by prostaglandin E_2 (PGE_2)

to permit effacement, dilatation and delivery to take place (Fig 1.3). That change is the process we now describe as 'cervical ripening'. The requisite loosening and degradation of the collagen bundles is now recognized as having much in common with an inflammatory process, which requires the participation of inflammatory mediators including prostaglandin E2 and cytokines (especially interleukin-8), the recruitment of neutrophils, and the synthesis of matrix metalloproteinases including collagenases and elastase (Fig 1.4).

Biological control of labour – triggering and maintenance

The process by which the labour process is triggered and maintained has been the subject of intensive investigations. The clinical drive to this area of research has been the desire:

- to better understand, prevent or suppress preterm labour with all its complications
- to improve our ability to correct abnormal uterine action and poor progress in labour
- to enhance our capacity to induce effective labour when dictated by clinical circumstances.

The following brief review oversimplifies what is a most complex set of interactions, but it may suffice as a basis for rational clinical intervention. It is now recognized that the trigger for parturition comes from the fetus rather than from the mother. The maturing fetal brain is thought to provoke the release of corticotrophin from the fetal pituitary gland (Fig 1.5). This may be considered analogous to the switching on of pituitary gonadotrophin production at the time of puberty. The fetal adrenal gland responds by releasing two main products, cortisol and dehydroepiandrosterone sulphate:

- Cortisol stimulates fetal pulmonary surfactant production to mature the lungs for extrauterine function and may also influence other organ systems. This is thought to result in changes in the composition of the amniotic fluid which provoke the release of prostaglandin E2 from the amnion. This may be important for a direct influence on the cervix, especially focused at the internal os as this is the portion of the cervix which lies in intimate contact with the fetal membranes. The internal os needs to ripen first to initiate cervical effacement. To do this the activity of the principal prostaglandin degrading enzyme PG dehydrogenase within the chorion must decline, a phenomenon which has recently been confirmed.
- Dehydro-epiandrosterone sulphate is metabolized in the placenta to enhance oestradiol levels which may provoke the release of prostaglandin $F_{2\alpha}$ from its richest source, the decidua, thereby exciting myometrial contractions.

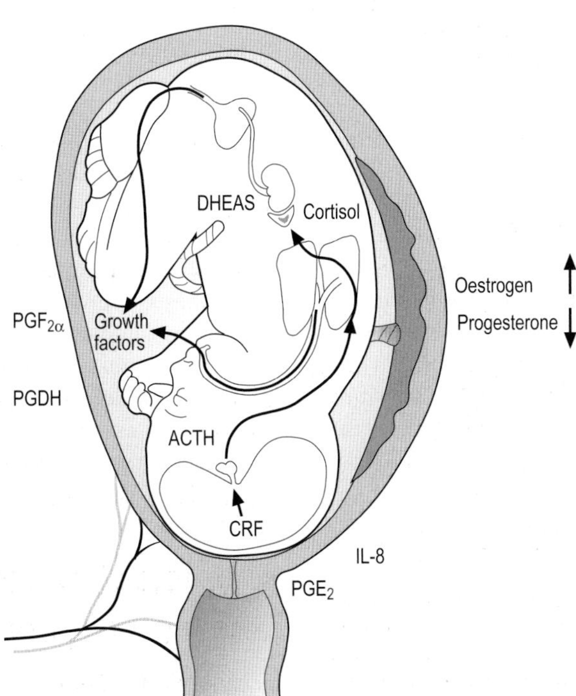

Figure 1.5 Fetal control of the onset of labour is thought to result from activation of its hypothalamo-pituitary-adrenal axis, which leads in turn to modification of placental steroid production and activation of prostaglandins in the decidua and cervix.

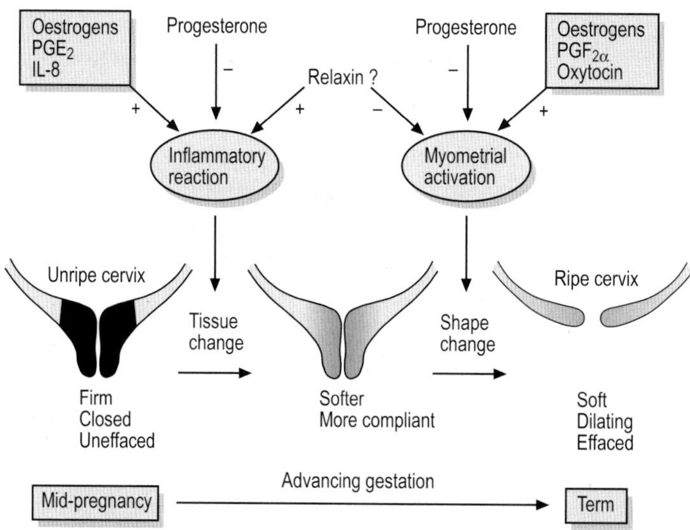

Figure 1.6 A schematic representation of the factors which bring about the softening and dilation of the cervix during the transition from pregnancy maintenance to parturition.

Progesterone remains the principal enigma. It is known to inhibit both myometrial contractility and the formation of gap junctions, and is also recognized as supporting the activity of prostaglandin dehydrogenase, but evidence for its withdrawal prior to parturition remains elusive. It seems likely that there is either a process whereby its activity at tissue level declines without a drop in circulating levels, or simply that its influence is overcome by other factors.

We can therefore postulate that a cascade of endocrine changes initiated by the fetal brain results in the activation of a variety of endocrine and inflammatory substances which have the effect of co-ordinating three key events:

- maturing essential fetal organ systems, notably the lungs, for the challenges of extrauterine life
- transforming the rigid cervix into a compliant and readily dilatable structure
- initiating the myometrial contractions which will ultimately drive the fetus through the birth canal.

Figure 1.6 summarizes the key biochemical components which are thought to control the inflammatory-type processes which convert the stroma of the cervix from a rigid structure to a soft and compliant one, and the activation of the myometrial contractility which ultimately brings about its effacement and dilatation.

This brief overview is of necessity simplistic. The control of the birth process requires the participation of a myriad of other factors, such as adhesion molecules and receptors for hormones and prostaglandins, as well as other hormones such as vasopressin and relaxin. Perhaps the most important recent change in thinking has been to see the whole process of parturition as an inflammatory-type event. This has vital consequences for our understanding of those pregnancies which do not follow the normal pattern of labour onset and progress, either because it is delayed or activated prematurely. The role of infection in the latter is gaining increasing importance and it seems likely that some women may be at increased risk of preterm labour on account of an increased susceptibility to infection from deficiency of endogenous antimicrobial substances (Fig 1.7).

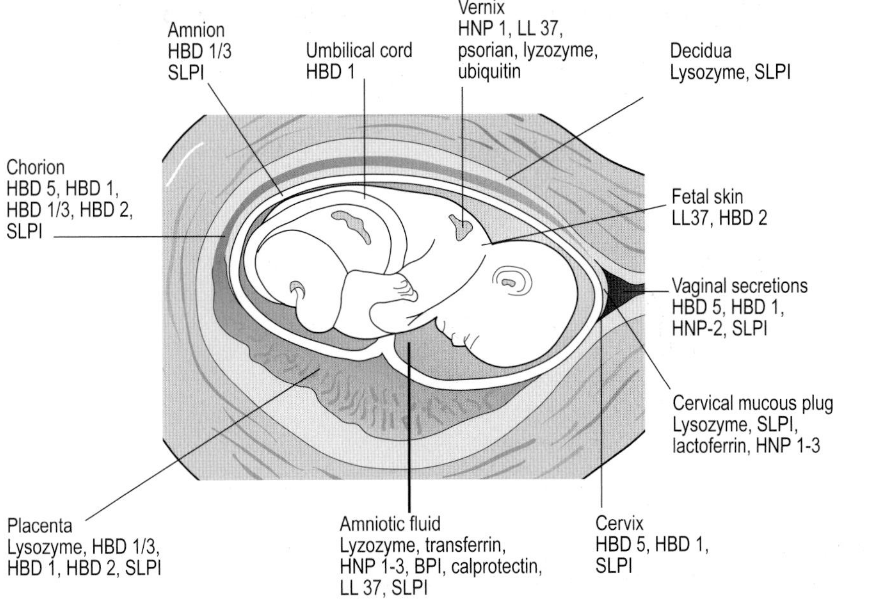

Figure 1.7 Some of the natural antimicrobial substances which may be important in resisting infection during pregnancy. A deficiency of these may predispose to preterm delivery (by permission of Dr Sarah Stock).

Bibliography

Calder AA, Greer IA. Physiology of labour. In: Phillip E, Setchell M, eds. Scientific foundations of obstetrics and gynaecology. Oxford: Butterworth, 1991.

Calder AA. Normal labour. In: Edmonds DK, ed. Dewhurst's textbook of obstetrics and gynaecology for postgraduates. Oxford: Blackwell, 1999.

Hunter W. Anatomy of the human gravid uterus. Birmingham: Baskerville, 1774.

Kerr JM. Operative midwifery. London: Bailliere, Tindal and Cox, 1908.

Smellie W. Treatise on the theory and practice of midwifery. London: D. Wilson, 1752.

Smellie W. Set of anatomical tables with explanations and an abridgement of the practice of midwifery. London: D. Wilson, 1754.

2

Obstetric risk management

Risk is defined as the potential for unwanted outcome.[1] *The Oxford English Dictionary* defines risk as the chance or possibility of loss or bad consequence. The *clinical risk incident* is defined as injury or harm to a patient as a result of care or treatment. *Near miss* is defined as an incident where there is potential for major harm or injury to a patient but the expected harm did not occur. This indicates that the systems may have to be scrutinized and better systems put in place to avoid near misses. *Serious clinical incident* is defined as a situation in which one or more patients are involved in an incident which is likely to:

- have an adverse effect on patients
- cause a major disruption to service
- attract press or media attention
- lead to a legal claim.

When we consider the issues of risk, clinical risk incident, near miss and serious clinical incident, questions arise as to why these occur and what deficiencies led to one of these events. When there is a train accident it might be due to a number of factors, such as: breaking the speed limit; brake failure; an untrained or inexperienced driver; a driver who fell asleep and did not see the signals; or it may be due to new territory; or faulty or new tracks and/or signals. One or several factors might have given rise to this accident and only a detailed enquiry and tests would reveal the cause(s). Similarly when there is a near miss or serious clinical incident the issue has to be investigated in detail to find out whether it is due to one or more factors. If the causes for that particular incident were not identified and rectified there may be recurrent near misses and serious clinical incidents. The Contingent Liability by Specialty

Table 2.1 Contingent liability by specialty: United Kingdom, 1997

Speciality	Value £ million
Accident and Emergency	2.3
Anaesthesia	2.9
General Surgery	2.1
Gynaecology	1.2
General Medicine	1.6
Paediatrics	2.9
Obstetrics	59.1
Orthopaedics	1.6
Cardiac Surgery	1.5
Others	6.0
Total	**81.2**

according to the Clinical Negligence Scheme for Trusts (CNST) for the year 1997 is provided in Table 2.1 and shows that some 70% of the total is for obstetrics.[2]

In 2004 potential claims over the next 10 years were estimated to be about £7.4 billion. Obstetrics leads to the largest claims and accounts for 50–60% of total liability bills. The large costs are due to payouts to manage children who have handicaps due to antenatal or intrapartum events which might have been avoided. Having a handicapped child is sadness for life and leads to disruption of family life as the extra parental care for the handicapped child reduces their time with the other children. The handicapped child suffering from various illnesses disturbs their sleep and may need repeated hospital admissions. Under the strain, marriage and family breakdown are not uncommon. Therefore, it is important to look at ways in which we can avoid medical negligence that might lead to a large financial burden to the state as well as a major emotional, physical and mental burden to the family.

Potential problem areas in obstetrics

The problem areas in the antenatal period relate to prenatal diagnosis, complications of invasive procedures and management of high-risk pregnancies.

Problems related to labour and delivery include meconium-stained liquor, fetal heart rate interpretation and fetal blood sampling, misuse of oxytocic drugs, mismanagement of previous caesarean section in labour, inappropriate use of forceps or vacuum, shoulder dystocia and inadequate analgesia during labour or delivery. In all of the preceding areas of practice there may be delays in diagnosis, decision making or action.

Postnatal issues relate to difficulties encountered with perineal tears and breakdown of perineal wounds or abdominal wounds, failure to advise or provide Rh immunoglobulin and Rubella immunization, misplacing results of neonatal screening tests for phenylketonuria and hypothyroidism, or inappropriate contraceptive advice.

Why do risks occur?

Risks tend to occur for a variety of reasons; the majority stem from system failures. The reasons include personal; trying to adopt short-cuts to carry out a procedure; poor communication and communication breakdowns; poorly defined responsibilities; inadequately trained staff; insufficient policies and guidelines related to management of cases and procedures. In centres where adequate policies and guidelines are in place, these may not be known to all staff on duty. Providing medical care is a multidisciplinary task and risk incidents tend to occur when there is a breakdown of care standards within the clinical team and poor co-ordination between departments.

A large Harvard study looked at adverse incidents by studying more than 30 000 hospital records of 51 randomly selected hospitals in an acute care setting in New York. Adverse events were identified in the treatment of 3.7% of cases.[3] Approximately 28% of these were considered to have resulted from negligent care or treatment. In the National Health Service in the UK a figure of 3–12% adverse incidents is estimated, although the figures quoted vary.[4] The risk incidents tend to vary in different disciplines and in different age groups – the elderly being more vulnerable to adverse risk incidents.

The National Health Service facts and figures suggest that there are an estimated 850 000 adverse incidents and errors that occur every year affecting 1 in 10 hospital admissions. One-third of adverse incidents may lead to patient disability and in a smaller proportion it may lead to permanent disability or death. The management of these adverse incidents or their sequelae costs approximately £2 billion a year in hospital stays alone. In addition, the clinical negligence cost to the health service was estimated by the British Medical Association as more than £400 million per annum.[5] Recently, the UK government has set up a National Patient Safety Agency (NPSA) to reduce these risks. The NPSA defined the problems and set targets.[6] The first of these targets set for the end of the year 2005 were as follows:

- to cut by 25% the number of risk incidents in obstetrics and gynaecology that lead to litigation
- to cut by 40% the number of serious prescribed drug errors
- to eliminate suicide by hanging from shower and curtain rails among mental health patients.

Clinical risk management

Aims

The aim of clinical risk management strategies within the hospital should be to reduce or eliminate harm to patients – which automatically leads to improved quality of care. Systems should be put in place to deal effectively with the injured patient including explanations, an apology and, if negligent, swift compensation.

The second aim in clinical risk management should be to protect the hospital and its medical, nursing and support staff. This should improve morale and the reputation of the hospital and limit depletion of valuable financial resources which could be diverted to clinical areas which are in need. It will also help to meet the clinical governance initiatives and to achieve the standards required by the CNST.[7]

Process

The process involves:

- identification of risk
- analysis of risk
- control of risk
- funding of risk.

In looking at the process one has to concentrate on organization of the service, the professional competence of the staff and the equipment available, and whether it is maintained in best working condition. Record keeping should be in good order to provide a co-ordinated service to that patient, so that the old records are available at any time to provide care and to help in analyzing any untoward risk that has happened in that particular case. Communication is a vital element in the risk management process. In many instances poor communication leads to misunderstanding of the facts by the patient or relatives and results in unnecessary medical litigation.

Risk management group

Risk management in an obstetric hospital is ideally administered by a group. Different hospitals have different configurations but the following is recommended:[8]

- lawyer with medical experience as chair
- senior midwife, to act as co-ordinator, collect the adverse incident statements and collate the information
- clinical director of obstetrics and gynaecology
- director of midwifery
- consultant anaesthetist and paediatrician

- consultant obstetrician and junior doctor (registrar)
- hospital legal officer.

In the absence of a lawyer committed to help the hospital, the lead obstetrician for the labour ward can chair the group. Such a group should have all the important people and any decision made will be multidisciplinary and can be disseminated to the rest of the staff in the midwifery, paediatric, anaesthetic and obstetric divisions. Analysis of cases will also help ascertain if there are any risk incidents which might lead to litigation so the hospital legal officer can take appropriate action.

The risk management group performs several tasks. They provide a review based on the adverse events and highlight cases of possible litigation. Advice on general management policies related to the events are discussed and disseminated to staff. Steps are taken to support the staff and the patients involved in the risk incident. All staff involved are asked to provide a report when the events are fresh in their minds. It is best for them to write a statement without looking at the hospital notes so that they are not influenced by what is written, but rather recollect the incident and give that statement.

The staff should not be called to give evidence in front of the risk management group which may intimidate and deter them from reporting adverse incidents. The group should act as a supportive organization rather than an inquisitorial group that finds fault in order to blame someone. The culture should be 'fact finding' rather than 'fault finding' and apportion responsibility with adequate guidance on how to prevent such problems in the future. The main purpose of this group should be to identify unsatisfactory practices and to put in place robust policies and guidelines that will eliminate or reduce such practices that lead to risk events.

Identification of risk

Risk needs to be identified and analyzed by several processes such as: incident reporting; audit of recurrent risk incidents; review of records for non-adherence to guidelines and protocol; audit of morbidity.

Incident reporting

Risk incidents should be identified by incident reporting and staff should be encouraged to report incidents in an open organizational culture of proportionate blame. All staff are encouraged to report any adverse incidents that they or their colleagues have come across. The midwife who is in charge of the labour ward or the theatre sister should take the major responsibility to ensure that risk incident report forms are completed and submitted. By having policies and guidelines that promote evidence-based practice the number of risk events can be reduced and deviation from guidelines that give rise to risk incidents can be identified. Even trivial risk incidents should be reported so that remedial action can be taken to prevent recurrences. Incidents of a larger magnitude, like near-miss incidents, should be reported and followed by open discussion in a multidisciplinary forum to find out how such near misses could be avoided. In many institutions there is a list of events that have been identified as incidents that need to be reported. Some of these include:

- admission to neonatal intensive care unit (NICU) for severe birth asphyxia
- neonatal convulsions
- shoulder dystocia
- intrapartum stillbirth
- birth trauma
- undiagnosed congenital malformation
- third degree perineal tear
- massive postpartum haemorrhage (PPH) – blood loss > 2 L.

Investigation of adverse events

Whenever there is a poor outcome or near miss event it should be identified and investigated. The staff involved and possibly non-clinical staff and parents should be interviewed. The purpose of the interview should be explained and confidentiality ensured. The relevant people should provide a detailed description of the sequence of events. Their statements should include the individual's role and that of their colleagues or other medical or paramedical staff who helped in the management of that particular case. The interview should include open questions so the staff will not be inhibited in explaining the situation. Answers to open questions might provide the explanation as to why certain actions were taken or not taken. They may also be able to say, with the benefit of hindsight, that a different action might have been taken, but due to a certain circumstance they acted differently.

In the open questioning process one asks whether they have suggestions for improvement in caring for such a case in the future. When dealing with a sensitive case there are often contradictory statements. Clarification should be sought so the facts of what happened can be established without confusion. If the individual would like to have a copy of the case notes it should be provided. However, it is best to provide a description of the case and to give reasons ('thinking behind the action') as to why a particular action was taken, especially if it was contrary to the policies and guidelines. After they complete their statement they could be encouraged to review the case notes in order to make sure the events stated and the relative time stated are accurate.

Audit of recurrent risk incidents

The incident reporting process identifies recurrent risk incidents. An audit should be set up to review the current practices related to these incidents. Goals should be established that will eliminate or reduce the risk based on the findings. An action plan can be developed in order to meet the goals, followed by information and education of staff in order to achieve the desired changes. Once adequate information has been provided, and the protocol or guidelines have been changed in order to improve practice, the changes introduced need to be monitored by a follow-up audit. This will provide the answer as to whether the changes introduced have reduced the risk frequency or the severity. If the risk frequency or severity has not been reduced then one has to re-assess the goals to see whether the situation could be improved. If the introduction of new policies, guidelines, education and training has improved the situation one should continue to monitor the incident on a regular basis to make sure that the improvement is maintained.

Review of records to identify potential risk events due to non-adherence to protocols and guidelines

Potential risk incidents can be identified by reviewing records from time to time to see whether there is compliance with agreed guidelines and protocols that are in place to avoid risk incidents. The Royal College of Obstetricians and Gynaecologists and Royal College of Midwives[9] have provided certain standards that need to be audited:

- Administration of steroids if delivery is less than 33 weeks.
- Consultant presence in potentially complicated caesarean sections like placenta praevia, abruptio placentae, preterm delivery less than 32 weeks, and multiple previous caesarean sections.
- Prophylactic antibiotics and thromboprophylaxis for caesarean section.
- Decision-to-delivery interval less than 30 minutes for cases with scalp blood pH less than 7.20, abruption, cord prolapse, scar dehiscence, and cases of prolonged bradycardia greater than 10 minutes.

Audit of morbidity

Risk management audit has to be cyclical in order to find out whether the standards in a particular practice are met; therefore national standards should be established. The purpose of this audit is to rectify any shortcomings by introducing new methods of technology or training programmes, and to show improvement in the next audit cycle so that the target can be met. Surgical morbidity in gynaecological practice is well documented.[10,11] Similar audits should be carried out in obstetrics and may include the following:

- bladder or ureteric injury
- vesico-vaginal fistula
- bowel injury (full thickness)
- haemorrhage or return to operating room because of postoperative haemorrhage
- blood transfusion and haematoma formation
- re-operation, for example drainage of abscess or re-implantation of ureter.

In addition to the immediate surgical morbidity, associated morbidity needs to be audited and this can take the form of the following:

- infection that requires prolonged use of antibiotics, including pyelonephritis but excluding lower urinary tract infection
- bowel problems such as ileus or obstruction
- thromboembolism
- re-admission – within 6 weeks related to the original surgery
- intensive care unit admission.

The above incidents may be rare and selected items may be recorded and audited. In obstetrics every near miss incident should be carefully identified and discussed with the whole team of care givers in order to identify the good and poor actions taken regarding each case. Common near miss incidents are obstetric hysterectomy and admission to intensive care unit, without which interventions the mother might have lost her life.[12–15]

Risk analysis

The risk might be minor, but happen several times in a week or a month, or it might be major but happen only once a year – i.e. the severity or magnitude of the risks might differ and the incidences vary. Therefore, analysis of the reported incidents and the outcome of audits should determine the severity of risk, the likelihood of recurrence and the cost–benefit analysis of controlling these risks. Based on this analysis priorities can be established and, if current funding is inadequate to contain the risk, then additional funding should be sought or consideration given to transfer the risk. This may include transfer of certain services to another hospital with special expertise or more staffing.

Risk control

Any risk identified should be controlled by having general and specific action plans. A multidisciplinary team may be necessary and whatever plans are put into place should be known to all staff. These processes or procedures should be included in all staff induction or orientation programmes. Specific action plans which are made should be included in protocols and guidelines and made accessible to staff in related work areas. With current information technology this may be made available on the hospital intranet. If there has been difficulty in adhering to protocols then remedial action should be taken and any new actions introduced should be notified and monitored for compliance. Such monitoring will also give information about good and competent clinical practice. The general and specific action plans will not materialize unless there is good communication and it cannot be audited unless there is good record keeping – both of which are essential for risk control.

Risk control may need re-organization of service and should include adequate staffing levels. Current recommendation is that there should be 1.5 midwives to 1 woman in labour, for all, or at least for the majority of the time. An experienced obstetrician, paediatrician and anaesthetist should be available within the delivery unit or at short notice. Hospitals with large delivery units are best served by a designated consultant who should be available for the delivery unit all day. Currently, the Royal College of Obstetricians and Gynaecologists have recommended a consultant on duty in the delivery unit during at least 40 working hours of the week.[9] The designated consultant of the labour ward should have overall responsibility for producing guidelines and protocols, standard setting and audit. The labour ward forum should include a multidisciplinary team with lay representation which should review major clinical problems and produce recommendations for their resolution. The final responsibility will rest with the lead obstetrician. Clear professional responsibilities should be the theme of intrapartum care – midwives and clinicians involved should know their roles. They should work coherently as a team with the anaesthetist and with members of other hospital disciplines.

Involved staff should receive education and be familiar with the operation and maintenance of the increasingly technical medical equipment on a labour ward. A designated person should look after and maintain medical equipment such as ventilators and resuscitators. The biomedical department of the hospital should check and maintain medical equipment on a regular basis.

Professional competence

This is a major issue in risk incidents and is part of clinical governance. Induction and orientation programmes should be mandatory for all levels of staff who work in a particular area. When they are new to the environment they should work under supervision for a period of time. Those working in the delivery unit should have adequate training in interpretation of fetal heart rate monitoring (CTG) and for deciding on appropriate action. They should be trained in skills and emergency drills for acute emergencies such as eclampsia, cord prolapse, postpartum haemorrhage and shoulder dystocia. All members of the team should have knowledge and skill in adult and neonatal resuscitation. Review of statistics and case discussions should take place in the unit to make sure that the emergencies are managed without serious morbidity or case fatalities. Adequate educational activities should be in place in order to maintain professional competence in the above areas.

Communication

Although the vast majority of communication in a delivery unit is verbal there should be written information regarding specific opinions, clinical condition of the patient, investigations needed and planned management. Where the patient is unable to speak in English there should be interpreters available so that the patient can participate in the management plan. There should be clear explanation of the plan of management and, where necessary, consent should be obtained in writing, especially if there are associated risks. Appropriate staff should be made available so that they can explain the procedure in detail. It is always useful for the senior clinician involved to give an honest explanation when things go wrong. Clear lines of communication and command are important to enable staff on duty to provide consistent information to the patient. In high-risk areas such as the labour ward, high dependency and intensive care units, there should be personal handover of cases at the senior level when there is change of staff. During this process those cases that need additional attention should be brought to the notice of all staff and be reviewed by the most senior person.

Record keeping

Legible record keeping is of paramount importance. The date and time should be accurately annotated along with the name of the individual, a legible signature and pager number. The record should be complete and contemporaneous. Because of potential medicolegal issues the mother and baby notes have to be stored for 25 years. The notes when transferred into another medium, such as microfilm, must be clearly legible and readily reproducible. Archival storage of CTGs is essential. Because they are recorded on thermal paper these tracings tend to fade. In cases that are likely to undergo litigation, the CTGs are often misplaced because of their educational interest and handling by many people.

Electronic storage is a good option and several companies produce equipment that electronically archives CTGs online. It is possible to store 4000 maternity records and 8 hours of CTGs for each case in one 'write many times read once' (WORM) disk. Hospitals should be encouraged to purchase and use them, so that the notes and CTGs can be easily retrieved. If this is not possible, the notes as well as the CTGs should be photocopied, certified and kept – photocopied CTGs do not fade. The policy decisions regarding place and format of storage should be reviewed periodically by the obstetrician involved with hospital administration. In addition to clinical notes it is important to store the protocols and guidelines which were in existence at that time, so that clinical management can be judged in the context of the protocols and guidelines at the time of the incident. This can be in hard copy or electronic format.

Conclusion

Success of clinical risk management cannot be quantified by immediate dividends and is difficult to judge in the short term. Avoidance of adverse outcome based on risk management principles should reduce medicolegal claims. The prime motive of risk management should be to improve the quality of care and this goes hand-in-hand with litigation risk reduction – the two goals being complementary. This can be achieved only by a culture of openness, clinical competence, professional development, good practice and good communication. All hospitals and services should have risk management as a mandatory agenda to improve quality of service.

References

1. Wilson RM, Runciman WB, Gibber RW. The quality in Australian healthcare study. Med J Austr 1995; 163:458–471.
2. www.nhsla.com/claims/schemes/CNST R2. *www.nhsla.com/claims/schemes/CNST*
3. Brennan TA, Leape LL, Laird N. Incidence of adverse incidents and negligence in hospitalised patients: results of the Harvard study. Part 1. N Engl J Med 1991; 324:370–377.
4. Chief Medical Officer 2000. An organisation with a memory: report of an expert group on learning from adverse events in the NHS. London: Department of Health, 2000.
5. *www.npsa.org.uk* or *www.doh.gov.uk/buildsafernhs*
6. Ceilia Hall – *www.news.telegraph*
7. CNST maternity clinical risk management standards. NSH litigation authority. April 2005; *www.nhsla.com/Riskmanagement/CnstStandards*
8. Arulkumaran S, Symonds EM. Intrapartum fetal monitoring – medico legal implications. The Obstetrician and Gynaecologist. Vol 1. London: RCOG Press, 1999:23–27.
9. Royal College of Obstetricians and Gynaecologists and Royal College of Midwives. Towards safer childbirth – minimum standards of the organisation of labour wards. Report of a joint working party. London: RCOG Press, 1999.
10. Baskett TF, Clough H. Perioperative morbidity of hysterectomy for benign gynaecological disease. J Obstet Gynaecol 2001; 21:504–506.
11. Tamizian O, Gilby J, Symonds I, Cust MP, Arulkumaran S. Immediate and associated complications of hysterectomy for benign disease. Aust NZ J Obstet Gynaecol 2002; 42:292–294.
12. Ng TI, Lim E, Tweed WA, Arulkumaran S. Obstetric admissions to the intensive care unit – a retrospective review. Ann Acad Med Singapore 1992; 21:804–906.
13. Drife JO. Maternal 'near-miss' reports? BMJ 1993; 307:1087–1088.
14. Baskett TF, Sternadel J. Maternal intensive care and near-miss mortality in obstetrics. Br J Obstet Gynaecol 1998; 105:981–984.
15. Baskett TF, O'Connell CM. Severe obstetric maternal morbidity: a 15-year population-based study. J Obstet Gynaecol 2005; 25:7–9.

Bibliography

American College of Obstetricians and Gynecologists. Committee Opinion No 353. Medical emergency preparedness. Obstet Gynecol 2006;108: 1597–1599.

Clements RV, ed. Risk management and litigation in obstetrics and gynaecology. London: RSM Press, 2001.

Forster AJ, Fung I, Caughey S, Oppenheimer L, Beach C, Shojania KG, van Walraven C. Adverse events detected by clinical surveillance on an obstetric service. Obstet Gynecol 2006;108: 1073–1083.

Hankins GDV, MacLennan AH, Speer ME, Strunk A, Nelson K. Obstetric litigation is asphyxiating our maternity services. Obstet Gynecol 2006;107: 1382–1385.

Hurwitz B. Clinical guidelines and the law: negligence, discretion and judgement. Abingdon: Radcliffe Medical Press, 1998.

Maresh M, ed. Audit in obstetrics and gynaecology. Oxford: Blackwell Scientific Publications, 1994.

Pearlman MD. Patient safety in obstetrics and gynecology: an agenda for the future. Obstet Gynecol 2006;108: 1266–1271.

Quality improvement in women's health care. American College of Obstetricians and Gynecologists. Washington, DC: ACOG, 2000.

Royal College of Obstetricians and Gynaecologists. Improving patient safety: risk management for maternity and gynaecology. Clinical Governance. Advice No. 2. London: RCOG, 2005.

Vincent C, ed. Clinical risk management. London: BMJ Publishing Group, 1995.

Wen SW, Huang L, Liston RM, Heaman M, Baskett TF, Rusen ID. Severe maternal morbidity in Canada, 1991–2001. Can Med Assoc J 2005;173: 759–763.

3

Assessment and management of labour

ON THE QUALIFICATIONS OF AN ACCOUCHER

'Those who intend to practice midwifery, ought first of all to make themselves masters of anatomy, and acquire competent knowledge in surgery and physick ... and of practising under a master, before he attempts to deliver by himself. He should also embrace every occasion of being present at real labours ... Over and above the advantages of education, he ought to be endued with a natural sagacity, resolution, and prudence; together with that humanity which adorns the owner, and never fails of being agreeable to the distressed patient'.

William Smellie
A Treatise on the Theory and Practice of Midwifery. London: D. Wilson, 1752, p446–447

Introduction

Throughout its long history the various authors of 'Munro Kerr' have stressed that, while the theme and title of the work has always contained the word 'operative', the foundation of safe and successful obstetrics rests on prevention of complications rather than on the operative dexterity which may be required to overcome them. This principle demands that all relevant factors pertaining to the expectant mother and her offspring are gathered, analyzed and recorded so that they can be viewed within the tapestry of the individual confinement. The attendants have a duty to be as fully informed as possible of the special characteristics of the two subjects of their care – mother and baby – so that the serious complications of pregnancy, and the hazards of labour and delivery, can be anticipated and thereby obviated as far as possible.

The concept of risk assessment has become increasingly important. While the attachment of labels such as 'high risk or 'low risk' to patients may be seen as simplistic, and in the view of some undesirable, it is beyond argument that a mental process designed to identify those maternities in which problems already exist is vital to ensuring the best outcome. It is a truism that life-threatening complications may arise with terrifying rapidity, even in the most hitherto benign circumstances. The old adage 'forewarned is forearmed' is especially applicable to obstetric practice. Birth attendants must therefore approach their responsibilities with as full an appreciation as possible of the special characteristics of each woman.

There is a fine line between over-emphasis of the clinical and medical features and acceptance that childbirth is in essence a normal, physiological process. However, failure to recognize those facets of a particular pregnancy which may presage trouble is a dereliction of clinical responsibility. Many clinical advances in recent years have been pilloried as leading to 'over-medicalization' of pregnancy and birth and have led to a backlash in several quarters. Pressure groups representing or purporting to represent patients' interests have been vocal in their criticism. Clinicians are portrayed as being obsessed with technical aspects of pregnancy and delivery to the neglect of human and emotional issues. The wise obstetrician must recognize these concerns and practice with sensitivity.

Failure to listen to such concerns inevitably results in conflicts which are in the interests of nobody. However irritating it may be to be lectured to by lay interests, it cannot be denied that charges of uncaring medical and obstetric arrogance are, on occasion, well founded and deserve to be addressed with due humility. On the other hand, if complicating features already beset an expectant mother or can be clearly seen to be at increased likelihood, an attitude of denial which often stems from the 'childbirth is not a medical process' lobby may itself add greatly to the dangers. The foregoing emphasizes the need for careful appraisal of every pregnant woman. The core principles of antenatal care can be summarized in three parts:

- defining the personal make-up of the individual patient – age, parity, medical, social, cultural and obstetric history
- a simple and standardized system of regular review – this defines the maternal condition in respect of symptoms, blood pressure, urinalysis, and the wellbeing and growth of the fetus and its orientation within the uterus
- appropriate identification of and response to deviations from normal as the pregnancy progresses.

Labour represents the high point of pregnancy. Most mothers approach labour with a mixture of emotions including excitement, apprehension and sometimes dread. It is the culmination of months of anticipation and expectation and its outcome may cover the entire spectrum from glorious fulfilment to catastrophic loss. The ultimate responsibility of obstetricians and midwives is to ensure as far as possible the former outcome. It is a paradox of modern society that as the human condition has become more and more sophisticated and the capabilities of our species have risen to ever greater heights, our ability to give birth remains fraught with imperfections and so much less straightforward than in most 'lesser' species. Nor is this a new phenomenon. The second book of Esdras in the *Apocrypha*, written more than 2000 years ago, has at chapter VII, verse 12:

> *'Then were the entrances of this world made narrow, full of sorrow and travail: they are but few and evil, full of perils and very painful.'*

The march of evolution has produced in *Homo sapiens* by far nature's most intelligent and capable species in all but perhaps one aspect – the efficiency of reproduction, especially in regard to childbirth.[1] This may be attributed to two main factors: one is our adoption of an upright, bipedal gait; the other our increased brain size. Furthermore, modern western society with all its technological advances is, if anything, even less likely to witness normal parturition than hitherto. Three influences are principally responsible for this:

- a disinclination of many modern mothers to endure the protracted and painful labours which were the common lot of previous generations
- a tendency of birth attendants to interfere with labour and delivery
- an ever higher expectation by parents for the birth of a perfect child.

While all of the above have been the object of criticism, none should occasion surprise or deserve condemnation. A medieval view, often supported by religious teachings, that women should simply endure all the anguish that labour might bring has happily, in the past 2 centuries, given way to more humane and enlightened attitudes. The benefits of this should not be underestimated. The days of mothers whose experience of a first labour were so harrowing that they would never entertain the prospect of another pregnancy have, we hope, receded.

While the expression 'interfering with nature' is usually pejorative, in the context of childbirth, nature is far from infallible. Doctors and, to a lesser extent, midwives are trained to interfere with nature in order to avoid or correct her imperfections. It can hardly be inappropriate for all concerned (parents, midwives, obstetricians, anaesthetists and neonatologists) to confirm the simple and indisputable goal of maternity care – the birth to a healthy, happy mother of a healthy offspring with the maximum potential to grow and develop fully.

Nevertheless, while progress in maternity care has indeed been characterized by more interference in the forms of effective methods of pain relief, induction and augmentation of labour, intrapartum fetal surveillance, operative vaginal delivery and caesarean section, it may be reasonable to hope that further improvements in the understanding of parturition may yield opportunities to ensure that labour and delivery becomes less complicated. We should not close our minds to the possibility that a greater proportion of mothers in future may be able to enjoy the fulfilment of normal childbirth which many continue to seek.

Assessment of labour

There are three imperatives in the assessment of the woman in labour:

1. Confirmation of the diagnosis of labour.
2. Timely identification of maternal or fetal problems which may influence its management, e.g. maternal distress, ketoacidosis, hypertension, fetal malpresentations, fetal hypoxia, placental or cord complications, state of the fetal membranes.
3. Setting the baseline from which subsequent progress of labour should be determined and recorded.

Diagnosis of labour

Labour is conventionally considered to have begun when regular, painful contractions are recognized. While this may be as useful a clinical definition as can be found, it presents a number of difficulties. Just as a fruit does not suddenly change from being unripe to ripe, the transition from pregnancy to labour is not a sudden event. The shift from pregnancy maintenance to parturition takes place across a period, perhaps as long as a month, which is sometimes described as 'prelabour'. This is

> *'If the os uteri remains close shut, it may be taken for granted, that the woman is not yet in labour, not withstanding the pains she may suffer.'*
>
> **William Smellie**
> *A Treatise on the Theory and Practice of Midwifery. London: D. Wilson, 1752, p189*

characterized by an increase in the frequency and amplitude of uterine contractions. The myometrium is never entirely quiescent and, indeed, has long been recognized to exhibit Braxton Hicks contractions which become more evident as term approaches. This may be a manifestation of the various physiological changes described in Chapter 1, such as the appearance of receptors for oxytocin and prostaglandins and the development of myometrial gap junctions. Prelabour is also the time when the cervix is ripening.

The need to establish a precise diagnosis of labour is crucial to good obstetric care. In normal labour at term, if we do not know when the process started we cannot measure how long it has lasted. Moreover, in cases of suspected preterm labour, an accurate diagnosis is vital to inform appropriate management. Recent history has witnessed the administration of so-called tocolytic agents to many women who, it is now accepted, were not in fact in preterm labour – as evidenced by the high rate of success of placebo therapy when appropriate trials were conducted. Reliance on assessment of uterine contractility is notoriously fallible, even with the help of an electronic tocometer. Rupture of the membranes or passage of a 'show' of blood/mucous is suggestive but no guarantee of labour. The gold standard for diagnosis of labour is to observe progressive change in cervical effacement and dilatation, but this requires a period of time to elapse between observations. A diagnosis of labour cannot be established until the cervix is effaced. Only after cervical effacement is well advanced can dilatation proceed.

In most instances the fact of established labour will be obvious when the mother is first assessed on arrival at hospital. Where there is uncertainty the situation will usually become clear within a few hours. When the diagnosis is uncertain, as it will be in about 20% of cases, it is appropriate to tell the woman that some hours may be required before she 'declares herself'. During this time she should be observed away from the labour ward if possible. The correct diagnosis of labour is paramount as all other decisions emanate from this point. As Kieran O'Driscoll put it:

'The most important single issue of care in labour is diagnosis. When the initial diagnosis is wrong, all subsequent care is likely to be also wrong'.[2]

Identification of maternal and fetal problems

At the same time as observing the signs and symptoms of the onset of labour, the attendants must also conduct a careful assessment to identify potential problems and departures from normal. The gestational age should be established based on the best available information. Routine assessment must include measurement of the mother's vital signs: pulse, blood pressure and temperature. The obstetric examination then focuses on the pregnant abdomen with assessment of the uterine size and its contents – the lie of the fetus, the level of the presenting part and a clinical assessment of the amniotic fluid volume. The fetal heart rate should be recorded, as well as the mother's perception of fetal movements. The frequency, duration and strength of uterine contractions must then be determined.

Vaginal examination

The single most important observation in the assessment of labour is the vaginal examination. However, as this may be distasteful and uncomfortable for the mother and carries risks, especially of introducing infection, it must be employed intelligently and sparingly. Other, simpler sources of information, especially abdominal palpation, should be exploited for the maximum information they can yield. Rectal examination is no longer widely practised since its disadvantages are now considered to outweigh its perceived advantages.

Vaginal examinations should be conducted every 3–4 hours except when a particular circumstance, for example non-progressive labour or fetal distress, indicates the need to reduce this interval. It is essential that vaginal examinations should not be wasted but should yield as much detailed information as possible. It is not enough simply to determine the degree of cervical dilatation, albeit this is most often the information of primary interest. Record should also be made of the degree of effacement of the cervix, whether or not it has become oedematous, and how well it is applied to the fetal presenting part. The position, station, degree of flexion, and the presence or absence of caput or moulding in cephalic presentations should be noted. Record the state of the fetal membranes, the condition and amount of the amniotic fluid if this is draining, and the presence of bleeding and/or passage of meconium. Finally, the appearance in the pelvis of unwelcome fetal parts such as hands, feet or limbs, and especially the umbilical cord, should be determined. These factors are summarized in Table 3.1.

Table 3.1 Factors to be assessed at vaginal examination in labour

Presentation	cephalic
	breech/foot
	shoulder/arm
	umbilical cord
Cervix	effacement
	dilatation
	oedema
	application to presenting part
Fetal head	station
	position
	flexion/deflexion
	caput
	asynclitism
	moulding
Membranes	intact/ruptured
Amniotic fluid	volume:
	– absent / scant / normal / abundant
	content:
	– clear
	– meconium (thin/thick)
	– blood

Assessment of progress

The crux of ensuring that progress in labour is appropriately assessed is to determine the reference points from which that progress proceeds. However imprecise our judgement of the start of labour may be, such a judgement should be made and a starting point recorded. Since it is exceptional for spontaneous labour to start with the attendants already present this point may be judged to have been several hours previously. The length of time the mother is thought already to have been in established labour is an important element of the clinical management. This is the first reference point. The second and more pragmatic reference point consists of the findings at the first vaginal examination during labour.

Partography

Graphical analysis of progress in labour whereby cervical dilatation is plotted against time is a comparatively recent science. It is based on the classical studies of Emmanuel Friedman in the United States[3] and the pragmatic innovations of Hugh Philpott in Southern Africa.[4,5] Friedman defined the norms of cervimetric progress in different types of labour, recognizing the important influence of parity. He defined the sigmoid curve followed during normal labours (Fig 3.1) with a shallow slope of relatively slow increase in dilatation in the 'latent phase' up to 3–4 cm, followed by the steeply sloping 'active phase' up to around 9 cm. He also suggested that the last centimetre or so of dilatation may be slower because the presenting part has to travel further down the birth canal till its widest part completes full dilatation, although this is rarely seen to be of clinical importance. Philpott developed the partogram with the object of assisting midwives in rural districts of Africa to make timely recognition of departures from normal labour progress, so that more skilled assistance could be summoned or that appropriate transfer of the patient should be effected.[4,5]

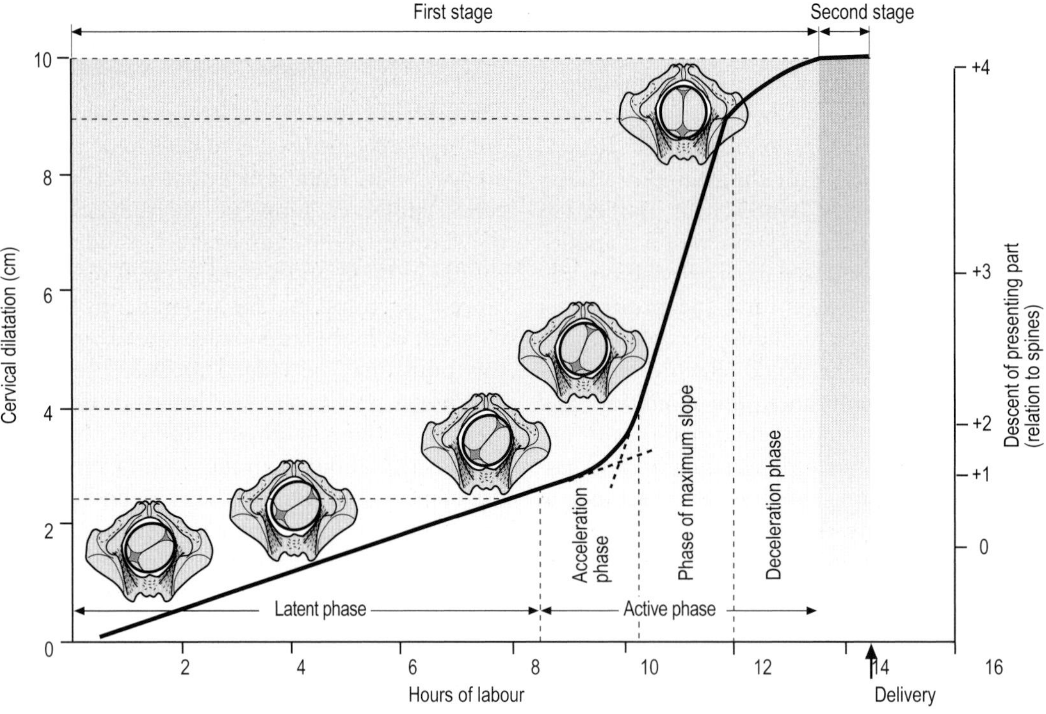

Figure 3.1 Friedman's curve.

The type of partograph varies widely in different services but its essential basis does not. The vertical axis of the graph plots cervimetric progress from 0 cm to 10 cm – conventionally taken to represent full cervical dilatation. The horizontal axis shows the passage of time in hours. Philpott's partograph showed two diagonal parallel lines whose slopes lay approximately between the gradual slope of Friedman's shallow latent phase and the steep slope of his active phase. The first of these – his 'alert line' – was followed at 4 hours delay by the 'action line' with guidance to the midwives as to the clinical response if the plotting of progress fell to the right of these landmarks. Using the partograph Philpott reduced prolonged labour, caesarean sections and perinatal deaths in Zimbabwe.[4,5] It is a tribute to the essential quality of his principles that the partograph is now a cornerstone of every effective obstetric service. The elements of Philpott's partograph were incorporated into the World Health Organization's partograph (Fig 3.2).[6,7]

The simplest partograph in common use is that devised in the National Maternal Hospital in Dublin as part of their policy of active management of labour.[2] This consists of a simple square matching 10 cm on the vertical axis with 10 hours on the horizontal for the first stage of labour. The action line is a simple diagonal running from 0 hours/0 cm to 10 hours/10 cm.

Management of labour

The essence of labour management may be summed up by asking three questions:

1 Is the mother well?
2 Is the fetus well?
3 Is the labour progressing?

Maternal wellbeing

Labour is a painful process but the degree of pain experienced varies widely between different mothers. High quality intrapartum care requires careful attention to the issue of pain relief which in itself now represents almost a

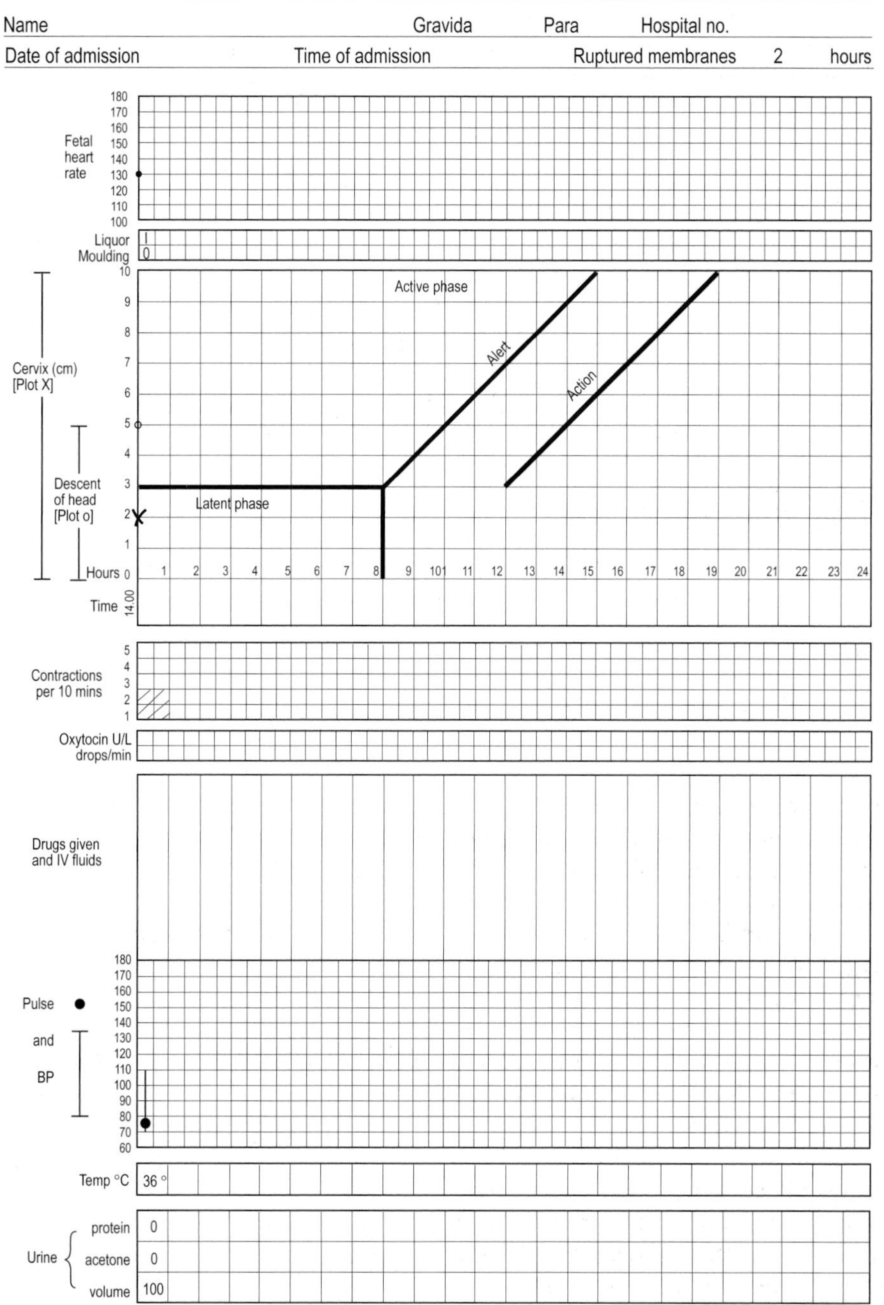

Figure 3.2 World Health Organization partograph.

separate obstetric discipline – much of which has been devolved to the obstetric anaesthetist. It is essential that the mother should understand the full range of options available to her and the implications of each for herself, her infant and her labour. Many will wish to avoid artificial forms of pain relief as far as possible and it is important that they should be supported if they wish to employ simpler methods. Ultimately, however, it is more likely that the mother's labour will be an unhappy experience if she has inadequate

'The mother being on her legs, causeth the inward orifice of the womb to dilate sooner than in bed, and her pains be stronger and frequenter, that her labour be nothing near so long.'

Francois Mauriçeau
Traité des Maladies de Femme Grosses. Paris, 1668

pain relief (see Chapter 25). During early labour the woman should be encouraged to move about and walk if she wishes. In general one tries to support what she wants to do, provided it is not harmful, rather than impose rigid practices upon her. Explanation, honest optimism, and encouragement for her and her partner are essential.

The broader aspect of maternal wellbeing concerns the need to identify abnormalities which constitute a serious health risk. These include the following: hypertensive disorders, including severe pre-eclampsia and eclampsia; medical disorders such as diabetes and cardiac, pulmonary and renal diseases; intrapartum haemorrhage or intrauterine sepsis. Careful attention to the observation of the maternal vital signs and urinalysis will generally be adequate for their early recognition.

Fetal wellbeing

The entire subject of fetal surveillance in labour is dealt with in the next chapter. It is sufficient here to emphasize that the condition of the fetus should continually be factored into the overall assessment and management of labour in conjunction with the other two concerns, maternal wellbeing and progress of labour.

Progress in labour

In the assessment of progress of labour it is essential to recognize that, in general, nulliparous and multiparous women are quite different in their behaviour in labour. Once labour is established (effaced cervix, ≥ 3 cm dilated) one should expect normal progress of ≥ 1 cm cervical dilatation per hour in nullipara and often a more rapid dilatation in multipara. It is the *progression* of labour, assessed at 2–4-hour intervals, which should be stressed rather than an arbitrary total duration of labour. It is in this context that the partograph plays such an important role.

Inadequate progress in labour

If partographic analysis shows inadequate progress in the first stage of labour one should consider the possible cause. Traditional teaching has pointed to the three main alternatives (the three Ps) as follows:

- faults in the passages
- faults in the passenger
- faults in the powers.

Faults in the passages

Obstruction in the passages may be from the soft tissues or the bony pelvis. A phenomenon, 'cervical dystocia', has been proposed indicating that the cervix is unduly rigid and consequently difficult to dilate even by adequate uterine contractions. Such a complication is probably extremely rare, although it may occur secondary to disease or treatment of the cervix. On rare occasions a large cervical fibroid may impede descent of the fetal presenting part.

Of greater importance is the issue of pelvic inadequacy, due either to its unusually small capacity or to an abnormal shape. The latter may be seen as a result of disease or injury, or simply the constitution of the mother. The issue of pelvic shape and capacity featured

'Watchful expectancy should not be allowed to degenerate into ignorant laissez-faire'

Chassar Moir
Munro Kerr's Operative Obstetrics. 7th edn. 1964, p131

much more prominently in the obstetrics of yesteryear than it does nowadays. Categorizing pelvic shapes into descriptive groups such as platypelloid, android or anthropoid used to be a prominent part of obstetric teaching but is no longer considered particularly useful, and x-ray pelvimetry no longer has any role in the management of labour. The decline in interest in such sophisticated anatomical analysis may derive in part from a much more straightforward approach to the complications of labour. If the labour is proving difficult as a result of pelvic abnormalities the solution nowadays lies in much readier resort to delivery by caesarean section than was felt justified in previous eras.

Faults in the passenger

The fetus may be the cause of dystocia in circumstances where the fetal dimensions, particularly those of the fetal head, presented to the birth canal are unduly large. This may occur in cases of macrosomia or where the attitude of the fetus results in the presentation of larger diameters than can be accommodated within the available pelvic space. This is particularly true where the fetal head is deflexed producing, at its worst, a brow presentation (mentovertical diameter = 13 cm) which is invariably incompatible with vaginal delivery in a fetus of normal size. More common are malpositions of the fetal head, especially occipito-posterior (occipito-bregmatic diameter = 11 cm) which may add to the duration and difficulty of labour. A third possible explanation lies in the fetus being structurally abnormal in conditions such as hydrocephalus.

Faults in the powers

Of the three causes of non-progressive labour, inadequate uterine action is the most common and generally the easiest to correct. In practice it is not uncommon for all three factors to be involved: the fetus may be large, the pelvis relatively small and the uterine contractions ineffective. The only one of these three factors that can be influenced is uterine action. If uterine contractions are inadequate there may be failure of the fetal head to descend, flex and rotate appropriately. As a result the fetal head deflexes and rotates occipito-posteriorly, thus presenting a greater diameter to the pelvis. If uterine action can be enhanced the fetal head may descend, flex and rotate occipito-anteriorly presenting a more favourable and narrower diameter to the pelvis.

If the membranes are intact, the first step toward correction of ineffective action is amniotomy. If, in 2 hours, this has not produced adequate uterine action then oxytocin augmentation is indicated. This is started with a 1–2 milliunit/min infusion which is doubled at 30-minute intervals. It is important here to stress again that the nulliparous and multiparous women should be viewed in separate categories. The vast majority of inadequate uterine action that does not respond to amniotomy occurs in the nulliparous woman and, provided the fetal heart rate is normal, the labour can be augmented with impunity. In the multiparous woman however, ineffective uterine action after amniotomy is uncommon and oxytocin augmentation should only be undertaken after very careful appraisal to rule out cephalopelvic disproportion.

Careful diagnosis of the onset of labour, one-to-one nursing care, partograph analysis of progress, and amniotomy and oxytocin to correct inefficient action constitute the main elements of active management of labour popularized at the National Maternity Hospital in Dublin.[2] In that institution progress of 1 cm/h is expected in the nulliparous woman. Others have used less stringent requirements for adequate uterine action and allow progress to fall below 0.5 cm/h, before moving to augmentation of uterine action. Whether one allows 2 or 4 hours of non-progressive labour before instituting augmentation will depend on the woman's wishes and perhaps the staffing levels in the obstetric unit.[8] Nonetheless, the principle of correcting inefficient uterine action early, even though the definition of 'early' may vary, is sound.[9,10] The dynamics of labour are more important than the mechanics and these depend upon the imponderables of fetal size, flexion and moulding of the fetal head, and the efficiency of uterine action. The only major factor in this equation that can be influenced by the

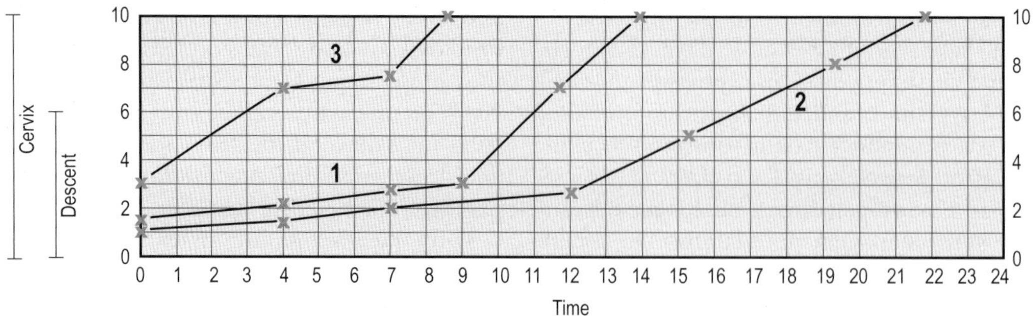

Figure 3.3 Abnormal labour patterns on partograph: (1) prolonged latent phase; (2) primary dysfunctional labour with prolonged latent and active phases; (3) secondary arrest.

obstetrician is to improve uterine action with oxytocin augmentation. As Ian Donald said: 'good contractions are worth half an inch of true conjugate'.[11]

A variety of patterns of cervimetric progress may be revealed by the partograph. These include:

- A prolonged latent phase followed by normal cervical dilatation in the active phase of labour.
- Primary dysfunctional labour or protraction disorder in which there is delay in the early part of the active phase between 3 and 6 cm. This is often a combination of relative disproportion due to deflexion of the fetal head and ineffective uterine action and many of these cases will respond to appropriate augmentation.
- A pattern of secondary arrest of labour usually shows normal progression until about 7 cm, at which point dilatation stops or is very slow. This is often due to cephalopelvic disproportion, particularly in the multiparous woman. However, in some nulliparous women this may be a combination of relative disproportion associated with ineffective uterine action and deflexion of the fetal head. In these cases careful augmentation with oxytocin may be justified in the hope that good uterine action will flex and rotate the fetal head, safely overcoming the relative cephalopelvic disproportion. These patterns are illustrated in Figure 3.3.

If, despite good uterine contractions, cervical dilatation remains slow; oedema of the cervix develops; there is little or no descent of the fetal head; and there is progressive development of caput and moulding, then the diagnosis of cephalopelvic disproportion is confirmed and delivery should be by caesarean section.

Second stage of labour

The details of assessment of progress in the second stage of labour are covered in Chapter 8, particularly with reference to assisted vaginal delivery. In the normally progressive second stage of labour the main role of the attendant is support and encouragement with minimal interference.

There are two phases to the second stage: the first, *passive phase*, in which uterine action alone brings the fetal head down to the pelvic floor and the second, *active phase*, during which maternal effort is added to complete descent and delivery of the fetal head.

The woman should be discouraged from bearing down until the fetal head has reached the pelvic floor (spines +3 to +4 cm). At this point, maternal effort should be productive in causing final descent and delivery of the fetal head. It is demoralizing, particularly in nullipara, for the woman to be directed to bear down when the fetal head is still in the mid-pelvis. She is likely to squander her best efforts in an unproductive attempt to bring the fetal head down to the pelvic floor, which at this level in the pelvis is better effected by uterine contractions.

The type of maternal effort should be left largely to the woman's instincts. Excessive coaching and loud encouragement to produce sustained Valsalva manoeuvres is inappropriate. This increases intra-thoracic pressure, decreases venous return and cardiac output, and may reduce utero-placental circulation. Along with the sustained increase of intrauterine pressure this may reduce intervillous blood flow to the extent that fetal heart rate abnormalities develop and operative intervention is provoked. Productive maternal effort is usually achieved by encouraging repeated 3–6-second bearing down efforts during uterine contractions.[12]

Maternal position during bearing down efforts should be of the woman's choosing. Although modern versions of the ancient birth chairs enjoyed a renaissance in recent times these have not been found to confer the advantages which were initially claimed.[13] However, in general, mothers should be encouraged to adopt a more upright posture. At all costs the supine, pushing uphill position should be avoided. Not only is there a mechanical disadvantage but the likelihood of aorta-caval compression leading to reduced utero-placental perfusion is increased.

Management of episiotomy and perineal trauma is outlined in Chapter 21.

Precipitate labour

Labours whose duration from onset to delivery are less than 1 hour are considered precipitate. While a short easy labour may be seen as a blessing for the mother such very rapid labours may carry special hazards as follows:

- If the rapidity is due to excessive or tumultuous uterine action this carries a risk of fetal hypoxia.
- Too rapid transit through the birth canal may incur risk of intracranial haemorrhage.

Rapid labours carry the risk of delivery in unsatisfactory circumstances, such as unexpectedly at home or during transit to the delivery unit. Fortunately it is in the nature of most such events that the delivery is straightforward. In these circumstances husbands, ambulance men, policemen and members of the public often earn plaudits for their heroic *accouchement* efforts.

References

1. Roy RP. A Darwinian view of obstructed labor. Obstet Gynecol 2003; 101:397–401.
2. O'Driscoll K, Meagher D, Robson M. Active management of labour: the Dublin experience. 4th ed. London: Mosby, 2003.
3. Friedman EA. Primigravid labor. A graphicostatistical analysis. Obstet Gynecol 1955; 6:567–589.
4. Philpott RH, Castle WM. Cervicographs in the management of labour in primigravidae. I: The alert line for detecting abnormal labour. J Obstet Gynaecol Br Cwlth 1972; 79:592–598.
5. Philpott RH, Castle WM. Cervicographs in the management of labour in primigravidae. II: The action line and treatment of abnormal labour. J Obstet Gynaecol Br Cwlth 1972; 79:599–602.
6. World Health Organization. The partograph. A managerial tool for the prevention of prolonged labour. Section I: The principal and strategy. Section II: A user's manual. Geneva: WHO, 1993.
7. World Health Organization. Partograph in management of labour. Lancet 1994; 343:1399–1404.
8. Arulkumaran S, Symonds IM. Psychosocial support or active management of labour or both to improve the outcome of labour. Br J Obstet Gynaecol 1999; 106:617–619.
9. Impey L, Boylan P. Active management of labour revisited. Br J Obstet Gynaecol 1999; 106:183–187.
10. Pattinson RC, Howarth GR, Mdluli W, Macdonald AP, Makin JD, Funk M. Active or expectant management of labour: a randomised clinical trial. Br J Obstet Gynaecol 2003; 110:457–461.
11. Donald I. Practical obstetric problems. 5th ed. London: Lloyd-Luke, 1979:606.

12. Bloom SL, Casey BM, Schaffer JI, McIntire DD, Leveno KJ. A randomised trial of coached versus uncoached maternal pushing during the second stage of labour. Am J Obstet Gynecol 2006; 194:10–13.

13. Stewart P, Hillan E, Calder AA. A randomised trial to evaluate the use of a birth chair for delivery. Lancet 1983; 1:1296–1298.

4

Fetal surveillance in labour

'By applying the ear to the mother's belly; if the child is alive you hear quite clearly the beats of its heart and easily distinguish them from the mother's pulse'.

François Mayor
Biblioth Universelle des Sciences et Arts. Geneva: 1818; 9:249

Labour is a very short period in the life of an individual but it poses the maximum threat to the fetus. Uterine contractions in labour sometimes reduce the circulation of blood to the placenta from the fetus by umbilical cord compression and always reduce maternal utero-placental circulation. At times there may be poor perfusion of the placenta on both the fetal and maternal sides of the placenta, e.g. fetal intrauterine growth restriction with small placenta and oligohydramnios. Identification of those at high or low risk is essential to offer appropriate surveillance. No fetus can be categorized at no risk such that all surveillance can be avoided. Despite appropriate surveillance, emergencies can arise that may compromise the fetus within a short period of time, as in cases of placental abruption, cord prolapse or uterine rupture. In such situations one takes action based on the clinical findings, even with minimal changes in the fetal heart rate, as the hypoxic insult can be sudden and severe, leading to rapid fetal deterioration if there is delay in delivery. The clinical situation is of overriding importance and fetal surveillance should aid management decisions to provide optimal care.

Appropriate surveillance

There are inadequate studies to provide evidence to support continuous electronic fetal heart rate monitoring (EFM) for low risk pregnancies. Currently available evidence suggests that EFM in low-risk pregnancy may reduce neonatal convulsions but will increase operative interventions.[1,2] The National Institute of Clinical Excellence (NICE) in the United Kingdom, and other national organizations, recommend intermittent auscultation for low-risk pregnancies and continuous EFM for high-risk pregnancies.[3–5] Should there be difficulty in performing intermittent auscultation as recommended (due to shortage of staff, difficulty in auscultation) or should the mother wish to have electronic fetal monitoring despite the fact the pregnancy is low risk, EFM should be performed. What may be low risk before labour may become high risk in labour.

Low risk pregnancy and intermittent auscultation

Low risk pregnancy is monitored by intermittent auscultation using a fetal stethoscope (Pinard or De Lee) or by using a Doppler device that will enable the mother and her partner to listen along with the attendant. NICE guidelines recommend that auscultation of the fetal heart rate (FHR) should be for 1 full minute soon after a contraction, every 15 minutes in the first stage and every 5 minutes in the second stage of labour. The practice of listening every 15 seconds and multiplying by four to calculate the rate per minute gives rise to the possibility of multiplying the error by four. Doppler devices are available that electronically calculate and provide digital display of the heart rate, hence negating the need to count the rate.

Monitoring the fetus with intermittent auscultation should ideally start by recording the latest time the woman felt fetal movements. The baseline FHR should then be auscultated and recorded. The attendant and mother can palpate the maternal abdomen for fetal movements and this observation is noted. Acceleration of the FHR > 15 beats above the baseline is a normal finding. Continued palpation allows uterine contractions to be felt. Auscultation immediately after the contraction should reveal if the FHR has a deceleration. Such 'intelligent auscultation' is almost equivalent to a CTG trace and will indicate the baseline rate, accelerations, and possibility of 'harmful' decelerations. In the presence of accelerations the baseline variability is likely to be normal and will indicate a non-hypoxic fetus.

The rationale for auscultation of the FHR after the contraction is for two reasons. The deceleration that returns to the baseline before the contraction abates is unlikely to be harmful to the fetus. In addition, it is irksome for the mother to place a fetal stethoscope during a contraction. There is also attenuation of the sound with thickening of the contracting myometrium. A Doppler device can be used during and soon after a contraction. Most of the harmful FHR decelerations are late, atypical variable and prolonged decelerations and should be identified by auscultation immediately after a contraction. Subsequent to the initial 'intelligent auscultation' the attendant can listen every 15 minutes in the first stage and every 5 minutes in the second stage of labour for 1 minute soon after a contraction. Should there be audible abnormality of the FHR (rise in baseline rate, decelerations), or

> *'One day whilst examining a patient near term and trying to follow the movements of the fetus with the stethoscope I was suddenly aware of a sound that I had not noticed before; it was like the ticking of a watch. At first I thought I was mistaken, but I was able to repeat the observation over and over again. On counting the beats I found that these occurred 143–148 times per minute and the patient's pulse was only 72 per minute.*
>
> **Jacques Alexandre Kergaradec**
> *Memoire sur l'auscultation, appliqué a l'etude de la grossesse. Paris: Mequignon-Marvis, 1822*

difficulty in auscultation, or should a high-risk factor become evident in labour (e.g. meconium or blood-stained liquor, need for oxytocin augmentation, bleeding), the process of intermittent auscultation should be converted to continuous EFM.

High-risk pregnancy and continuous EFM

Those identified as high risk (Table 4.1) during the antenatal period or in labour should be offered continuous EFM. EFM is the recording of the fetal heart rate in a continuous manner using a transabdominal ultrasound transducer to pick up fetal heart wall movements, or by obtaining the fetal electrocardiogram (ECG) using a scalp electrode on the fetal scalp after the membranes have ruptured. A toco transducer, which perceives the anterior thrust of the abdominal wall due to the antero-posterior expansion of the uterine fundus with contractions, is worn by the mother midway between the umbilicus and the uterine fundus to record the uterine contractions. The FHR is recorded on the upper 'cardio' channel and the contractions are recorded on the lower 'toco' channel of the recording graph paper and this cardiotocograph (CTG) displays the FHR in relation to the contractions.

Table 4.1 Factors that would recommend EFM

Maternal	Fetal
Pre-eclampsia	Intrauterine growth restriction (IUGR)
Diabetes	Prematurity
Prelabour rupture of membranes (> 24 hours)	Prolonged pregnancy (> 42 weeks)
Previous caesarean section	Breech presentation
Antepartum haemorrhage	Abnormal fetal function tests
Maternal medical disorders	Oligohydramnios/ meconium stained liquor
Induced labour	Multiple pregnancy

There are four features in the fetal heart rate trace recorded by electronic fetal heart rate monitors; baseline rate, baseline variability, accelerations and decelerations. These are described below.

Baseline fetal heart rate

Each fetus will exhibit its own baseline rate. It is deduced by drawing a line where the FHR is steady without the transient changes of acceleration and deceleration. The normal baseline rate at term is 110–160 beats per minutes (bpm).

Baseline variability

Baseline variability is the 'wiggliness' of the baseline and is a reflection of the integrity of the autonomic nervous system and its influence on the heart rate. The ascending limb is due to the sympathetic and the descending limb is due to the parasympathetic activity of the fetal autonomic nervous system. The baseline variability is assessed by measuring the bandwidth of the 'wiggliness' seen during a 1-minute segment of the FHR trace. The normal baseline variability is 5–25 bpm. When it is < 5 bpm the baseline variability is reduced – which may be due to fetal sleep, drugs that act on the central nervous system, hypoxia, brain haemorrhage, infection, chromosomal or congenital malformation of the brain or heart.

Accelerations

Accelerations are a sudden rise of the FHR from the baseline by > 15 beats for a duration of > 15 seconds. These are usually associated with fetal movements. Two such accelerations in a 15-minute CTG trace are termed *reactive* and this usually indicates a non-hypoxic fetus.[6] It is very unusual for the neonate to be acidotic at birth if the FHR trace was reactive just before delivery.[7]

Decelerations

Decelerations are a sudden fall of the baseline rate of > 15 bpm for > 15 seconds. The shapes of the decelerations and relationship to contractions vary. Decelerations indicate a transient stress to the fetus. Based on the shape and timing of decelerations to the contractions, one can identify the cause of the stress.

Early decelerations are 'mirror images' of contractions and are associated with head compression in the late first and second stages of labour (Fig 4.1). There is a slow reduction in FHR as the intensity of contraction increases – the lowest FHR or nadir of the deceleration is at the peak or acme of the contraction. There is slow recovery of the FHR to the baseline rate as the contraction abates and returns to the baseline. Since they are reflective of head compression and vagal stimulation they should be seen only in the late first stage or second stage of labour. Early decelerations are not due to hypoxia and they do not decelerate > 40 bpm below the baseline rate.

Variable decelerations show a precipitous fall and quick recovery of the fetal heart rate that varies in shape, size and timing in relation to contractions. They are due to cord compression and are baroreceptor mediated. They can also be due to head compression but those due to cord compression have a momentary slight increase in the baseline rate just before and after the deceleration. These pre and post humps are described as 'shouldering' (Fig 4.2). Variable decelerations due to cord compression may be relieved by amnioinfusion.[8]

Atypical variable decelerations (Fig 4.3) In a pregnancy, more than one mechanism of stress may operate on the fetus. There may be cord compression due to oligohydramnios, maybe associated with placental insufficiency, so that with contractions the fetus may also exhibit late decelerations. When both mechanisms operate (cord compression and uteroplacental insufficiency) there may be a merger of variable and late decelerations. These can present as variable decelerations with late recovery of the FHR to the baseline rate after the contractions or as a biphasic or combined deceleration where a late deceleration follows

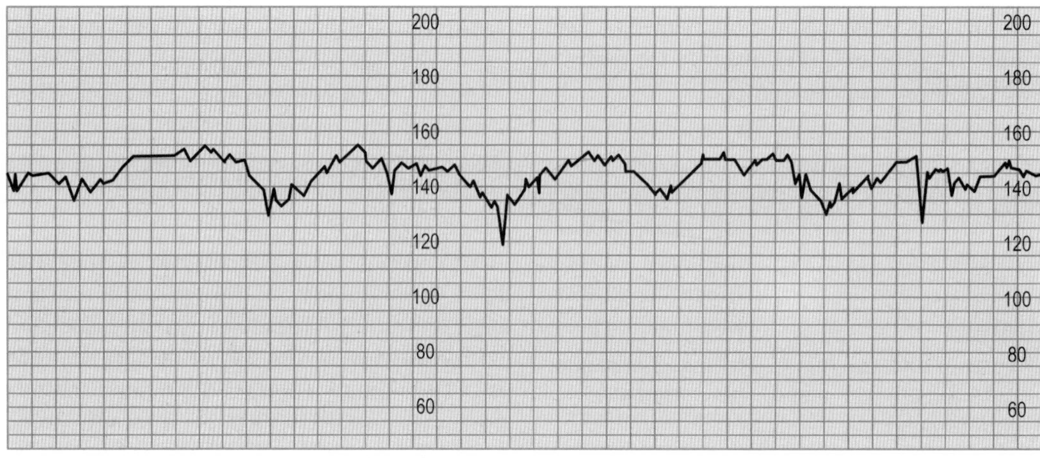

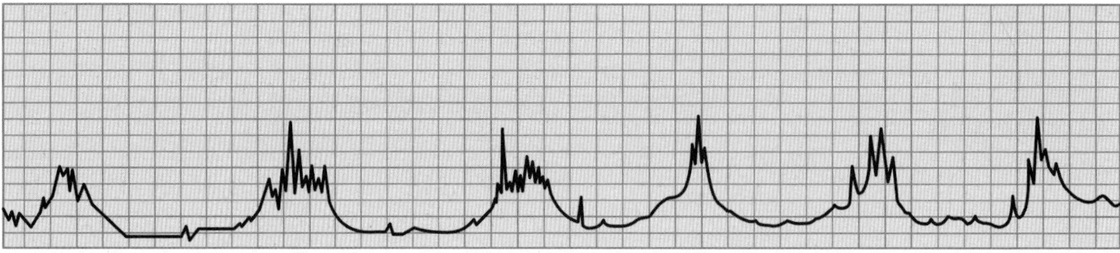

Figure 4.1 Early decelerations.

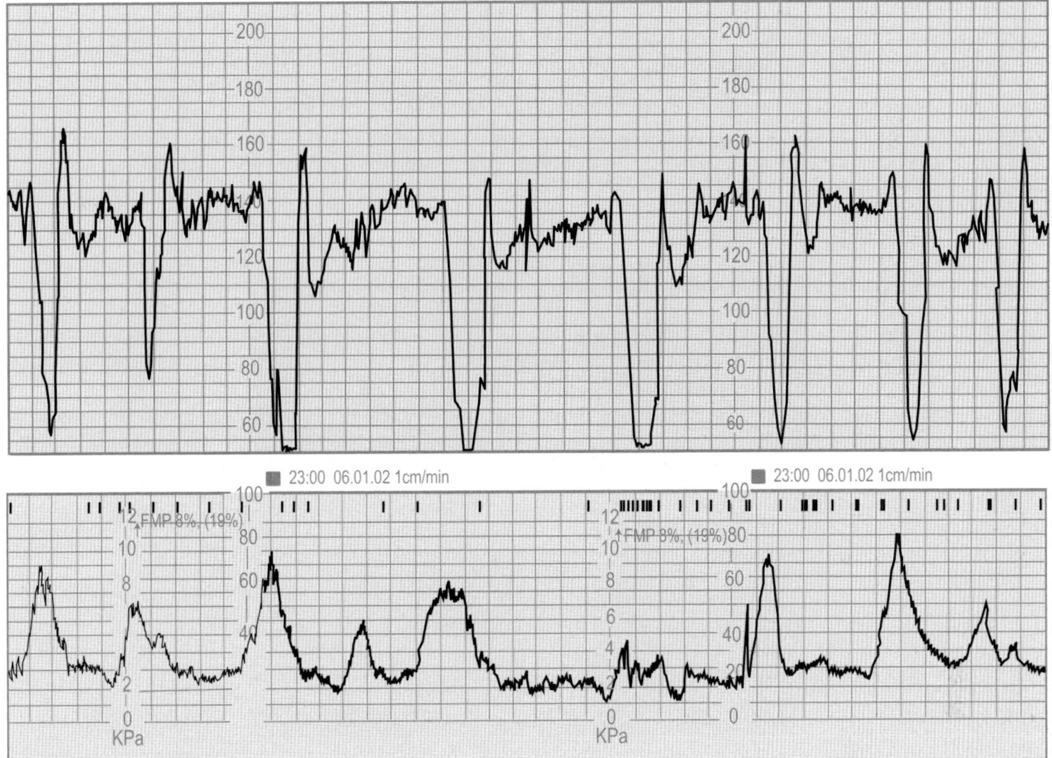

Figure 4.2 Simple variable decelerations with 'shouldering'.

immediately after a variable deceleration before it reaches the baseline. Variable decelerations with duration > 60 seconds and depth > 60 beats, and those with absence of baseline variability during and between variable decelerations, or overshoot of the returning heart rate, or the absence of shouldering after being present initially, are classified as atypical variable decelerations. Atypical variable decelerations are considered an abnormal feature in a CTG trace, whilst simple variable decelerations are considered a suspicious feature.[3]

Late decelerations start towards the end or soon after the contraction peaks and the rate does not recover until well after the contraction has ceased. When blood flow and oxygen supply to the intervillous space are critically reduced the fetal heart rate slows – an effect mediated via chemoreceptors. Typical late decelerations are shown in Figure 4.4.

The combination of late decelerations (however subtle) with persistent tachycardia and reduced baseline variability is the most predictably bad of all fetal heart rate patterns and is almost invariably associated with fetal hypoxaemia (Fig 4.5).

Fetal behavioural state in the CTG – 'cycling'

Non-hypoxic fetuses have alternate *active* and *quiet* sleep epochs on the CTG and this is referred to as 'cycling'. During the active sleep epoch there are several accelerations and good baseline variability. During the quiet epoch there are no or occasional accelerations and the baseline variability may be reduced to < 5 bpm. The quiet period can be 15–40 minutes and rarely more than 90 minutes unless

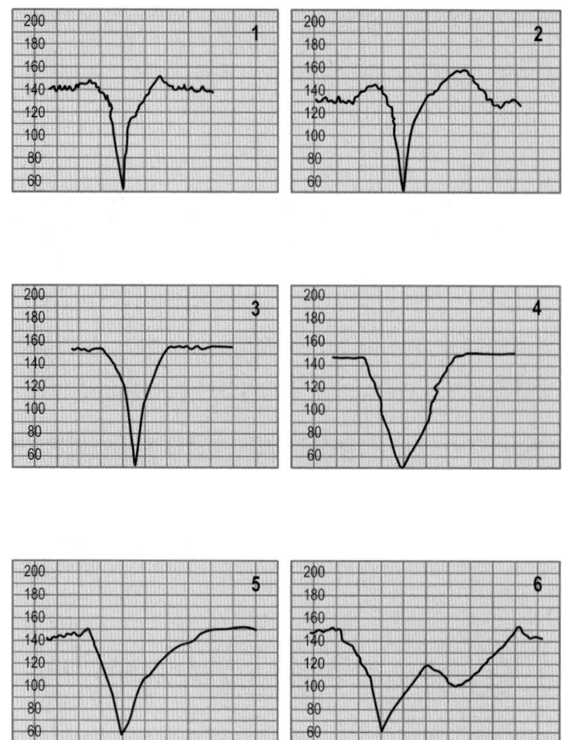

Figure 4.3 (1) Typical variable deceleration with shouldering; (2) atypical variable deceleration with overshoot; (3) atypical variable deceleration with loss of shouldering; (4) atypical variable deceleration showing loss of variability, and a depth of deceleration of 60 beats for > 60 seconds; (5) atypical variable deceleration with late recovery; (6) atypical variable deceleration with a variable and late component.

influenced by medication.[9] In the late first stage of labour the CTG may show a long quiet epoch when the head is deeply in the pelvis or after a narcotic is given for pain relief. Occasionally, a healthy fetus that has accelerations and good baseline variability may show segments of reduced variability and shallow decelerations during the quiet epoch but this period does not usually last for > 40 minutes, and rarely > 90 minutes, and seems to be associated with fetal breathing episodes.[10]

The absence of cycling indicates the possibility of an insult or injury that may have already happened or it may be that the fetus is hypoxic. If the trace was reactive and cycling and then becomes abnormal one may be able to identify the time of the insult. If the trace is abnormal from the time of admission then the insult/injury may have already taken place and the timing of injury may be difficult to ascertain. A reactive heart rate pattern of a fetus that exhibits cycling from early labour to near full dilatation is shown in Figure 4.6.

Cycling with an active followed by a quiet sleep pattern suggests that the baby is well oxygenated and likely to be neurologically normal. Absence of cycling may be due to drugs, infection, cerebral haemorrhage, chromosomal or congenital malformation or previous brain damage. A previously brain damaged fetus may or may not show cycling but the cord pH may be normal if there are accelerations. Such infants may exhibit signs of neurological damage later on in life.

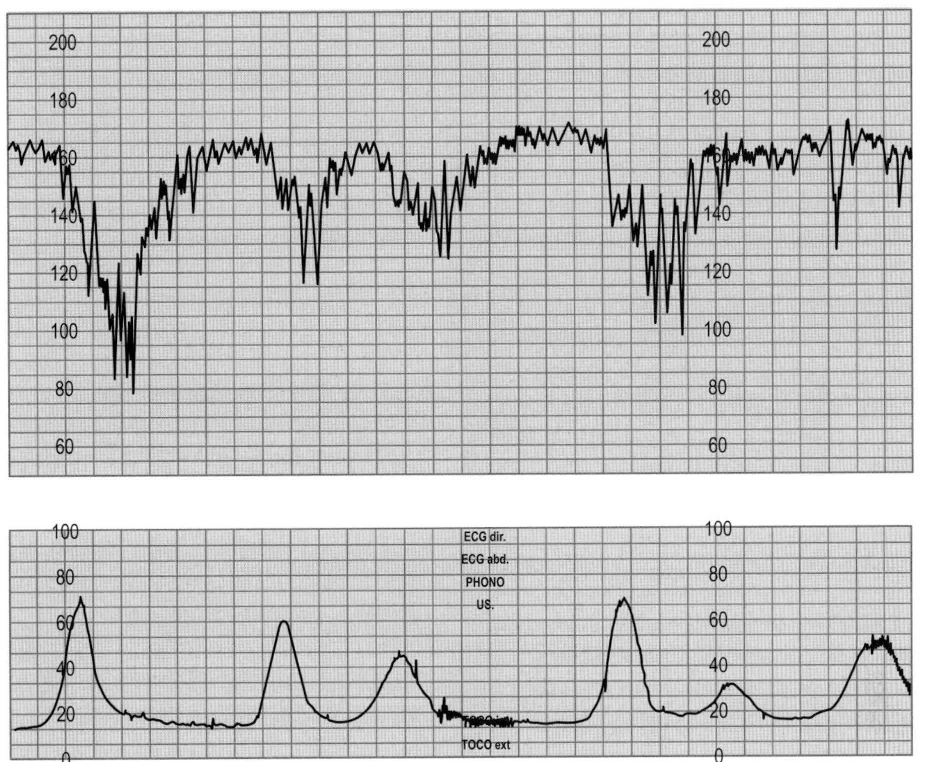

Figure 4.4 Late decelerations. The deceleration starts at or beyond the acme of the uterine contraction, is uniform in shape and does not recover until well after the contraction is over.

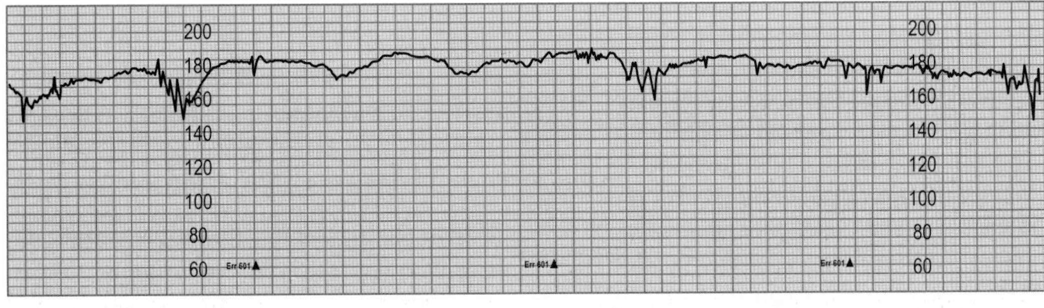

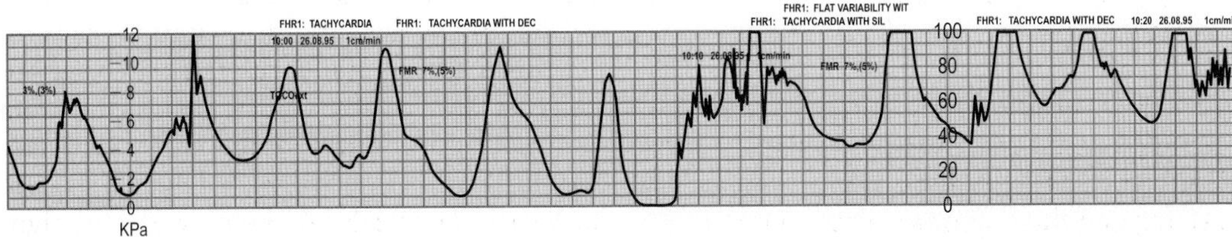

Figure 4.5 Combination of late decelerations, persistent tachycardia and reduced baseline variability – the fetal heart rate pattern most consistently associated with fetal hypoxaemia.

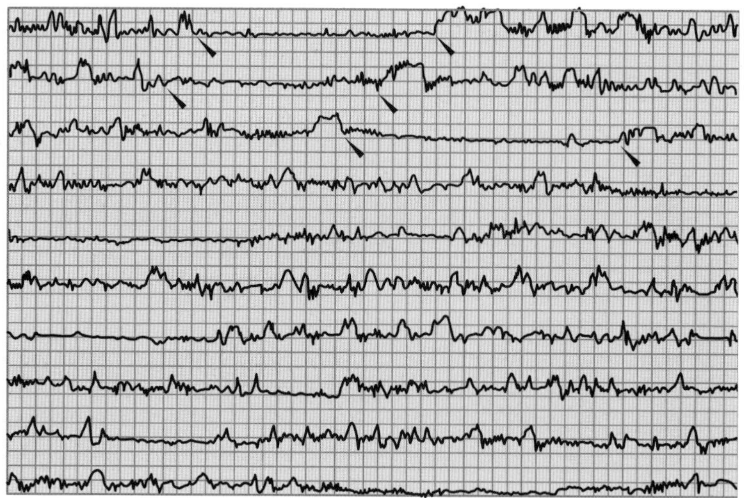

Figure 4.6 Active epochs with accelerations and good baseline variability, alternating with quiet epochs with hardly any acceleration and reduced baseline variability, can be seen in a CTG trace from the beginning to the end of labour.

'The foetal pulsation is much more frequent than the maternal pulse ... being about 130 or 140 in the minute; however, it is not necessarily observed to beat always at this rate ... This variation may depend upon a variety of inherent vital causes in the foetus ... An obvious explanation, however, is muscular action on the part of the foetus; and we shall very generally observe the pulsation of the foetal heart increased in frequency after such. The external cause which we shall find most frequently to operate on the fetal circulation, is uterine action, particularly when long continued, as in labour'.

Evory Kennedy
Observations on Obstetric Auscultation. Dublin: Longman, 1833

Identification of individual features of CTG trace and their classification

The NICE guidelines have provided a framework to categorize the CTG as normal, suspicious or pathological.[3] Once the trace is categorized as suspicious or pathological by the attendant he/she has to seek the possible cause and take action. Action may be one or more of the following: observation and continue with labour, hydration, stopping oxytocin, repositioning the mother, tocolysis, fetal scalp blood sampling, or delivery by the most appropriate route. This decision will depend on the parity, the cervical dilatation, rate of progress of labour, and risk factors based on the past and current obstetric history. The mother should be told of the issues involved and the possible actions needed, which should be based on informed choice and with her consent.

Classification of the individual features of the FHR trace[3]

See Table 4.2.

Classification of the cardiotocograph[3]

- *Normal* – all four features are reassuring.
- *Suspicious* – one of the features is non-reassuring.
- *Pathological* – ≥ 2 non-reassuring features; ≥ 1 abnormal feature.

The course of action necessary may vary even within the pathological category. If there is one feature that is abnormal, simple remedial actions and observation may be adequate. On the other hand if three features are abnormal the remedial action may be one or more of the following: stopping oxytocin, hydration, repositioning the woman, tocolytics if indicated, fetal scalp blood sampling (FBS) for pH, and/or delivery as thought to be appropriate depending on the clinical situation.

Sinusoidal pattern

Sinusoidal pattern is a description of the trace where the FHR appears like a sine wave form (Fig 4.7) but has none of the other features of baseline variability, accelerations or decelerations. Sinusoidal pattern was first described in fetuses with severe anaemia – pathological sinusoidal pattern.[11] Fetuses that are healthy and thumb sucking, as observed in an ultrasound examination, can also exhibit a physiological sinusoidal pattern.[12] The following are the known reasons for fetal anaemia that could give rise to a sinusoidal pattern.

Blood group antibodies that cross the placenta

In Rhesus iso-immunization higher concentration of antibodies can give rise to in utero anaemia. Maternal blood tests will reveal the presence of Rhesus antibodies and the concentration of antibodies can be measured. Presence of anti-Kell and anti-Duff antibodies can cause fetal anaemia. ABO blood group antibodies usually cause neonatal jaundice rather than fetal anaemia. Lewis a and b antibodies are not known to cause fetal anaemia.

Haemoglobinopathy

Alpha-thalassaemia in the fetus results in anaemia that may be associated with a sinusoidal pattern. Usually the mother presents in early third trimester with oedema and signs of pre-eclampsia. Ultrasound examination may

Table 4.2 Features of the FHR trace

	Baseline rate (bpm)	Variability (bpm)	Decelerations	Accelerations*
Reassuring	110–160	≥ 5	None Early	Present
Non-reassuring	100–109 161–180	< 5 for ≥ 40 min but < 90 min	Variable Single prolonged < 3 min	
Abnormal	< 100 > 180	< 5 for > 90 min Sinusoidal pattern for > 10 min	Atypical variable Late Single prolonged deceleration > 3 min	

* The absence of accelerations with an otherwise normal CTG is of uncertain significance.

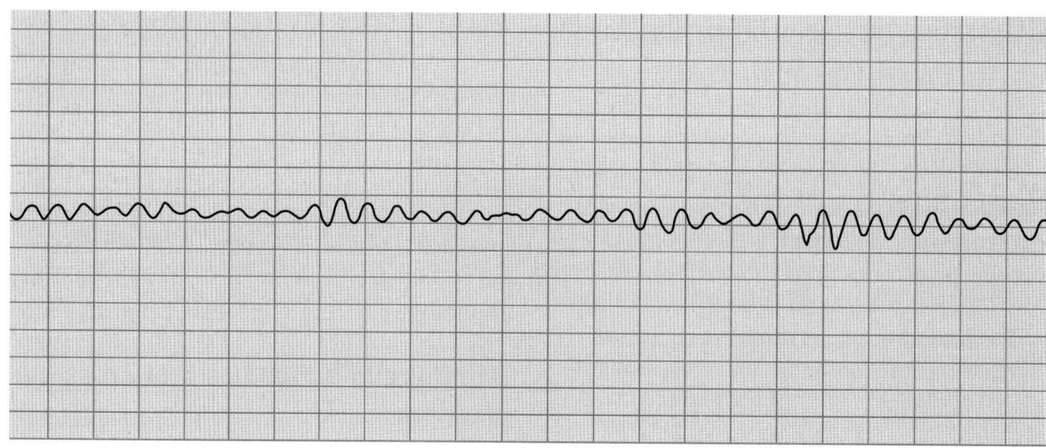

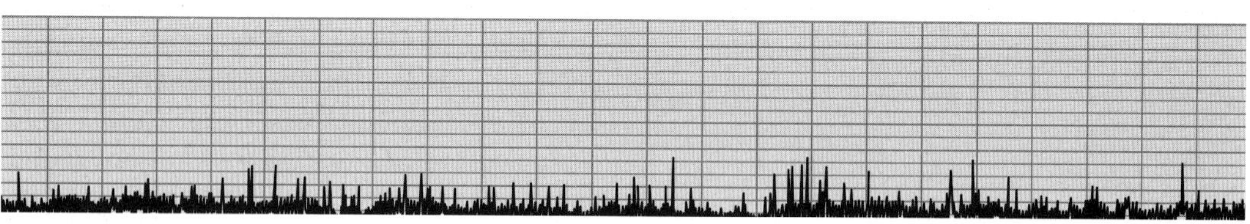

Figure 4.7 Sinusoidal pattern.

reveal polyhydramnios, hyperplacentosis and hydrops fetalis ('Bart's hydrops' due to four gene deletion). In these cases the mother may be a known thalassaemia carrier. Termination of pregnancy should be offered as the fetus with Bart's hydrops does not survive.

Fetal infection

Parvo virus infection is known to cause fetal anaemia. If a mother comes with a history of reduced or no fetal movements after a flu-like infection, an ultrasound examination would be useful in the presence of a sinusoidal pattern. A fetus appropriate for gestational age with reduced movement and with poor tone (open palm), or a hydropic fetus with ascites is suggestive of fetal anaemia and its consequences. Referral to a fetal medicine unit would be necessary to make a definitive diagnosis and possible therapy by intrauterine transfusion.

Feto-maternal transfusion

This is a well known cause of fetal anaemia and may show a pseudosinusoidal pattern (Fig 4.8). The Kleihauer–Betke test should identify fetal cells in maternal blood to confirm that the cause of anaemia is feto-maternal haemorrhage.

Monitoring uterine contractions

Interpretation of the FHR pattern in labour is not complete without relating it to uterine contractions. Uterine contractions are monitored by palpating the uterus between the uterine fundus and the umbilicus. By counting the number of contractions over a 10-minute period the frequency of uterine contractions can be accurately assessed. The duration of contractions can be assessed to some degree of accuracy by palpation but the baseline pressure and the amplitude or strength of contraction cannot. The observed uterine activity is usually charted in specific boxes provided on the partogram. There are five boxes and depending on the number of contractions over 10 minutes the boxes are shaded. If the

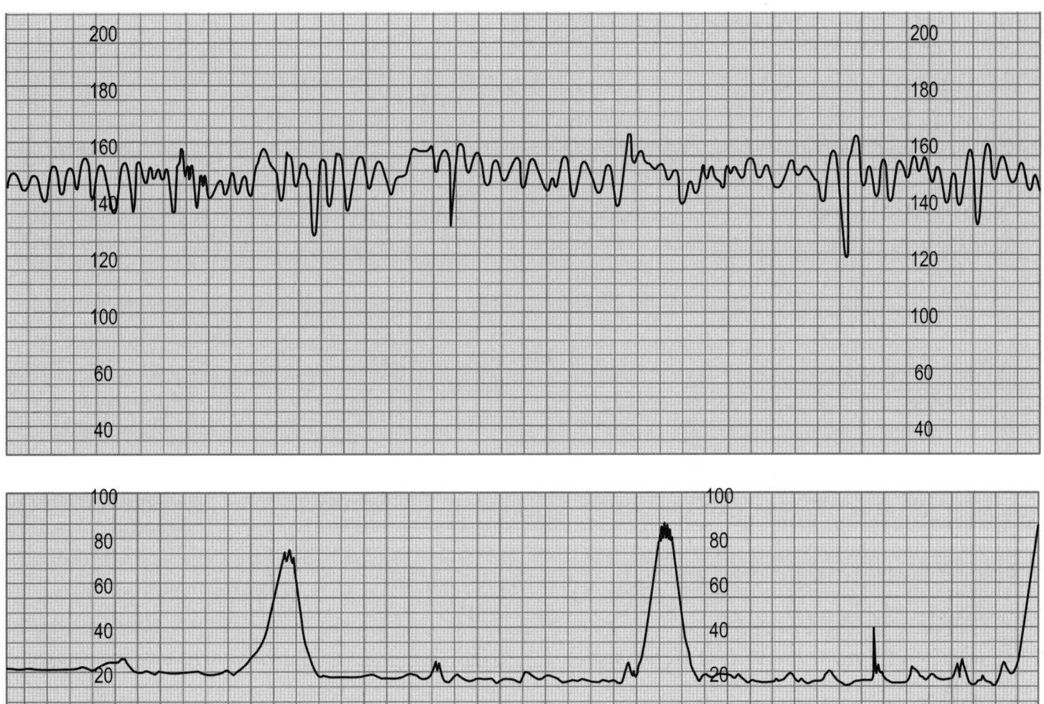

Figure 4.8 Pseudo sinusoidal pattern.

contractions last for < 20 seconds, dots are used; if the duration is 20–40 seconds oblique lines are drawn; and if it is > 40 seconds the boxes are completely shaded (Fig 4.9).

External tocography is performed by placing a transducer firmly across the abdomen over the uterus, midway between the uterine fundus and the umbilicus. With uterine contraction the upper part of the uterus expands anteriorly pushing the diaphragm or button on the toco transducer to produce the contraction curves. The baseline pressure can be set to 20 mmHg by using an automatic adjustment switch or by turning the toco knob on the machine. The contraction curves recorded will help to calculate the frequency and the duration accurately but not the baseline pressure or the amplitude of the uterine contractions. To accurately determine the baseline pressure and amplitude of contraction a pressure measuring catheter needs to be placed in utero after the membranes have ruptured.

Intrauterine catheters were initially fluid filled but went out of favour because of the inaccuracies associated with blockage by vernix and blood clots. Transducer tipped catheters are easy to insert and in recent times disposable transducer tipped catheters are available. The use of these catheters helps to

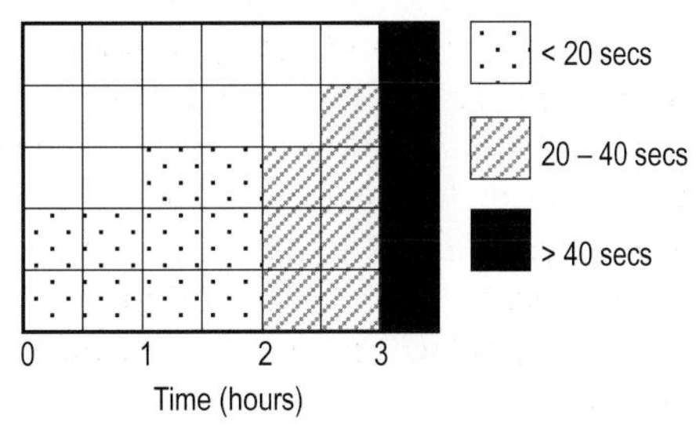

Figure 4.9 Quantification of uterine contractions by clinical palpation. Frequency per 10 min is recorded by shading the equivalent number of boxes. The type of shading indicates the duration of each contraction.

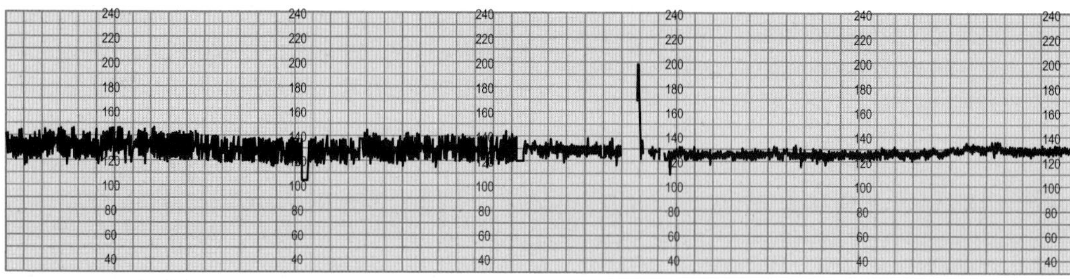

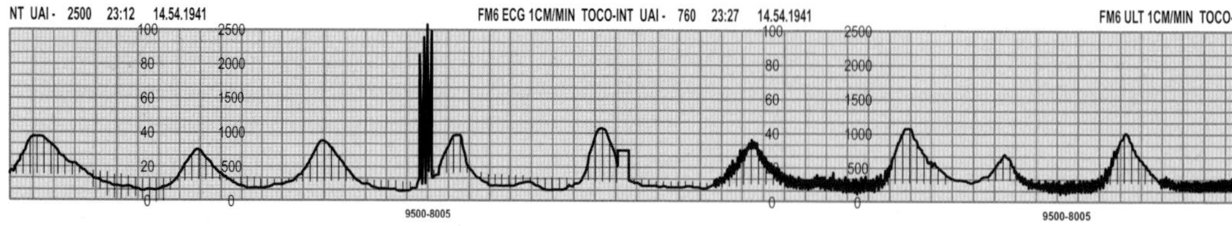

Figure 4.10 Quantification of uterine activity.

record the baseline pressure, frequency, duration and amplitude of contractions accurately. Equipment is available that can calculate the area under each contraction above the baseline pressure and quantify the uterine activity in kiloPascals every 15 minutes and annotate on the CTG trace[13] (Fig 4.10). The uterine activity in normal nulliparous and multiparous labour was studied[14,15] with a view to utilizing these values for induction and augmentation of labour. Despite the sophistication and knowledge obtained, randomized controlled trials did not show any benefit in using intrauterine catheters for induced or augmented labour when compared with external tocography.[16,17] Palpation of uterine contractions is the norm in low-risk labour and external tocography in high-risk labour. Current evidence does not recommend routine use of internal tocography.

'The discharge of meconium pending labour, in cases where the head presents, is dwelt upon by some as proving the death of the child. But its palpable insufficiency in this respect has been so well pointed out by Dr. Denman and indeed must be so obvious to every practical man, that it is deemed unnecessary to dwell upon it here, further than to state that it merits no confidence whatsoever, as a proof of the death of the fetus'.

Evory Kennedy
Observations on Obstetric Auscultation. Dublin: Longman, 1833

Meconium stained amniotic fluid

Meconium is the passage of bowel contents which usually occurs after birth but can happen in utero. The appearance of meconium in the amniotic fluid usually starts at term and the incidence increases with the period of gestation and is considered a function of maturing peristalsis.[18] An alternative explanation given is that the meconium is passed due to hypoxia causing relaxation of the fetal anal sphincter. It is rare to find meconium stained fluid in the preterm period. When it is found preterm it is usually due to infection and can be associated with listeriosis.[18,19]

It is not common to find meconium in cases of acute hypoxia, like cord prolapse or placental abruption. The chance of developing acidosis is greater in the presence of thick compared with light meconium stained fluid in the presence of an abnormal FHR pattern.[20] It is also known that when the FHR is abnormal in the presence of meconium, acidosis develops faster compared with clear fluid.[21] Hence, the presence of meconium is an indication for continuous EFM. If the FHR is reactive and normal the chance of acidosis is minimal and there is no need to do FBS to establish the fetal condition. On the other hand, if the CTG becomes abnormal in the presence of meconium FBS should be considered at an earlier stage. In clinical practice the presence of thick meconium with scanty fluid is of concern, as oligohydramnios may be due to reduced placental function.

An additional concern is the possibility of meconium aspiration during labour or at the time of birth. Meconium aspiration has no correlation to fetal acidaemia. No clear mechanism as to why the fetus aspirates meconium is known.[22] It is postulated that it may be associated with hypoxic episodes in utero. Care is taken when suctioning the oropharynx and nasopharynx at birth to prevent stimulation that may cause the fetus to aspirate, although available evidence does not support this practice.[23] Paediatricians look for signs of meconium below the vocal cords and, if present, carry out gastric and bronchial lavage to minimize the chances of meconium aspiration syndrome – a chemical pneumonitis that can be fatal. Amnioinfusion has been practised successfully in some centres to dilute the meconium in the amniotic fluid and reduce in utero meconium aspiration.[24] However, a large randomized control study showed no benefit with amnioinfusion for this purpose.[25]

Fetal scalp blood sampling (FBS)

Pre-terminal CTG patterns such as prolonged bradycardia, or a trace with markedly reduced baseline variability and late or atypical variable decelerations, warrant immediate delivery without FBS. Obvious clinical situations such as placental abruption, scar rupture or cord prolapse also prompts the need to take immediate action without FBS. Barring these situations the changes in the CTG may be of concern but do not necessarily indicate fetal hypoxia and acidosis. The parity, cervical dilatation, progress of labour and other obstetric risk factors such as the presence of meconium, intrauterine growth restriction, etc. may dictate the need for intervention and delivery, or close observation in anticipation of vaginal delivery, or possible instrumental delivery, or the need to do FBS. With an abnormal CTG a policy of awaiting spontaneous delivery or instrumental delivery in a short time may be acceptable in a multipara in the late first stage of labour who has been progressing well, whilst a caesarean section may be more appropriate if there is thick meconium in a primigravid who is 3–4 cm dilated. FBS may be considered if the woman is 5–6 cm dilated without any risk factors. Careful consideration of the clinical situation and good interpretation of the CTG is likely to reduce the number of cases that need FBS.

Results of continuous electronic fetal monitoring from the Cochrane reviews suggest that the relative risk of having a caesarean section with electronic fetal monitoring without the use of FBS is 1.72 (1.38–2.15) and that this could be reduced to 1.24 (1.05–1.48) with appropriate use of FBS.[26] The cut-off values in Table 4.3 are considered for action based on FBS.

If the result of the last FBS was closer to 7.25, or the CTG is getting worse, or there are additional risk factors like meconium, perform the FBS within an hour. Depending on the decline of the FBS and the progress in labour a clinical decision may then be made whether to allow more time or whether it is better to deliver the fetus.

FBS is contraindicated in known cases of HIV, hepatitis B carriers, suspected or confirmed cases of intrauterine infection, and in those with bleeding disorders. The discomfort to the mother, inconvenience for the operator and the difficulties in obtaining samples has made clinicians look for alternate methods. The intermittent nature of FBS is also a

Table 4.3 Actions based on FBS levels

pH	Condition	Action
< 7.20	Acidosis	Immediate delivery
7.20–7.25	Pre-acidosis	Consider another FBS in 30 minutes
> 7.25	Normal	Observe the CTG and if it does not improve consider another FBS based on the clinical situation and the evolving CTG pattern

disadvantage, as at times several samples are needed to make a clear decision. The alternate methods that are used in place of FBS or as an adjunct are described below.

Alternate or adjunctive methods of assessing fetal health

Fetal stimulation tests

Stimulation of an adult brought unconscious to an emergency department is a standard procedure and the level of arousal is considered a marker of the level of insult to the central nervous system. Extending the same principle, investigators have shown that fetal heart rate acceleration in response to an external stimulus is likely to be associated with a fetus that is not acidotic. Clarke et al showed that the fetal scalp pH was greater than 7.20 when it responded with a FHR acceleration to the stimulation of fetal scalp blood sampling.[27] The type of stimulation was extended to the use of Allis tissue forceps applied to the scalp[28,29] and then to a vibroacoustic stimulus through the maternal abdomen.[30,31] When the fetus responded with an acceleration the fetal pH was > 7.20, but when there was no response about 50% of the fetuses were acidotic. Concern was raised about stress to the fetus by the vibroacoustic stimulus because of prolonged periods of tachycardia following such stimulus in some fetuses.[32] Measurement of catecholamines in the umbilical cord blood during indicated cordocentesis has not shown any such increase after vibroacoustic stimulation.[33] Fear of auditory damage has been alleviated by follow-up testing at 4 years of age.[34,35]

Despite such reassurance the method has not found favour in many countries except North America. A meta analysis reviewed the likelihood ratios and 95% confidence intervals (CI) for some of the available observational studies on vibroacoustic stimulation tests.[36] Absence of FHR acceleration (positive test to detect acidaemia) had a likelihood ratio and 95% CI of 5.06 (2.69–9.50). Presence of an acceleration (negative test to exclude acidaemia) had a likelihood ratio and 95% CI of 0.32 (0.19–0.55). Thus, although the presence of acceleration is reassuring, the absence of acceleration requires verification of the fetal condition by fetal scalp blood sampling. Nonetheless, the fetal scalp stimulation test with Allis or similar forceps remains one of the simplest and most available clinical tests to help clarify a non-reassuring FHR pattern.

Fetal pulse oximetry

Pulse oximetry is used in intensive care and anaesthesia to monitor oxygen saturation in the adult. The same principle has been adapted for use to monitor the fetus in labour. Oxygen saturation is very variable in the fetus and the normal range fluctuates between 30% and 80%.[37] The sensors are placed apposed to the fetal cheek and held in position by the design which exerts counter pressure on the lower uterine segment to press the sensing surface against the fetal skin. Fetal scalp oximetry sensors that can be secured to the scalp have become available. Based on animal experiments and observational studies in the human fetus, the threshold value for action has been identified as 30% over a period of 10 minutes.[38] A number of prospective studies have assessed the feasibility and usefulness of this methodology in busy labour ward settings.[39]

A multi-centre controlled trial of fetal pulse oximetry in the intrapartum management of non-reassuring fetal heart rate patterns studied 1010 women.[40] When randomized, 502 had monitoring by CTG and 508 had CTG and pulse oximetry. Caesarean section (CS) for non-reassuring FHR pattern was 10.2% in the CTG arm compared with 4.5% in the CTG and pulse oximetry arm; a reduction of > 50% (p = 0.007). However, there was no reduction in overall CS rate; it was 26% in the CTG arm compared with 29% in the CTG pulse oximetry arm. The study concluded that if SpO_2 was > 30% the fetus is unlikely to be hypoxic but the use of pulse oximetry did not reduce the overall caesarean rate. Further randomized trials are in progress to evaluate its usefulness in clinical practice.

Fetal ECG waveform analysis

Animal experimental work consistently shows elevation of the ST segment or rise in the T wave with increasing hypoxia.[41,42] It has been observed that the degree of hypoxia prior to such changes depends on the myocardial glycogen in each species. Myocardial glycogen is mobilized to glucose in response to catecholamine release associated with hypoxic stress and the ST changes are due to entry of glucose into the cells with potassium (K^+). The fetal ECG signal is obtained with the help of a spiral electrode applied to the scalp of the fetus.[43,44] A maternal skin electrode is needed and computer software in the ST waveform analyzer (STAN 21 or 31- Neoventa, Goteborg, Sweden) formulates a sample ECG from 30 received complexes and analyses the T/QRS ratio.

The computer analysis of ECG to identify the baseline rise or episodic rise of T/QRS ratio is based on identifying the lowest T/QRS ratio for that fetus. This is done by the computer calculating the lowest T/QRS for 20 minutes by a moving window method (e.g. 4.20–4.40 h, 4.21–4.41 h and so on). The lowest T/QRS ratio for the previous 3 hours is considered for calculating the rise in T/QRS ratio. Therefore, the event log requires 20 minutes before automatic ST analysis can begin. During the first 20 minutes of use and when there is a decrease in signal quality with discontinuous T/QRS ratios (there should be at least 10 signals in a 10-minute window for computer analysis), manual data analysis is required. If the machine is disconnected from the woman, and then reconnected within 3 hours, the computer retains the lowest 20-minute T/QRS ratio in memory from the previous 3 hours for that fetus. This enables it to provide the analysis with change in T/QRS ratio once the equipment is reconnected.

In addition to rise in the T/QRS ratio (Fig 4.11) there may be changes in the ST segment – these are known as biphasic ST waveform (Fig 4.12). If the ST waveform changes are above the isoelectric line it is called biphasic grade I, if it cuts the isoelectric line it is biphasic grade II and if the changes are below the isoelectric line it is grade III. The change is due to repolarization of the ventricle and is a function of the flow of current from endocardium to epicardium. These changes are seen often in a preterm fetus and may be due to the thickness of the myocardium; hence, ST analysis is not used in fetuses less than 36 completed weeks. In addition to chronic hypoxia it may be seen in the initial phases of acute hypoxia, in cases of myocardial dystrophy and with maternal fever and infection.

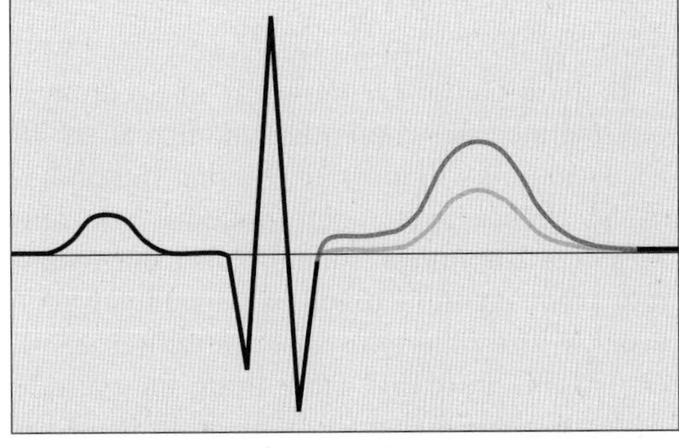

Figure 4.11 Fetal ECG waveform analysis. The rise in ST segment and increase in T wave height with hypoxia, adrenaline surge and anaerobic metabolism.

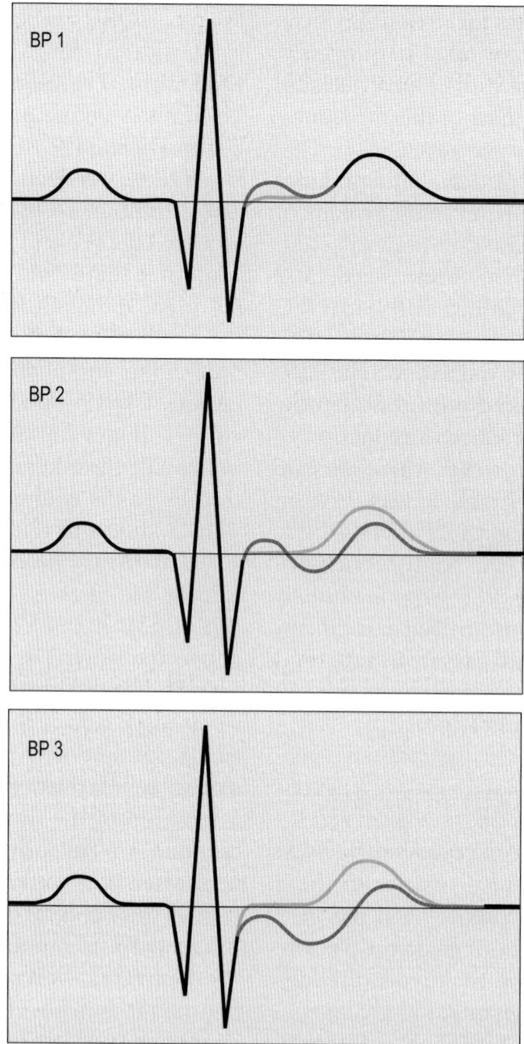

Figure 4.12 Fetal ECG waveform analysis. BP1 biphasic grade 1 (ST change is above the isoelectric line). BP2 biphasic grade 2 (ST change cuts the isoelectric line). BP3 biphasic grade 3 (ST change is below the isoelectric line).

If the biphasic events occur in a continuous manner the computer will flag it as an ST event and will indicate whether the biphasic ST changes were continuous for > 5 minutes or > 2 minutes. If the biphasic events are more than a couple it will be flagged as an ST event. More than two episodes with a suspicious CTG trace and more than one episode with an abnormal trace is an indication for intervention.

Significant ST events identified by the ST analyzer are flagged and described according to the *type* (e.g. baseline T/QRS rise, episodic rise in T/QRS, continuous biphasic patterns > 2 or 5 minutes, or episodes of biphasic patterns) and *magnitude* of change. These STAN events need to be correlated with the CTG, which needs to be visually interpreted. If one is unable to categorize the CTG as suspicious or abnormal then fetal scalp blood sampling may be required to resolve the situation.

Two randomized controlled trials[45,46] are included in the Cochrane review.[47] These studies conclude that operative delivery for fetal distress and the incidence of fetal metabolic acidosis are reduced by the combined analysis of the FHR and ST waveform. An additional benefit was fewer indicated fetal scalp blood samples.

Fetal scalp lactate measurements

In the fetus a short period of prolonged bradycardia reduces the circulation through the placenta, causing CO_2 to accumulate in the circulation and a decline in pH – respiratory acidosis. However, when the circulation returns to normal the CO_2 is transferred through the placenta, resulting in the rapid return of the pH to normal. In the fetus pre-acidaemia is likely to be of respiratory origin. If the circulation continues to be slow, due to prolonged bradycardia, it will affect oxygen transfer to the fetus. This will result in anaerobic metabolism that takes place within the cell and leads to accumulation of lactic acid.

The metabolic acidosis caused by excess lactate is metabolized very slowly and takes an estimated 2–4 hours to clear. The build-up of lactate appears to be related to hypoxia > 10 minutes. The duration of hypoxia will determine the lactate levels. Because lactate takes hours to clear the metabolic acid remains long after hypoxia is corrected.

A prospective randomized study compared lactate with pH analysis at fetal scalp blood sampling and found no significant differences in caesarean section rates, or cord artery pH.[48] One benefit of lactate analysis is that only 5 μl of blood is required, compared with 35 μl for most automatic pH and blood gas analyses.

Scalp blood lactate correlates well with umbilical arterial and venous lactate, indicating that it could be used for clinical decision making.[49] The surrogate measures considered for subsequent neurological outcome of the newborn such as Apgar scores, cord arterial pH and base deficit, have good correlation to cord blood lactate levels.[50,51] The use of lactate or pH and base deficit has similar sensitivity, specificity and predictive values for perinatal complications.[52]

Near infrared spectroscopy

Direct measurement of cerebral oxygenation is an attractive concept and near infrared (NIR) spectroscopy – a 'non-invasive' technique – has been evaluated.[53,54] Optic bundles in a silicone mold are placed against the fetal head via the cervix to measure the absorption characteristics of oxygenated and de-oxygenated haemoglobin. The NIR light at wavelength 750–1000 nm is transmitted through the scalp, skull and brain and the reflected light is measured to calculate the absorption.[55] The results indicate a positive correlation between the mean cerebral oxygen saturation and the umbilical artery acid–base measurements.[56] However, the machine is large and the technique needs further refinement before clinical trials can start.

Intrapartum maternal pyrexia and neonatal encephalopathy

There are several risk factors for neonatal encephalopathy and maternal pyrexia is being increasingly identified as a major determinant. A study from Western Australia reported an odds ratio for neonatal encephalopathy of 3.82 for maternal pyrexia, compared with 4.29 for persistent occipito-posterior position and 4.44 for an acute intrapartum event.[57] Intrapartum fever is also associated with epidural use.[58] In a series of 4915 low-risk term labours, after controlling for epidural use the odds ratio for neonatal encephalopathy with intrapartum pyrexia was 4.7 (1.3–17.4).[59] There was also a higher incidence of metabolic acidosis (odds ratio 2.91; 1.14–7.39), and admission to neonatal intensive care (odds ratio 1.78; 1.1–2.89).

Not only the incidence of neonatal encephalopathy but the incidence of cerebral palsy is increased in women who have pyrexia exceeding 38°C in labour, with an odds ratio as high as 9.3 (CI 2.7–31.0).[60]

Based on these reports it is important to treat pyrexia in labour although it may not always have an infective origin. Steer and his group have been working on measuring fetal temperature in labour for over a decade. Using special sensors they measured maternal and fetal temperature and showed that fetal temperature was one degree higher than the maternal temperature. They also showed that it is possible to reduce the fetal temperature by lowering the maternal temperature.[61]

Conclusions

Every labour has an inherent risk to the mother or the fetus. Prospectively we label pregnancies as low and high risk and plan to provide appropriate care. The woman and her partner's wishes need to be considered and the plan of care formulated according to their request after discussion. Mothers at low risk should be offered intermittent auscultation, as continuous EFM carries an increased risk of obstetric interventions. EFM has been in use over the last four decades but has not reduced perinatal mortality and morbidity based on available studies. Most studies have been in low-risk labours and are under-powered to show any difference in the rare outcome measures of hypoxic ischaemic encephalopathy, cerebral palsy, or intrapartum deaths. The 4th Confidential Enquiries into Stillbirths and Deaths in Infancy (CESDI) [62] highlighted that in 1995, there were about 1 in 1600 intrapartum deaths in babies weighing > 1500 g with no chromosomal or congenital malformation. The report concluded that about 50% of the deaths could have been avoided if there was proper interpretation of CTG and prompt action. Other reviews have reached similar conclusions.[63,64] This highlights the need for a clear understanding of CTG interpretation and additional methods of intrapartum surveillance. The need is urgent as recent studies based on neuro-imaging suggest that 27% of cerebral palsy in term infants may be due to intrapartum asphyxia.[65]

In order to overcome the difficulties in interpretation of CTGs new technologies have been introduced. A recent large randomized trial on pulse oximetry has shown the method to be of little value in intrapartum surveillance. However, none of these can be used in isolation – only as adjuncts to CTG monitoring. Hence, learning CTG interpretation is vital for anyone providing care for high-risk women in labour, and it has to be considered in the clinical context of each individual case. The following points are useful when CTG is used for fetal surveillance:[67]

- Accelerations and baseline variability are hallmarks of fetal health
- Accelerations without baseline variability should be considered suspicious
- Periods of decreased variability without decelerations may represent quiet sleep
- Hypoxic fetuses may have a normal baseline FHR of 110–160 bpm with no accelerations and baseline variability of < 5 for > 40 minutes
- In the presence of baseline variability < 5 bpm even shallow late decelerations < 15 bpm are ominous in a non-reactive trace
- Abruption, cord prolapse and scar rupture can cause acute hypoxia and should be suspected and managed clinically (may give rise to prolonged decelerations/bradycardia)
- Fetal hypoxia and acidosis may develop faster with an abnormal trace when there is scanty fluid with thick meconium, intrauterine growth restriction, intrauterine infection with pyrexia, bleeding and/or pre- or post-term labour
- In preterm fetuses (especially < 34 weeks), hypoxia and acidosis can increase the likelihood of respiratory distress syndrome and may contribute to intraventricular haemorrhage, warranting early intervention in the presence of an abnormal trace
- Hypoxia can be made worse by oxytocin, epidural analgesia and difficult operative deliveries
- During labour, if decelerations are absent, asphyxia is unlikely although it cannot be completely excluded
- Abnormal patterns may represent the effects of drugs, fetal anomaly, fetal injury or infection and not only hypoxia.

References

1. Thacker SB, Stroup DF, Chang M. Continuous electronic heart rate monitoring for fetal assessment during labor (Cochrane review). The Cochrane Library 2004;1. Chichester: John Wiley.
2. Thacker SB, Stroup DF, Chang M. Continuous electronic heart rate monitoring for fetal assessment during labor (Cochrane review). The Cochrane Library 2002;2. Oxford: Update software UK.
3. National Institute of Clinical Excellence. Royal College of Obstetricians and Gynaecologists. The use of electronic fetal heart rate monitoring. Evidence Based Clinical Guideline No. 8. London: RCOG Press, 2001.
4. Society of Obstetricians and Gynaecologists of Canada. Clinical Practice Guideline No. 112. J Obstet Gynaecol Can 2002; 24:342–348.
5. American College of Obstetricians and Gynecologists. Practice Bulletin No. 70. Obstet Gynecol 2005; 106:1453–1461.
6. Kubli FW, Hon EH, Khazin AF, Takemura H. Observations on heart rate and pH in the human fetus during labour. Am J Obstet Gynecol 1969; 109:1190–1206.
7. Beard RW, Filshie GM, Knight CA, Roberts GM. The significance of the changes in the continuous fetal heart rate in the first stage of labour. J Obstet Gynaecol Br Commw 1971; 78:865–881.
8. Miyazaki FS, Nevarez F. Saline amniotic infusion for relief of repetitive variable decelerations: a prospective randomized study. Am J Obstet Gynecol 1985; 153:301–303.
9. Spencer JAD, Johnson P. Fetal heart rate variability changes and fetal behavioural cycles during labour. Br J Obstet Gynaecol 1986; 93:314–321.
10. Schifrin B, Artenos J, Lyseight N. Late-onset fetal cardiac decelerations associated with fetal breathing movements. J Matern Fetal Neonat Med 2002; 12:253–259.
11. Modanlou HD, Freeman RH. Sinusoidal fetal heart rate patterns; its definition and clinical significance. Am J Obstet Gynecol 1982; 142:1033–1038.
12. Nijhuis JG, Staisch KJ, Martin C, Prechtel HFR. A sinusoidal like fetal heart rate pattern in association with fetal sucking. Report of 2 cases. Eur J Obstet Gynecol Reprod Biol 1984; 16:353–358.
13. Steer PJ. The measurement and control of uterine contractions. In: Beard RW, ed. The current status of fetal heart rate monitoring and ultrasound in obstetrics. London: RCOG Press, 1977.
14. Gibb DMF, Arulkumaran S, Lun KC, Ratnam SS. Characteristics of uterine activity in nulliparous labour. Br J Obstet Gynaecol 1984; 91:220–227.
15. Arulkumaran S, Gibb DMF, Lun KC, Ratnam SS. The effect of parity on uterine activity in labour. Br J Obstet Gynaecol 1984; 91:843–848.
16. Chua S, Kurup A, Arulkumaran S, Ratnam SS. Augmentation of labor: does internal tocography produce better obstetric outcome then external tocography? Obstet Gynecol 1990; 76:164–167.
17. Arulkumaran S, Ingemarsson I, Ratnam SS. Oxytocin titration to achieve preset active contraction area values does not improve the outcome of induced labour. Br J Obstet Gynaecol 1987; 94:242–248.
18. Miller FC. Meconium staining of the amniotic fluid. Clin Obstet Gynecol 1979; 6:359–365.
19. Buchdahl R, Hird M, Gibb DMF. Listeriosis revisited: the role of the obstetrician. Br J Obstet Gynaecol 1990; 97:186–189.
20. Arulkumaran S, Yeoh SC, Gibb DMF. Obstetric outcome of meconium stained liquor in labour. Singapore Med J 1985; 26:523–526.
21. Steer PJ. Fetal distress. In: Crawford J, ed. Risks of labour. Chichester: John Wiley, 1985:11–31.
22. Wiswell TE, Bent RC. Meconium staining and meconium aspiration syndrome. Unresolved issues. Pediatr Clin North Am 1993; 40:955–981.
23. Vain NE, Szyld EG, Prudent LM, Wiswell TE, Aguilar AM, Vivas NI. Oropharyngeal and nasopharyngeal suctioning of meconium stained neonates before delivery of their shoulders: multicentre, randomised controlled trial. Lancet 2004; 364:597–602.
24. Hofmyer GJ. Amnioinfusion for meconium stained liquor in labour (Cochrane Review). Cochrane Library, 2004. Chichester: John Wiley.

25. Fraser W, Hofmeyr G, Lede R, et al. Amnioinfusion for the prevention of the meconium aspiration syndrome. N Engl J Med 2005; 353:909–917.

26. Neilson JP. Fetal scalp blood sampling as adjunct to heart rate monitoring, In: Enkin MW, Keirse MJ, Renfew MJ, Neilson JP, eds. Pregnancy and childbirth module of the Cochrane database of systematic reviews. Cochrane Collaboration, Issue 2. Oxford: Update software UK, 1995.

27. Clarke SL, Gimovsky ML, Miller FC. Fetal heart rate response to scalp blood sampling. Am J Obstet Gynecol 1983; 144:706–708.

28. Clarke SL, Gimovsky ML, Miller FC. The scalp stimulation test: a clinical alternative to fetal scalp blood sampling. Am J Obstet Gynecol 1984; 148:274–277.

29. Arulkumaran S, Ingemarsson I, Ratnam SS. Fetal heart rate response to scalp stimulation as a test for fetal wellbeing in labour. Asia Oceania J Obstet Gynecol 1987; 13:131–135.

30. Edersheim TG, Hutson JM, Druzin ML, Kogut EA. Fetal heart rate response to vibratory acoustic stimulation predicts fetal pH in labor. Am J Obstet Gynecol 1987; 157:1557–1560.

31. Ingemarsson I, Arulkumaran S. Reactive FHR response to sound stimulation in fetuses with low scalp blood pH. Br J Obstet Gynaecol 1989; 96:562–565.

32. Spencer JAD, Deans A, Nicolaidis P, Arulkumaran S. Fetal response to vibroacoustic stimulation during low and high fetal heart rate variability episodes in late pregnancy. Am J Obstet Gynecol 1991; 165:86–90.

33. Fisk NM, Nicolaidis P, Arulkumaran S. Vibroacoustic stimulation is not associated with sudden fetal catecholamine release. Early Hum Dev 1991; 25:11–17.

34. Arulkumaran S, Skurr B, Tong H. No evidence of hearing loss due to fetal acoustic stimulation test. Obstet Gynecol 1991; 78:283–285.

35. Nyman M, Barr M, Westgren M. A four year follow up of hearing and development in children exposed to in utero vibro-acoustic stimulation. Br J Obstet Gynaecol 1992; 99:685–688.

36. Skupski DW, Rosenberg CR, Eglinton GS. Intrapartum fetal stimulation tests: a meta-analysis. Obstet Gynecol 2002; 99:129–134.

37. Chua S, Yeong SM, Razvi K, Arulkumaran S. Fetal oxygen saturation during labour. Br J Obstet Gynaecol 1997; 104:1080–1083.

38. Kuhnert M, Seelbach-Goebel B, Di Renzo GC, Howarth E, Butterwegge M, Murray JM. Guidelines for the use of fetal pulse oximetry during labour and delivery. Prenatal Neonatal Med 1998; 3:423–433.

39. Chua S, Rhazvi K, Yeong SM, Arulkumaran S. Intrapartum fetal oxygen saturation monitoring in a busy labour ward. Eur J Obstet Gynecol Reprod Biol 1999; 82:185–189.

40. Garite TJ, Dildy GA, McNamara H. A multicenter controlled trial of fetal pulse oximetry in the intrapartum management of non-reassuring fetal heart rate patterns. Am J Obstet Gynecol 2000; 183:1049–1058.

41. Rosen KG, Dagbjartsson A, Henriksson BA, Lagercrantz H, Kjellmer I. The relationship between circulating catecholamines and ST waveform in fetal lamb electrocardiogram during hypoxia. Am J Obstet Gynecol 1984; 149:190–195.

42. Greene KR, Dawes GS, Lilja H, Rosen KG. Changes in the ST waveform of the lamb electrocardiogram with hypoxia. Am J Obstet Gynecol 1982; 144:950–957.

43. Lilja H, Arulkumaran S, Lindecrantz K. Fetal ECG during labour; a presentation of a microprocessor based system. J Biomed Eng 1988; 10:348–350.

44. Arulkumaran S, Lilja H, Lindecrantz K, Ratnam SS, Thavarasah AS, Rosen KG. Fetal ECG waveform analysis should improve fetal surveillance in labour. J Perinat Med 1990; 187:13–22.

45. Amer-Wahlin I, Hellsten C, Noren H, et al. Carditocography only versus cardiotocography plus ST analysis of fetal electrocardiogram for intrapartum fetal monitoring: a Swedish randomised controlled trial. Lancet 2001; 358:534–538.

46. Westgate J, Harris M, Curnow JSH, Greene KR. Randomised trial of cardiotocography alone or with ST waveform analysis for intrapartum monitoring. Lancet 1992;2:194–198.

47. Neilson JP. Fetal electrocardiogram (ECG) for fetal monitoring during labour. The Cochrane Library, Issue 2, 2003. Oxford.

48. Westgren M, Kruger K, Ek S, Gruwevald C, Kublickas M, Naka K. Lactate compared with pH analysis at fetal scalp blood sampling. a prospective randomised study. Br J Obstet Gynaecol 1998; 105:29–33.

49. Kruger K, Kublickas M, Westgren. Lactate in scalp and cord blood from fetuses with ominous fetal heart rate patterns. Obstet Gynecol 1998; 92:918–922.

50. Nordstrom L, Achanna S, Naka K, Arulkumaran S. Fetal and maternal lactate increase during active second stage of labour. Br J Obstet Gynaecol 2001; 108:263–268.

51. Nordstrom L. Fetal scalp and cord blood lactate. Best Pract Res Clin Obstet Gynaecol 2004; 18:467–476.

52. Kruger K, Hallberg B, Blennow M. Predictive value of fetal scalp blood lactate concentration and pH as a marker for neurologic disability. Am J Obstet Gynecol 1999; 181:1072–1078.

53. O'Brien PM, Doyle PR, Rolfe P. Near infrared spectroscopy in fetal monitoring. Br J Hosp Med 1993; 49:483–487.

54. Peebles DM. Cerebral haemodynamics and oxygenation in the fetus: the role of intrapartum near-infrared spectroscopy. Clin Perinatol 1997; 24:547–565.

55. Peebles DM, Edwards AD, Wyatt JS, et al. Changes in human fetal cerebral hemoglobin concentration and oxygenation during labor measured by near-infrared spectroscopy. Am J Obstet Gynecol 1992; 166:1369–1373.

56. Aldrich CJ, D'Antona D, Wyatt JS, Spencer JAD, Peebles DM, Reynolds EOR. Fetal cerebral oxygenation measured by near-infrared spectroscopy shortly after birth and acid-base status at birth. Obstet Gynecol 1994; 84:861–866.

57. Badawi N, Kurinczuk JJ, Keogh JM, et al. Intrapartum risk factors for newborn encephalopathy: the Western Australian case-control study. BMJ 1998; 317:1554–1558.

58. Fusi L, Steer PJ, Maresh MJ, Beard RW. Maternal pyrexia associated with the use of epidural analgesia in labour. Lancet 1989; 1:1250–1252.

59. Impey L, Greenwood C, MacQuillan K, Reynolds M, Sheil O. Fever in labour and neonatal encephalopathy: a prospective cohort study. Br J Obstet Gynaecol 2001; 108:594–597.

60. Grether JK, Nelson KB. Maternal infection and cerebral palsy in infants of normal birth weight. JAMA 1997; 278:207–211.

61. Banerjee S, Steer PJ. The rise in maternal temperature associated with regional analgesia in labour is harmful and should be treated. Int J Obstet Anaesth 2003; 12:280–286.

62. Confidential Enquiry into Stillbirths and Deaths in Infancy. 4th Annual Report. London: Maternal and Child Health Research Consortium, 1997.

63. Westergaard HB, Kanghoff-Roos J, Larsen S, Borch-Christensen H, Luidmark G. Intrapartum death of normal formed fetuses in Denmark and Sweden in 1991. A perinatal audit. Acta Obstet Gynecol Scand 1997; 76:959–963.

64. Mattatall FM, O'Connell CM, Baskett TF. A review of intrapartum deaths, 1982 to 2002. Am J Obstet Gynecol 2005; 192:1475–1477.

65. Hagberg B, Hagberg G, Beckung E, Uvebrant P. Changing panorama of cerebral palsy in Sweden. VII. Prevalence and origin in the birth year period 1991–1994. Acta Paediatrica 2001; 90:271–277.

66. Bloom SL, Spong CY, Thom E, et al. Fetal pulse oximetry and cesarean delivery. N Engl Med J 2006; 388:2195–2202.

67. Arulkumaran S, Ingemarsson I, Montan S, et al. Traces of you: fetal trace interpretation. Nederland, Philips Medical Systems, 2002. Ref. 4522 981 88671/862.

Acknowledgements

The authors acknowledge Mr Donald Gibb and Elsevier for permission to reproduce in Chapters 4 and 5 some of the Figures from *Fetal Monitoring in Practice*, 2nd edn. Oxford: Butterworth 1997.

5

Fetal asphyxia

'Abnormal parturition, besides ending in death or recovery, not infrequently had a third termination in other diseases ... a delay of only a few moments in the substitution of pulmonary for the ceased placental respiration would lead to the apprehension that even the want of a few breathings, if not fatal to the economy, may imprint a lasting injury upon it.'

William John Little
On the influence of abnormal parturition, difficult labours, premature birth, and asphyxia neonatorum, on the mental and physical condition of the child, especially in relation to deformities. Trans Obstet Soc London 1861–62; 3:293–344.

The main contributor to litigation in obstetrics relates to fetal surveillance in labour. The Clinical Negligence Scheme for Trust (CNST) has introduced maternity standards in order to achieve better care for women and the newborn.[1] The National Patient Safety Agency (NPSA) has placed obstetrics as number one priority in their list, with the goal of reducing adverse outcome by 50% in the next few years.[2] The fourth Confidential Enquiry into Stillbirths and Deaths in Infancy (CESDI) report examined intrapartum deaths of babies over 1500 g with no chromosomal or congenital malformation.[3] They concluded that 50% of deaths were avoidable and another 25% were potentially avoidable. A considerable number of asphyxial injuries could be prevented if the problem is recognized and acted upon promptly. With the advent of magnetic resonance imaging (MRI), animal experimentation started to look at different types of hypoxia, changes in fetal heart rate (FHR) patterns and associated brain injury.[4] The type of brain injury seen on MRI correlates with the type of cerebral palsy. A recent study from Sweden suggests that up to 28%[5] rather than the conventional 10% of cases[6] of cerebral palsy may be related to intrapartum asphyxia. Although asphyxial injures are few in number, in terms of medical negligence they account for about 30% of claims and for about 60–70% of compensation paid out by the CNST. This chapter examines the cardiotocograph (CTG) patterns associated with injuries due to birth asphyxia that lead to litigation and how these could be reduced.

Hypoxaemia, hypoxia and asphyxia

The definitions of the terms hypoxaemia, hypoxia and asphyxia used in this chapter are provided below. *Hypoxaemia* is reduced oxygen in the blood and *hypoxia* is reduced oxygen in the tissues secondary to continuing hypoxaemia. *Asphyxia* is hypoxia and metabolic acidosis in the tissues. The fetus reacts to hypoxaemia by extracting more oxygen from the blood and this period is associated with reduced fetal movements and absence of fetal heart rate accelerations. With hypoxia there is a catecholamine surge causing vasoconstriction in non-essential organs (skin, muscle, bone, liver, intestines and kidneys), and an increase in cardiac output by raising the heart rate. This vascular redistribution mechanism maintains the oxygen requirements to the tissues. If the hypoxia is sustained, there is further deprivation of oxygen and the cells undertake anaerobic metabolism, converting glucose into lactic acid rather than CO_2 and water.

This state of hypoxia and metabolic acidosis results in asphyxia and is the final step before cellular and organ failure. The time needed to build up hypoxia and acidosis sufficient to cause asphyxia will vary from fetus to fetus depending on its 'physiological reserve' and also on the extent to which the blood supply to and from the placenta is disrupted. The disruption of oxygen supply may be a complete acute cessation due to placental abruption, or it may be intermittent in the form of cord compression in labour, or due to placental insufficiency. Lack of oxygen due to reduced placental perfusion associated with intrauterine growth restriction leads to hypoxaemic hypoxia, whilst that due to cord compression leads to ischaemic hypoxia, and these two mechanisms can co-exist. The fetal heart rate (FHR) patterns associated with hypoxia and acidosis are discussed below.

FHR patterns related to hypoxia and acidosis

The features of the CTG (baseline rate, baseline variability, accelerations and decelerations) described in Chapter 4 may occur in various combinations in a given FHR trace. One study has suggested that 50% of the fetuses may get acidotic in 90 minutes with late decelerations; in 120 minutes with variable decelerations; and in 190 minutes with reduced baseline variability.[7] Expanding this philosophy further and combining all four features of the FHR, certain patterns have been described to estimate the rate with which hypoxia and acidosis evolve.[8] Obviously this is not an exact science, as the rate with which acidosis will develop depends not only on the type of FHR pattern observed but also on the 'physiological reserve' of the fetus. In the presence of a similarly abnormal CTG, those fetuses that are growth restricted, those with infection, or with scanty thick meconium stained fluid, develop hypoxia and acidosis at a faster rate compared with a fetus that is appropriately grown and with a normal amount of clear amniotic fluid.[9,10]

The following patterns are described with cerebral palsy or with abnormal neurological outcome and may prove clinically useful in deciding the timing of intervention when taken in consideration with the clinical picture.[11]

1 Acute hypoxia usually presents with prolonged bradycardia < 80 bpm.[12]
2 Subacute hypoxia presents with steep decelerations reducing the FHR to

< 80 bpm and which last longer than the time the FHR is at the normal baseline rate. The above two patterns usually present with acute clinical events such as placental abruption, cord prolapse or scar rupture, or in the late first or second stage of labour. At times the cause is not known and may be related to occult cord compression.

3 Gradually developing hypoxia may be manifest by the development of tachycardia, reduced variability and absence of accelerations.

4 Longstanding hypoxia may show a pattern with reduced baseline variability and shallow late decelerations in a non-reactive trace.

Acute hypoxia

Prolonged bradycardia or deceleration < 80 bpm leads to acute hypoxia and if it is associated with placental abruption, cord prolapse and uterine scar rupture warrants immediate delivery. Uterine hyperstimulation causing bradycardia can be dealt with by acute tocolysis (see Chapter 26). Important considerations in other cases are the cardiotocograph (CTG) prior to the bradycardia and to potentially influencing associations such as thick meconium stained amniotic fluid, intrauterine growth restriction (IUGR), infection, and antepartum haemorrhage – in which acidosis can develop rapidly.

A FHR < 80 bpm for longer than 6 minutes, prolonged bradycardia/prolonged deceleration, can lead to rapid acute hypoxia and acidosis. A prolonged deceleration < 3 minutes is considered suspicious and > 3 minutes is abnormal. Causes of transient bradycardia include hypotension (e.g. regional anaesthesia), dorsal position of the mother, uterine hyperstimulation, artificial rupture of the membranes and vaginal examination. In these cases remedial actions should be undertaken, such as maternal repositioning; correction of hypotension; stopping oxytocin and acute tocolysis for hyperstimulation with prostaglandins whilst awaiting recovery of the fetal heart rate. Pressure on the head at crowning with maternal bearing down in the second stage may also be associated with bradycardia, and if it does not recover within 6 minutes delivery should be facilitated. At times the cause for bradycardia is not known and the fetal heart rate may not recover, despite the usual resuscitative measures, necessitating immediate delivery. The longer the bradycardia the greater is the chance for fetal acidosis. The pH is likely to decline more rapidly in high-risk clinical situations such as thick meconium, oligohydramnios, IUGR, intrauterine infection and in cases where the CTG was suspicious or pathological before the onset of bradycardia. In such cases if the bradycardia does not recover by 6 to 7 minutes delivery should be undertaken as soon as feasible.

The placenta acts as the lungs for the fetus in utero. Carbon dioxide is eliminated and oxygen is absorbed through the placenta. For optimal gas exchange there should be adequate circulation on the maternal and fetal sides of the placenta. With the normal fetal heart rate (FHR) of about 140 bpm for 10 minutes there are 1400 circulations through the placenta that help transfer carbon dioxide out of the fetal circulation and absorb adequate oxygen for the fetus. When the FHR is 80 bpm there will be only 800 circulations in 10 minutes and the fetus will miss 600 circulations. The amount of carbon dioxide excreted becomes less and accumulates within the fetus, leading to the formation of carbonic acid with a decline in pH – respiratory acidosis. With increasing duration of bradycardia the oxygen transferred to the fetus is also reduced, leading to anaerobic metabolism and accumulation of metabolites giving rise to metabolic acidosis. This has an additive effect to the already existing respiratory acidosis. If the fetal heart rate returns to normal within a short period of time the number of circulations through the placenta will normalize, allowing the respiratory acidosis to be corrected by transferring the carbon dioxide to the maternal circulation. This is a quick process whilst reversal of metabolic acidosis takes longer. If conservative measures fail, and the fetal heart rate does not return to normal within 6–9 minutes, delivery of the fetus and establishing neonatal respiration will quickly reverse the respiratory acidosis and, with time, the metabolic acidosis.

Subacute hypoxia

Prolonged decelerations with the FHR below the baseline for a longer time than at the normal baseline rate leads to subacute hypoxia, i.e. the development of hypoxia and acidosis, but less rapidly compared with acute and prolonged bradycardia. When such fetal heart rate decelerations are frequent and profound the evolution of hypoxia and acidosis can be rapid. It is difficult to quantify the duration for which the FHR should be below the baseline rate and the duration for which it should be at the correct baseline to prevent hypoxia and acidosis. It will depend on the 'physiological reserve' of each fetus. One could consider that the build up of hypoxia and acidosis is likely to be greater if the duration of the FHR at the normal baseline rate is one-third or less of the total time. Initially this will result in slow elimination of carbon dioxide leading to respiratory acidosis, but as time passes, oxygen transfer will be critically reduced and metabolic acidosis will ensue.

The series of traces in Figures 5.1–5.5 show the subacute hypoxia pattern with atypical variable decelerations and the final outcome in a fetus with severe metabolic acidosis. The end of the trace was bradycardia for 10 minutes and the baby was delivered at that stage by forceps (Fig 5.5).

Gradually developing hypoxia

In gradually developing hypoxia decelerations appear, followed by absence of accelerations, a rise in the baseline rate, and a reduction in baseline variability. As always one should consider the clinical picture of parity, cervical dilatation, rate of progress and high-risk

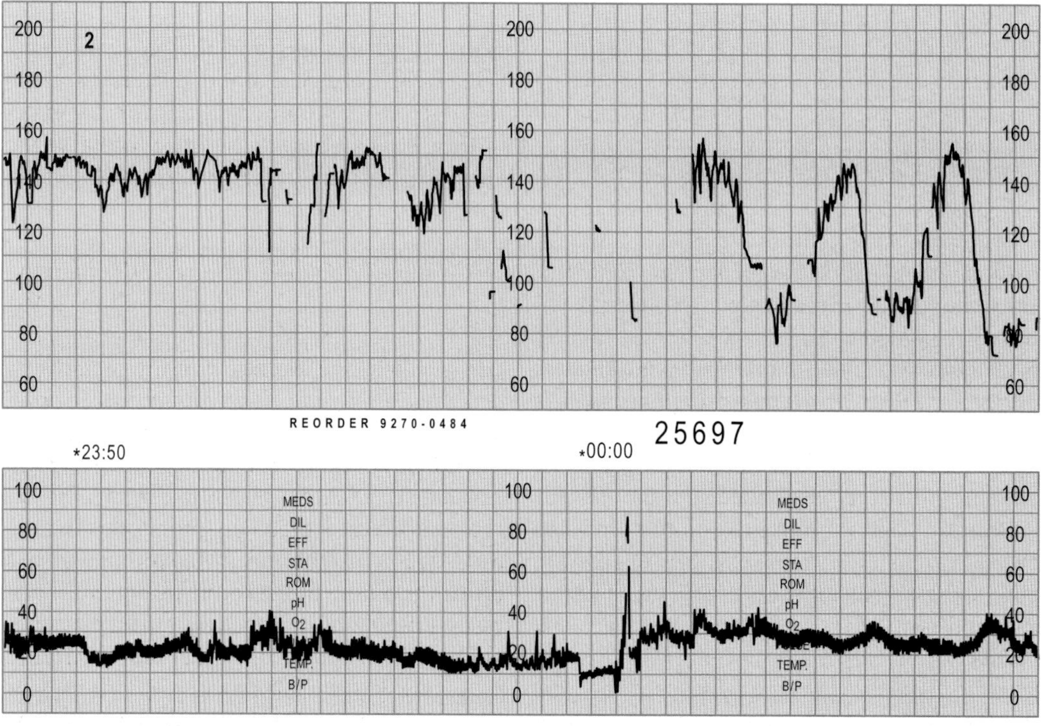

Figure 5.1 Decelerations start as shallow and then get steeper and wider lasting for 2 minutes and recovering to the baseline rate of 140 bpm for only 30 seconds.

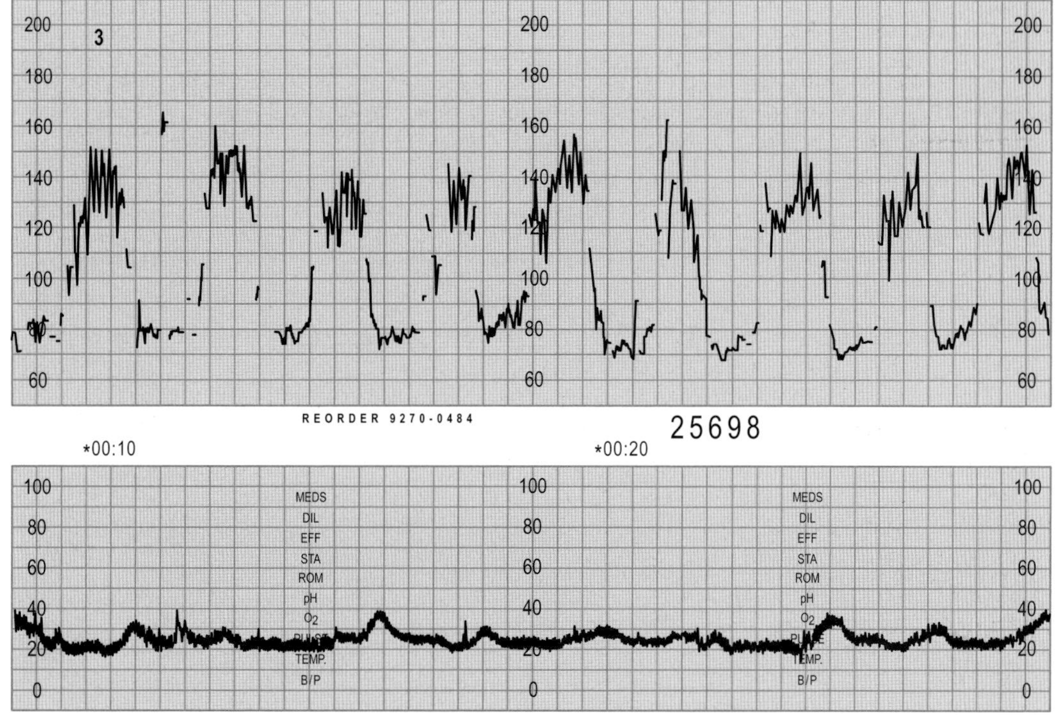

Figure 5.2 Prolonged decelerations with saltatory baseline variability during short period of recovery.

factors and institute conservative measures (e.g. stopping oxytocin, hydration, change of maternal position), or perform fetal blood sampling (FBS), or consider delivery.

Figures 5.6–5.8 exhibit the pattern seen with gradually developing hypoxia: decelerations progressively become more pronounced, accelerations disappear, there is a rise in the baseline rate and finally a reduction of the baseline variability. The decelerations are variable, suggestive of cord compression.

Longstanding hypoxia

In cases with longstanding hypoxia there are no accelerations, the baseline variability is markedly reduced and there are shallow late decelerations, often < 15 bpm. These characteristic features of hypoxia are seen even though the fetus may have a normal baseline rate. The absence of accelerations and 'cycling' suggests that the fetus may have already sustained asphyxial injury, or is hypoxic, or is affected by some other insult such as infection. Figure 5.9 is an FHR trace with features suggestive of longstanding hypoxia.

Vascular ischaemic injury

A cerebral vascular injury such as haemorrhage or thrombosis can give rise to neurological deficits. A vascular ischaemic injury of the brain may take place due to vascular malformation in the brain vessels associated with pressure on the fetal head. At times a vascular thrombosis may form due to coagulation disorders. In many the cause is unknown. The time of this occurrence may be recognizable on the CTG as a sudden rise in the baseline rate with absence of accelerations and reduced variability of the FHR.[13] These infants may present with hemi-paretic cerebral palsy although the baby may show normal pH and blood gases at birth.[14,15]

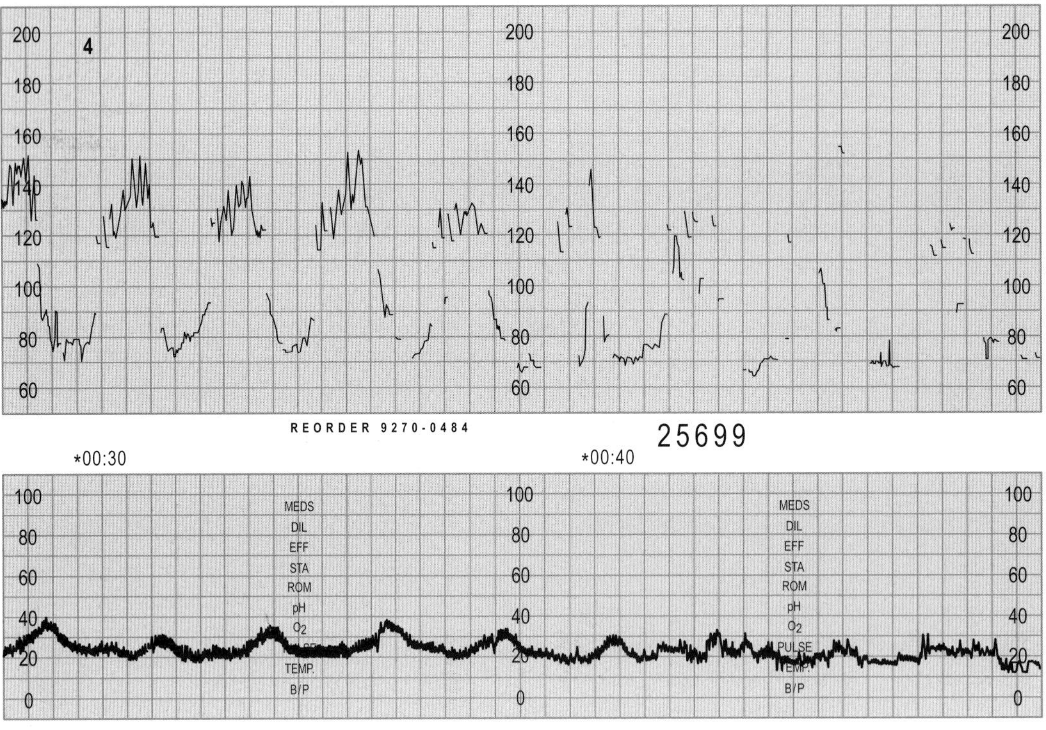

Figure 5.3 The baseline rate drops from 150 bpm to 120 bpm with prolonged decelerations.

In cases of prolonged bradycardia, if the fetal heart rate recovers, returns to the normal baseline rate, and shows reactivity with accelerations and cyclicity, then ischaemic neurological injury is unlikely. On the other hand, if the FHR does not recover at the time of delivery or has returned to but shows a shift in the baseline rate, with reduced baseline variability and no reactivity or cyclicity, then it is suggestive of a vascular injury of a localized area, or ischaemic injury of basal ganglia region of the brain.

In cases of ischaemic injury the neonate may have convulsions several hours after birth. The CT or MRI scan may show a segmental or localized infarct in the brain, rather than a diffuse injury in the cortical area or cerebral oedema or injury in the basal ganglia area – which are the features of intermittent or acute asphyxial injury.[16,17]

When the fetus is subjected to hypoxaemia there is a preferential redistribution of blood perfusion to the essential organs of heart, brain and adrenals in preference to skin, muscle and other viscera like the gut and kidneys.[18,19] However, when there is severe mechanical compression of the head, as in some cases of the second stage of labour, there may be hardly any blood flow to the brain. This has been shown in animal experiments.[20] With near infrared spectroscopy reduction in oxyhaemoglobin in relation to deoxyhaemoglobin has been shown in human fetuses.[21] If these episodes are prolonged it may give rise to asphyxial brain injury with low Apgar scores and subsequent neurological disorders, including cerebral palsy. However, because there was no generalized metabolic acidosis, the insult being confined to the brain, the cord pH at birth may be normal.

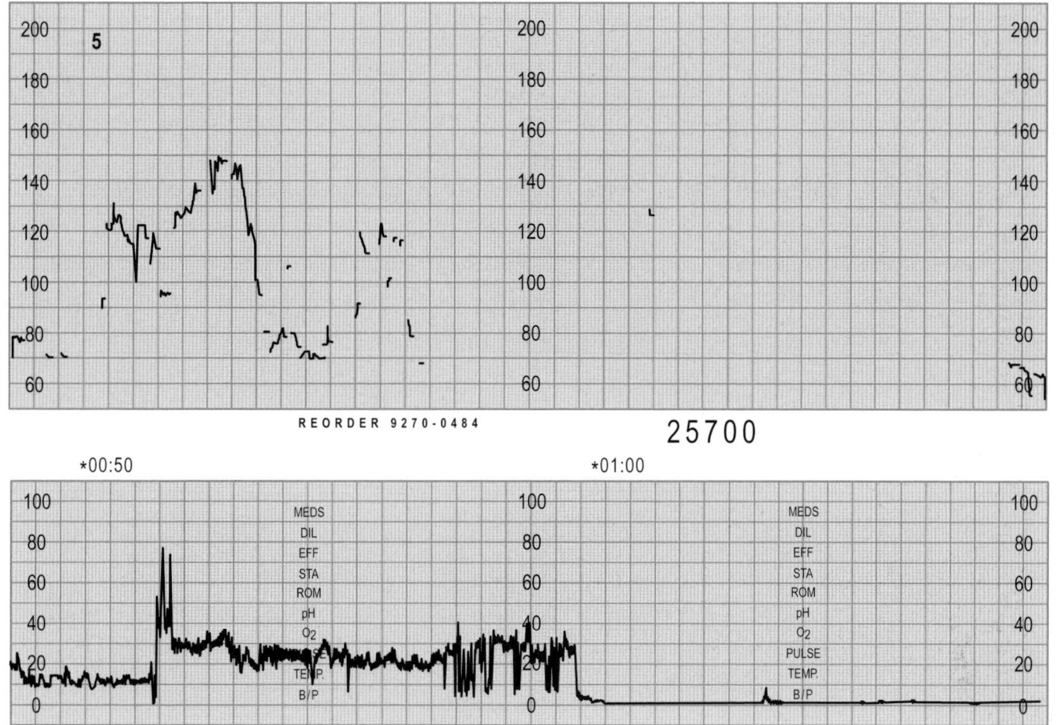

Figure 5.4 Prolonged bradycardia following decelerations.

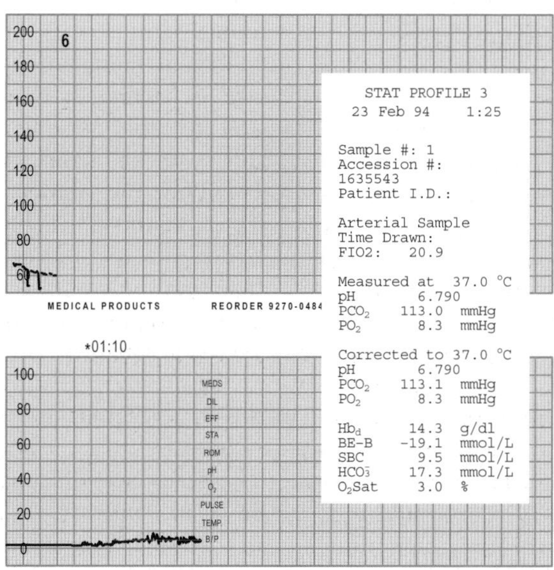

Figure 5.5 Time of delivery is annotated and the strip shows a low pH and high base excess.

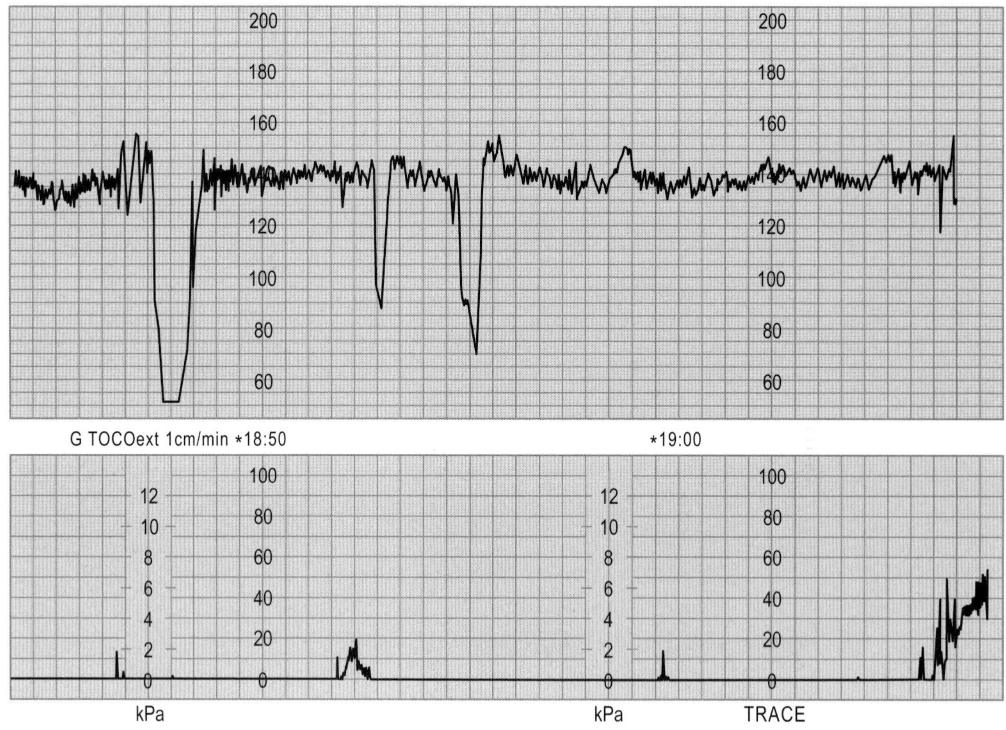

Figure 5.6 The trace shows a baseline rate of 140 bpm with simple variable decelerations, normal baseline variability and accelerations. It has been misinterpreted as early decelerations.

Correlation of CTG patterns with observed brain injury

Animal experimental models have been used to correlate the different types of asphyxial injuries seen in the MRI with the resultant neurological outcome seen in the infant.[4] Severe fetal bradycardia (acute hypoxia CTG pattern) leads to poor circulation, causes fetal asphyxia and renders the whole brain ischaemic. Different tissues have varying susceptibility to hypoxia-asphyxia based on their metabolic demands. Animal experiments suggest that there is damage to the putamina and lentiform nuclei within 10 minutes of profound lack of perfusion; to the central gyri, hippocampus and calcarine regions in 20–30 minutes; and to the whole cerebrum by 30 minutes – if the animal fetus is resuscitated before death.[22]

Unlike complete circulatory obstruction and ischaemia, if there is partial ischaemia and hypoxia, autoregulation results in vasodilatation to maintain cerebral blood flow. However, the border zones, which are the distal regions of the blood flow, may become under-perfused and be damaged if unable to maintain the metabolic needs. It is estimated that neurons in this region may become irreversibly damaged in 30 minutes. Because of the preferential autoregulation mechanism the vital regions of the brain will not be ischaemic whilst the border zones are affected. The period for which the autoregulation process can continue, without affecting the rest of the brain, before final collapse is estimated to be 30–60 minutes.

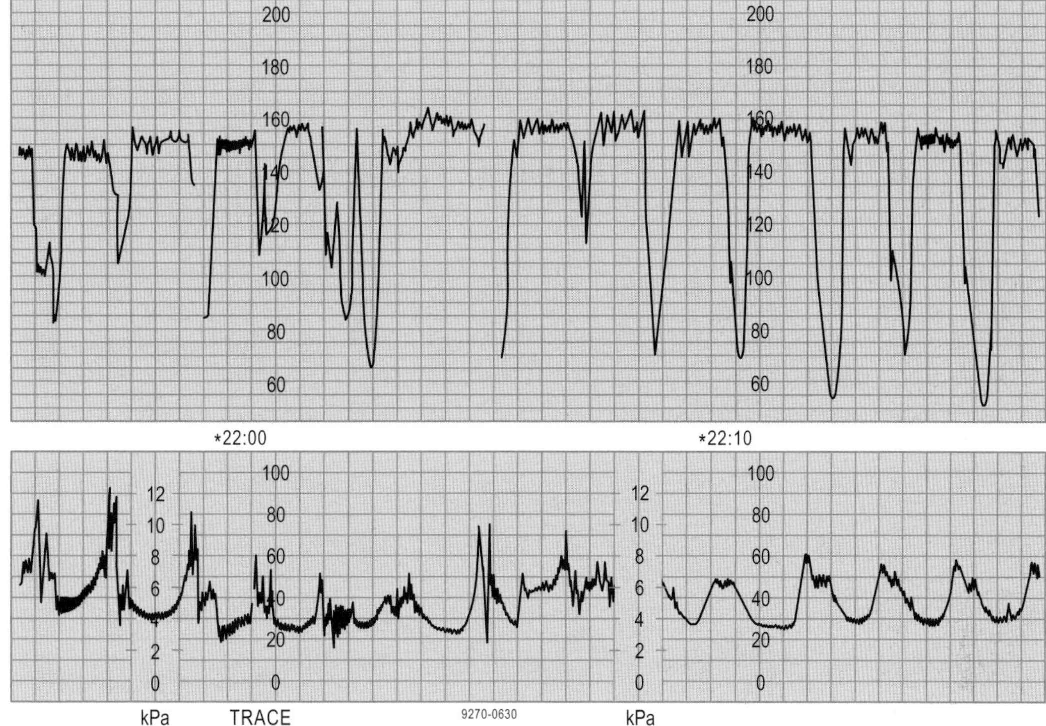

Figure 5.7 Rise in baseline rate to 150 bpm, reduced baseline variability and no accelerations.

Intermittent reduction in blood flow leading to increasing hypoxaemia and hypoxia is likely with profound intermittent deceleration seen with subacute hypoxic CTG pattern, and during the terminal stages of gradually developing hypoxic patterns. In the sheep model, carotid artery occlusion for 30–40 minutes results in ischaemia and necrosis in the parasagittal cortex, basal ganglia and thalamus.[23] Parasagittal cortical injury similar to the watershed damage seen in human newborns can be produced by prolonged gradual obstruction of the iliac artery for periods of 1–2 hours. The experiment showed some variation from animal to animal, but in general there needed to be at least 30 minutes of partial asphyxia for parasagittal damage, and the damage was greater if the process continued for > 60 minutes. Basal ganglia lesions were common with bradycardia lasting 30 minutes. When this period was longer than 30 minutes white matter damage in the watershed areas was seen. The odds of damage in the watershed area were significantly increased when prolonged bradycardia of 1 hour was compared with a period of less than 1 hour. Animal experiments have shown that 50 minutes of partial asphyxia, followed by 3–4 minutes of total asphyxia, results in cortical and basal ganglia damage. The MRI pictures of brain damage after prenatal, perinatal and postnasal asphyxia have been well described.[24]

Medicolegal implications

To establish negligence, *causation* and *liability* has to be proven. The following features are sought for evidence of causation: abnormal

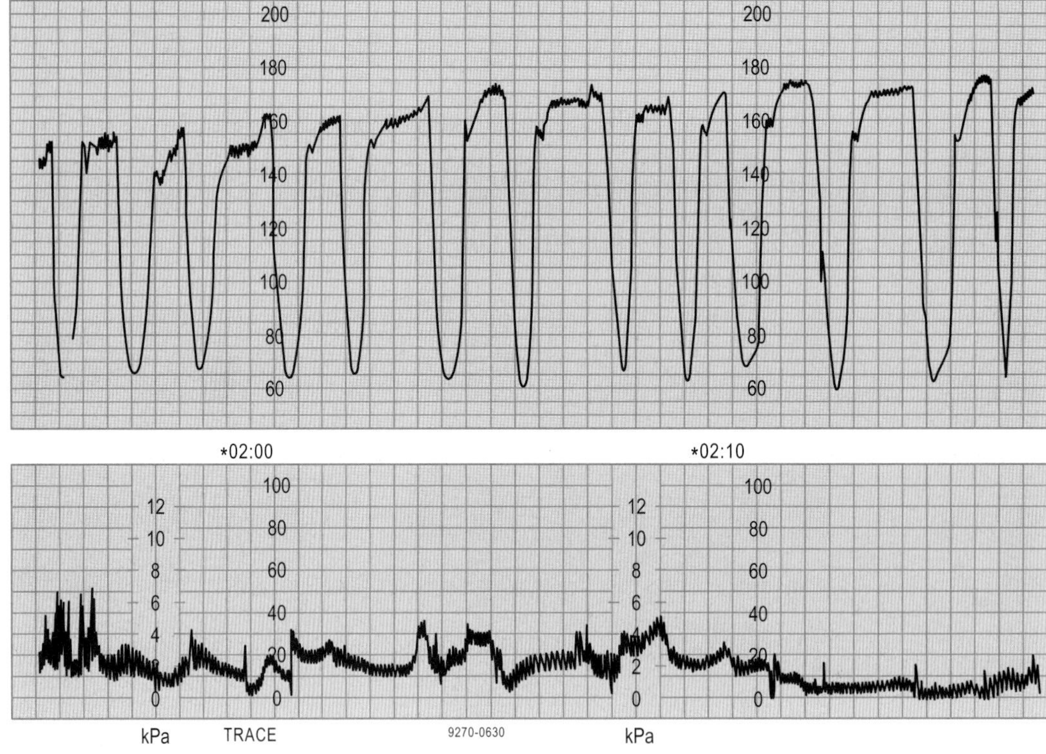

Figure 5.8 Rise in baseline rate to 170 bpm with no baseline variability.

> *'One has to consider that the anomaly of the birth process, rather than being the causal etiological factor, may itself be the consequence of the real perinatal etiology.'*
>
> **Sigmund Freud**
> *Die Infantile Cerebrallähmung. Vienna, 1897*

CTG, low Apgar score, low cord arterial pH, need for assisted ventilation, admission to neonatal intensive care unit (NICU), hypoxic ischaemic encephalopathy (HIE) and subsequent neurological damage. However, several metabolic disorders may cause neurological disability and an abnormal CTG and inappropriate management may be coincidental. The following list of essential and additional criteria has been proposed to help determine whether birth asphyxia can be considered causative:[25]

Essential criteria:

- Evidence of metabolic acidosis in cord umbilical artery (UA) or early neonatal (NN) samples: pH < 7.0 and base deficit > 12 mmol/L
- Early onset of severe or moderate neonatal encephalopathy in infants > 34 weeks
- Cerebral palsy of a spastic quadriplegic or dyskinetic type.

Additional criteria:

- A sentinel hypoxic event occurring immediately before or during labour
- A sudden rapid sustained deterioration in FHR pattern
- Apgar score < 7 for more than 5 minutes
- Early evidence of multisystem involvement
- Early imaging evidence of acute cerebral involvement.

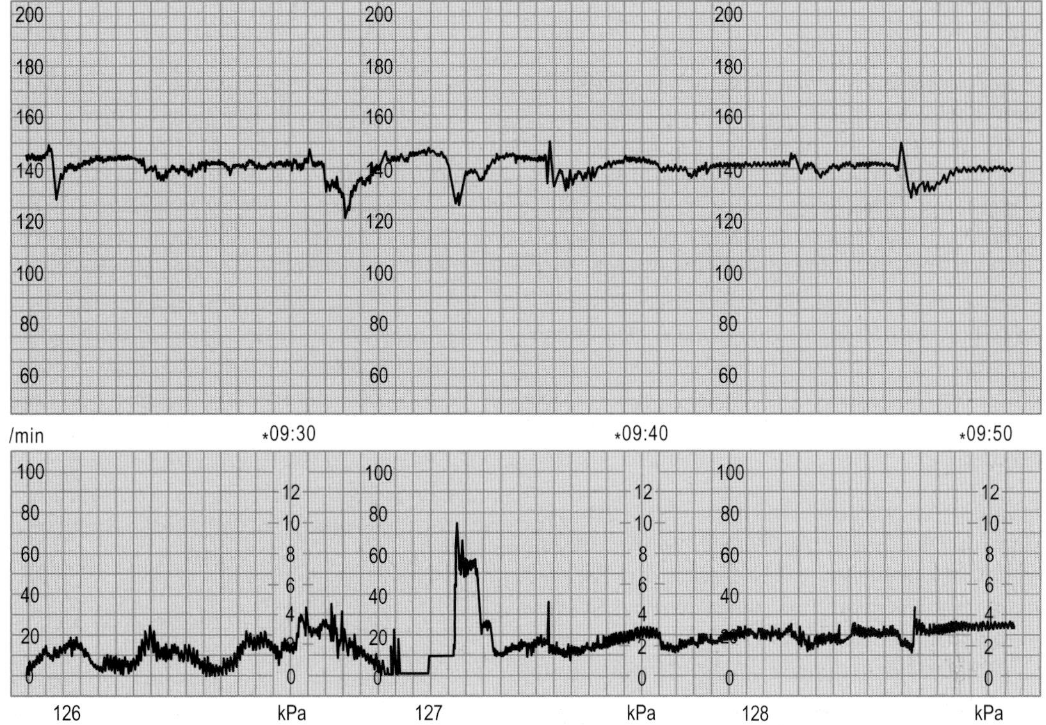

Figure 5.9 A CTG with the baseline rate in the normal range, with no accelerations, minimal baseline variability and shallow decelerations suggestive of pre-existing hypoxia.

The above criteria emphasize the need to correlate the neurological outcome described by the paediatric neurologist to the MRI pictures, the CTG trace, and the clinical history prior to and soon after delivery. There may be difficulties in correlating these criteria in a given case and hence the need to establish why some of the above criteria are present, whilst others are not.

Causation

A discrepancy between a low Apgar score (≤3) at birth and good pH values in umbilical artery and/or venous blood makes it difficult to establish causation. The surrogate measures of the newborn at delivery that indicate the possibility of adverse neurological outcome in later life are umbilical cord arterial pH and blood gases – more specifically the base deficit that indicates whether the acidosis was respiratory or metabolic, the latter being associated with poor outcome. There are several reasons for low Apgar scores, such as congenital malformation; prematurity; infection; and effects of medication given to the mother. Other surrogate markers of possible adverse neurological outcome are the need for resuscitation, assisted ventilation, neurological behaviour in the first few days, categorization of the neurological state as hypoxic ischaemic encephalopathy (HIE) grades 1 to 3, in addition to imaging evidence (CT or MRI scanning) of ischaemic or hypoxic insult.

It is not uncommon to find two or three of these surrogate markers in a case and not all the features. Occasionally a baby is born with a good pH and base excess of the cord arterial and venous blood whilst the baby has a low Apgar score, needs resuscitation and assisted ventilation, and develops abnormal neurological behaviour in the immediate newborn period. This may be due to acute cord compression with no circulation beyond the point of compression for some time. The portion of the cord distal to the compression connected to the placenta will maintain the pH whilst the cord proximal to the compression, closer to the fetus, is likely to have a low blood pH because of the continuing fetal metabolism. Depending on the duration of the insult the baby may exhibit abnormal neurological behaviour seen after birth and have long-term sequelae.

Liability

If causation is established in a case with an abnormal CTG and poor outcome the issue of liability needs to be resolved. If appropriate action was taken in a timely manner in the presence of an abnormal CTG one is not liable. Medical expert opinion should state that the care given did not fall short of what was expected by a responsible body of medical opinion. Liability is generally judged by Bolam's Principle:

> *'The test is the standard of the ordinary skilled man exercising and professing to have the specialist skill, A man need not possess the highest expert skill at risk of being found negligent …'*

In recent times Bolithos' Principle has been applied:

> *'If it can be demonstrated that the professional opinion is not capable of withstanding logical analysis, the judge is entitled to hold that the body of opinion is not reasonable or responsible.'*

Therefore, it is important that the argument put forward to defend 'appropriate and timely action' needs to be accurate and logical. This involves a review of the type of insult suffered by the fetus and whether timely action was taken. The pattern of CTGs already discussed ascribes certain speeds with which asphyxia may set in, and it has to be shown that the attendant did carry out the appropriate action in a timely manner.

The 'timing of injury' needs to be judged to derive liability and this is not always possible based on the CTG. In the presence of an abnormal CTG how long one can wait before intervention, and whether the delay worsens the injury without further changes in the CTG, needs to be assessed by the medical expert. The classification of various CTGs representing acute, subacute, gradually developing or longstanding hypoxia may be useful to help answer these questions. A final conclusion can be reached if the duration of the CTG pattern fits in with what was found on the neonatal MRI by the neuroradiologist and the damage in the child as described by the paediatric neurologist. Having ascertained the possible mechanism and timing of injury, the expert witness has to decide whether appropriate and timely action was taken. If there was delay in taking action because of non-recognition of an abnormal pattern, or there was delay in taking action after recognizing the pattern was abnormal, then liability is confirmed.

Reducing adverse outcomes

From a review of the CESDI report[3] and medicolegal cases, adverse outcomes can be attributed to common themes: inability to interpret FHR traces, inappropriate or delayed action, mistakes due to lack of understanding of the technology, and poor communication. Record keeping is also essential but often poor. These risks can be reduced by education and training, supervision, incident reporting, audit and risk management. Some of these aspects are discussed in Chapter 2, but those that are specific to fetal asphyxia are reviewed below.

Inability to interpret CTG traces

In many cases the attendants do not have the knowledge to interpret the CTG. This may be due to inadequate training and failure to maintain standards. In-house education, refresher courses and training material are essential. There are commercial systems available that can highlight abnormal features which occur on the CTG. Further trials are in progress to have a computer assisted system that can incorporate the clinical picture and prompt the clinician with management options. The importance of considering the clinical picture in planning management is essential. Earlier action is needed in the presence of intrauterine growth restriction, preterm, post-term, intrauterine infection, and thick meconium with scanty amniotic fluid. Injudicious use of oxytocin, epidural and difficult operative delivery can give rise to further compromise when the CTG is abnormal. Emphasis should be laid on observations of reactivity (accelerations) and cycling (quiet and active sleep cycles) that indicates a non-hypoxic fetus with a normal behavioural pattern. A non-reactive trace with baseline variability < 5 bpm and shallow decelerations (< 15 beats) that last for > 90 minutes suggests the probability of pre-existing hypoxia. Within the clinical context such a trace should almost always prompt early delivery.

Inappropriate action

In the presence of placental abruption, cord prolapse or scar rupture delivery should take place when the diagnosis is made. In prolonged bradycardia < 80 bpm, the pH may decline by 0.01 every 2–3 minutes and delivery should ideally be within 15 minutes or as soon as feasible. Special arrangements should be in place in each unit to deliver these cases as a category 1 caesarean section – within 30 minutes. Systems should be in place to activate an 'immediate CS code' to summon the theatre staff and anaesthetist needed to carry out the procedure immediately.

With prolonged decelerations lasting more than 90 seconds, which have a transient recovery (< 30 seconds) to the baseline rate, early delivery – within 30–60 minutes – is warranted. Fetal scalp blood sampling (FBS) is inappropriate in such situations and is likely to cause delay and compromise the baby. In situations with an abnormal CTG due to uterine hyperstimulation, especially that due to prostaglandins, or in cases of spontaneous labour with an abnormal fetal heart rate pattern where an operating theatre is not immediately available, a bolus dose of a tocolytic drug such as terbutaline 0.25 mg diluted in 5 ml saline given by slow intravenous injection[26] or subcutaneously may abolish the uterine contractions and help improve the fetal condition despite the delay (see Chapter 26).

Non-recognition of technical errors

The CTG records the fetal heart rate pattern. When the monitor is attached it is essential to make sure that it is the movement of the fetal heart that is picked up by the ultrasound transducer to the ECG signal via the electrode. This is done by auscultating the fetal heart prior to application. On the ultrasound mode the monitor can record the same or double the maternal heart rate by picking up the pulsations of various maternal vessels. Slippage of the ultrasound transducer from tracking the fetal heart to the maternal pulse during labour can occur on rare occasions.[27] With the fetal ECG electrode, accidental recording of maternal ECG would provide the same rate as the mother. The whole CTG should be reviewed from time to time for sudden changes in the rate. Care should be taken when monitoring the second twin after delivery of the first twin.

When the trace is technically unsatisfactory it is important to auscultate and record the findings in the notes or on the CTG paper. If feasible, a scalp electrode should be used to get a trace of better technical quality. Attention should be paid to monitoring the uterine contraction pattern when the fetal heart rate is abnormal.

Record keeping

CTGs are recorded on thermosensitive paper which tends to fade after 3–4 years. Despite every effort CTG traces tend to go missing, especially if there was an adverse outcome. In a study of obstetric accidents 18 of 64 cases of possible litigation had lost FHR traces.[28] In another six cases the CTG could not be interpreted. Legally these traces need to be kept for 25 years. The fetal monitoring companies produce systems that have automatic online download of the CTG and archival capability in magneto-optic discs and the hard drives. There are 'write once, read many times' (WORM) disks that can each archive 4000 patient records with 8 hours of trace and clinical notes. Not only is each archive good storage, but it can help in teaching, research and audit. Storage of such disks can be on a shelf instead of using a warehouse to store 100 000 case notes (4000 cases × 25 years). These systems come with overview monitors that can be kept at a central station or in an adjacent room.

Education and training

Education and training are essential and have been emphasized in the CESDI report and subsequent CNST recommendations. Twenty years ago what was a 1 hour lecture on CTG before starting practice has changed to at least one full day of education. Several books, CDs and websites are available. In-house training with review of the unit's own cases is the best way of reinforcing knowledge in addition to regular education programmes.

There is a constant influx of new doctors and midwives on any labour ward. Some are there soon after they qualify and others may be there after working outside an obstetric unit. Immediate attention is needed to evaluate the trace if it looks abnormal and to take action if necessary. Hence, a senior person with adequate knowledge of CTG should be available to allay anxiety, to educate, to take appropriate action, and to avoid unnecessary operative delivery. In some countries a consultant is available on the labour ward floor for 24 hours each day. In the UK attempts are made to provide consultant cover for 24 hours – at least in larger units.

Incident reporting and audit

Incident reporting of adverse outcomes and audit of poor outcome – low Apgar scores, low cord arterial pH, need for assisted ventilation, admission for neonatal intensive care, and HIE – is essential to find out whether there is a system failure such as education and training, induction of personnel, supervision and inadequate staffing levels. All potential litigation cases need to be thoroughly evaluated by a risk management team. Findings of the risk management team and their recommendations need to be disseminated to prevent further recurrence (Chapter 2).

Conclusions

The main reasons for litigation when there is injury related to asphyxia are: parents want to know what happened and why; to prevent recurrence; that the staff involved should account for their actions; for recovery of costs determined by injury, pain and suffering; actual losses experienced and costs of future care. Obstetric litigation is distressing to all involved. Parents of a handicapped child would always prefer to have a normal child rather than considerable financial remuneration given for child care. Their life is stressful and sad watching the child suffering. We have to do everything possible to eliminate or reduce such occurrences. There is no conflict between improving clinical care, minimizing clinical error and reducing obstetric litigation. They are complementary and can be achieved by research, audit, education and training and risk management – the components of clinical governance to improve health care.

References

1. www.nhs.org.uk/CNST
2. www.nhs.org.uk/NPSA
3. Confidential Enquiry into Stillbirths and Deaths in Infancy. 4th Annual Report. London: Maternal and Child Health Research Consortium, 1997.
4. Pasternak JF. Hypoxic-ischemic brain damage in term infant – lessons from the laboratory. Pediatr Clin North Am 1993; 40:1061–1072.
5. Hagberg B, Hagberg G, Beckung E, Uvebrant P. Changing panorama of cerebral palsy in Sweden. VII. Prevalance and origin in the

birth year period 1991–1994. Acta Paediatrica 2001; 90:272–277.

6. Blair E, Stanley FJ. Intrapartum asphyxia: a rare cause of cerebral palsy. J Pediatr 1988; 12:515–519.
7. Fleischer A, Schulman H, Jagani N, Mitchell J, Randolph G. The development of fetal acidosis in the presence of an abnormal fetal heart rate tracing. I. The average for gestational age fetus. Am J Obstet Gynecol 1982; 144:55–60.
8. Phelan JP, Kim JO. Fetal heart rate observations in the brain-damaged infant. Semin Perinatol 2000; 24:221–229.
9. Lin CC, Mouward AH, Rosenow PJ, River P. Acid-base characteristics of fetuses with intrauterine growth retardation during labor and delivery. Am J Obstet Gynecol 1980; 137:553–559.
10. Steer PJ. Fetal distress. In: Crawford J, ed. Risks of labour. Chichester: John Wiley, 1985:11–31.
11. Baskett TF, Arulkumaran S. Intrapartum care. London: RCOG Press, 2002:17–29.
12. National Institute of Clinical Excellence and Royal College of Obstetricians and Gynaecologists. The use of electronic fetal heart rate monitoring. Evidence Based Clinical Guideline No 8. London: RCOG Press, 2001.
13. Schifrin BS. The CTG and the timing and mechanism of fetal neurological injuries. Best Pract Res Clin Obstet Gynaecol 2004; 18:467–478.
14. Micahelis R, Rooschuz B, Dopfer R. Prenatal origin of congenital spastic hemiparesis. Early Hum Dev 1980; 4:243–255.
15. Nelson KB, Grether JK. Potentially asphyxiating conditions and spastic cerebral palsy in infants of normal birth weight. Am J Obstet Gynecol 1998; 179:507–513.
16. Rosenbloom L. Dyskinetic cerebral palsy and birth asphyxia. Dev Med Child Neurol 1994; 36:285–289.
17. Stanley FJ, Blair E, Hockey A, Patterson B, Watson L. Spastic quadriplegia in Western Australia: a genetic epidemiological study. I. Case population and perinatal risk factors. Dev Med Child Neurol 1993; 35:191–201.
18. Berger R, Garnier Y, Lobbert T, Pfeiffer D, Jensen A. Circulatory responses to acute asphyxia are not affected by the glutamate antagonist lubeluzole in fetal sheep near term. J Soc Gynecol Invest 2001; 8:143–148.
19. Richardson BS, Carmichael L, Homan J, Johnston L, Gagnon R. Fetal cerebral, circulatory, and metabolic responses during heart rate decelerations with umbilical cord compression. Am J Obstet Gynecol 1996; 175:929–936.
20. O'Brien WF, David SE, Grissom MP, Eng RR, Golden SM. Effect of cephalic pressure on fetal cerebral blood flow. Am J Perinatol 1984; 1:223–226.
21. Aldrich CJ, D'Antona D, Spencer JA, et al. The effect of maternal pushing on fetal cerebral oxygenation and blood volume during the second stage of labour. Br J Obstet Gynaecol 1995; 102:448–453.
22. Williams CE, Gunn AJ, Synek B, Gluckman PD. Delayed seizures occurring with hypoxic-ischemic encephalopathy in the fetal sheep. Pediat Res 1990; 27:561–568.
23. Myers RE. Four patterns of perinatal brain damage and their conditions of occurrence in primates. Adv Neurol 1975; 10:223–232.
24. Sie LT, van der Knapp MS, Oosting J, de Vries LS, Lafebar HN, Valk JMR. Patterns of hypoxic-ischaemic brain damage after prenatal, perinatal and postnatal asphyxia. Neuropaediatrics 2000; 31:128–136.
25. McLennan A. A template for defining a causal relation between acute intrapartum events and cerebral palsy: international consensus statement. BMJ 1999; 40:13–21.
26. Ingemarsson I, Arulkumaran S, Ratnam SS. Single injection of terbutaline in term labor. Effect on fetal pH in cases with prolonged bradycardia. Am J Obstet Gynecol 1985; 153:859–864.
27. Gibb DMF, Arulkumaran S. Fetal monitoring in practice. 2nd ed. Oxford: Butterworth Heinemann, 1997:10–19.
28. Ennis S, Vincent CA. Obstetric accidents: a review of 64 cases. BMJ 1990; 300:1365–1367.

6

Induction of labour

'The spontaneous onset of labour is a robust and effective mechanism which is preceded by the maturation of several fetal systems, and should be given every opportunity to operate on its own. We should only induce labour when we are sure that we can do better.'

Alec Turnbull, 1976

Historical Background

The human race has for centuries found reasons to interfere with pregnancy by trying to hasten its conclusion. Often this consisted of attempts to procure the abortion of unwanted pregnancies, but other more positive motives arose from the desire to relieve the mother of a life-threatening pregnancy or to achieve a mechanically more favourable vaginal delivery of a smaller premature baby through a constricted birth canal. Through time, as a better perception of fetal and maternal risks developed alongside more efficient methods of labour induction, the indications shifted more commonly to serve the interest of the fetus perceived to be in jeopardy.

The first reliable technique to be used widely in obstetric practice was amniotomy – artificial rupture of the membranes. Although this procedure had probably been employed much earlier it first entered the medical literature in 1756 when Thomas Denman (1733–1815) of the

Historical Background

Middlesex Hospital of London wrote extolling its virtues. As a result it became known within Europe as the 'English method'.

Another mechanical method was devised in 1861 by Robert Barnes (1817–1907) of London, using a hydrostatic bag placed through the cervix and filled with water with a view to labour induction.[1] A similar approach was later taken by Camille Champetier de Ribes (1848–1935) in Paris[2] and by James Voorhees (1869–1929) in New York .[3] More than a century later modern obstetricians would follow the same principle using a Foley catheter, but by now understanding that the modus operandi *was the local release of prostaglandins.*

Amniotomy alone, however, is only effective in very favourable circumstances. It was not until oxytocin was identified and made available for clinical application that any degree of reliability in labour induction could be achieved. Even then it was in use for almost 60 years before it could be employed with any degree of confidence. Sir Henry Dale (1875–1968) made the first observation that posterior pituitary extract caused uterine contractions.[4] He gave samples to the obstetrician William Blair Bell (1871–1936) who began to use it for induction of labour.[5] Nevertheless, because the preparations consisted of crude extracts of the posterior pituitary of variable purity and potency, and because these were initially given as intramuscular injections with a poor degree of control, it was hardly surprising that there were instances of fatal hyperstimulation of the uterus. In the 1920s the eminent American obstetrician, Joseph Bolivar de Lee (1869–1942), famously addressed a meeting of the American College of Obstetricians and Gynecologists and was scathing in his condemnation of oxytocin. He held up in one hand a ruptured uterus and in the other a dead fetus and declared 'It biteth like the adder, it stingeth like the asp'. This quotation from chapter 23 verse 32 of the book of Proverbs in reality is a caution against the dangers of ethyl alcohol which, it is ironic to note, has been used by obstetricians to inhibit rather than to promote uterine contractility.

It was not until the latter half of the 20th century that reliable preparations of oxytocin became available following its chemical characterization as an octapeptide and its synthetic elaboration.[6–8] There followed a period of controversy during which Geoffrey Theobald advocated a dilute intravenous infusion of oxytocin as a 'physiological drip', i.e. a dilute intravenous infusion.[9] This was motivated by the desire to maximize the safety of the drugs but it had the drawback of reducing its potency and reliability. Nevertheless, it is now recognized that the claim that this was a physiological approach was ill-founded. It was not until the late 1960s that Alec Turnbull and Anne Anderson advocated the more pharmacologically sound approach of oxytocin 'titration' whereby the dose rate was steadily increased until the uterus responded by contracting effectively, at which point the dose rate was held steady.[10] It was later recognized that as uterine contractions became established in response to oxytocin, sensitivity to the hormone increased and as labour progressed the dose rate could be reduced again. Hitherto oxytocin had also been administered for absorption from the buccal mucosa, 'buccal pitocin', but this was largely abandoned in favour of intravenous titration.

The availability of an effective method of labour induction had a dramatic effect on obstetric practice. In retrospect there was over-exuberance on the part of obstetricians to widen the indications for labour induction by amniotomy followed by oxytocin titration, since this was clearly more efficient than any previously available approach. Induction rates rose dramatically in the United Kingdom and other countries and became the object of widespread criticism in the lay press. In some hospitals, labour was induced in excess of 50% of patients for what were thought to be justifiable reasons. It can now be seen to have been an excessive swing of the clinical pendulum beyond what was justified. As commonly happens in medical practice, enthusiasm for innovation outstripped sound clinical judgement.

It was against this background that a significant new development in the practice of labour induction emerged – the clinical availability of prostaglandins. These agents, the existence of which was first suspected in the 1930s, took more than 30 years to reach the point of clinical application, largely as a result of work by Sune Bergstrom and his colleagues at the Karolinska Institute in Stockholm.[11] By around 1975 it was clear that prostaglandins added an extra dimension to induction of labour, particularly since they not only provoked uterine contractions but also had a positive effect on cervical ripening.[12–13] As with oxytocin, a variety of different routes were explored, including oral, intramuscular and intravenous, before it was recognized that local delivery, within the reproductive tract, required a lower dose and greatly reduced unpleasant side effects. Although prostaglandin $F_{2\alpha}$ is a potent myometrial stimulant it has little effect on cervical ripening, whereas prostaglandin E_2 influences both components of labour. Extra-amniotic and intracervical routes proved effective, especially for cervical ripening, but the slightly greater efficiency of these routes has not been sufficient to justify the inconvenience to patient and clinician. Simply introducing PGE_2 into the vagina has become the route of choice.[14]

The most recent chapter in the use of prostaglandins for labour induction has been the widespread use of misoprostol, a synthetic analogue of PGE_1, which was developed as a cytoprotective agent for the upper gastrointestinal tract. This agent, which has never been subjected to the conventional testing for toxicity and other pharmacological issues normally required in drug development and licensing, has been employed so widely across the globe for induction of labour and abortion to good effect that it has effectively by-passed 'the system'. The drive for this has been its cost, which is a mere fraction of the cost of conventional PGE_2 preparations.[15] Moves are now underway to regularize the situation by producing misoprostol in a form which will meet with the approval of the regulatory authorities.

Indications for induction of labour

As mentioned above, induction of labour has for decades been a source of controversy among obstetricians who have occupied a spectrum from those who have used the intervention only very sparingly to those who have used it with excessive zeal. The watchword for appropriate induction of labour is when the clinician genuinely perceives that the interests of the mother or baby, or both, are better served by procuring delivery than by allowing the pregnancy to continue. In essence he or she must judge that the risks if the pregnancy continues outweigh the risks if the pregnancy is interrupted. Each pregnancy should be assessed in respect of the 'obstetric balance'(Fig 6.1). The perceptive clinician will immediately recognize that such a view is unduly simple for two reasons:

First, it is not only a matter of deciding that induction of labour will magically transport the fetus from an intrauterine to an extrauterine environment. While that is the objective its accomplishment may expose both the mother and the infant to additional risks. There is no virtue in intervening by inducing labour to avoid a perceived risk if the nature of the labour which results is such as to risk greater jeopardy for either party.

Second, an intervention which may be in the interests of one partner in the pregnancy may coincidentally run counter to the interests of the other. For instance, induction of labour in a mother with severe pre-eclampsia may be extremely beneficial in reducing the risks which she faces, while at the same time exposing the offspring to the risks of prematurity – although in many such cases the fetus in utero is in as much jeopardy as the mother. Conversely, induction of labour in a diabetic mother, which would more commonly serve the interests of the fetus, may increase the hazards faced by the mother.

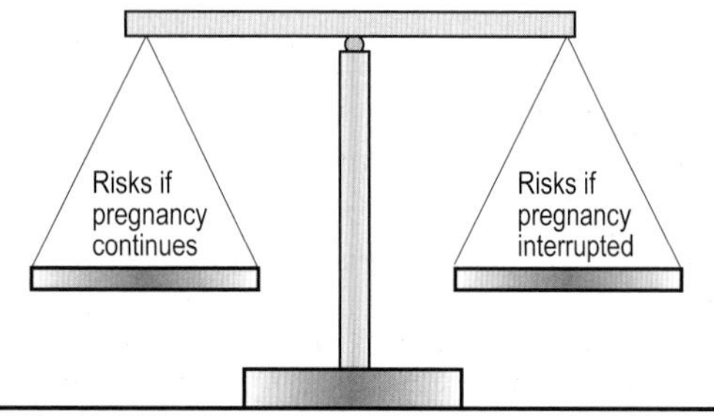

Figure 6.1 The obstetric balance.

A list of common indications for induction of labour is set out below, but this should not be regarded as a rigid set of recommendations:

- prolonged pregnancy
- pre-eclampsia/hypertension
- premature rupture of the membranes
- maternal diabetes
- multi-fetal pregnancy
- poor fetal growth – placental dysfunction
- history of precipitate labour
- fetal jeopardy from various causes (e.g. rhesus immunization)
- social and geographic considerations (e.g. availability of partner, distance from hospital).

Each pregnancy must be considered on its own merits, taking account of the risks and benefits to mother and baby deriving from specific complications. In considering the obstetric balance it should be remembered that for most pregnancies the balance remains tipped against intervention throughout the pregnancy, until spontaneous onset of labour leads to delivery without intervention. In the minority of cases in which the balance has shifted in favour of intervention, account must be taken of the additional elements of risk which that intervention itself may introduce.

In some women it is clear that the pregnancy in question is obviously beset by specific and immediate risks. These include the fetus affected by severe Rhesus immunization or facing imminent demise from placental insufficiency. There are other circumstances in which a specific condition is known to carry an increased likelihood of fetal compromise such as diabetes and pre-eclampsia, but where the danger is assumed from the existence of the maternal condition rather than from direct evidence of fetal jeopardy. There may be even less specific risks where delivery is considered appropriate, the most obvious of which is prolonged pregnancy. It is recognized that the longer the pregnancy progresses beyond the expected date of delivery the greater the likelihood of fetal demise but this indication can be seen as being one based on epidemiological rather than specific evidence pertaining to the individual pregnancy.[16] In most clinical services, however, prolonged pregnancy emerges as the commonest reason for labour induction. Figure 6.2 outlines a paradigm to be followed when the question of interruption of pregnancy arises.

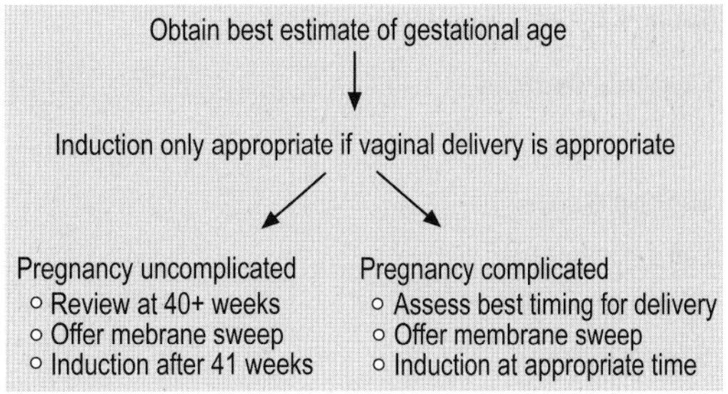

Figure 6.2 A paradigm to be followed when the question of interruption of pregnancy arises.

Methods of induction

Before considering the specific methods of labour induction it is important to establish some underlying principles.

The first is to obtain the most reliable information concerning gestational age. This may already be available from reliable menstrual data and an ultrasound examination in early pregnancy, but if such information is lacking the clinician must be circumspect, recognizing that an error in determining the gestational age may have a major impact on the outcome.

The second important principle is to recognize that not all women will respond to intervention in the same way. Nulliparous and multiparous women are likely to display different responses to induction and these must be anticipated. More importantly it must be recognized that some labours can be induced with ease while others may prove extremely resistant to induction. In this respect, and regardless of gestation, the biggest single factor is the proximity to the spontaneous onset of labour. Because the transition from the state of pregnancy maintenance to established labour is a gradual one (see Chapter 1), it is obvious that if a particular woman is programmed to be in labour tomorrow, labour induction today is likely to be simple. In contrast if, even at or beyond term, spontaneous labour remains a distant prospect then induction is almost inevitably fraught with difficulty. The most useful predictor of this is the degree of cervical ripening. Indeed, the original study on which Bishop based his cervical scoring system correlated the score to the interval before spontaneous labour began.[17] A high score presaged a short delay before the onset of labour, a low score indicated that it remained a distant prospect. The former was shown to be favourable for induction of labour, the latter unfavourable.

In practice the application of a scoring system based on Bishop's concept provides a reliable prediction of how successful labour induction is likely to be, but also of what method is most suitable (Fig 6.3). If the cervical score (Table 6.1) is high, labour is imminent and can usually be successfully induced by amniotomy alone or even simply sweeping the membranes digitally from the inner aspect of the lower uterine segment. For intermediate scores amniotomy followed by intravenous oxytocin may be appropriate, although

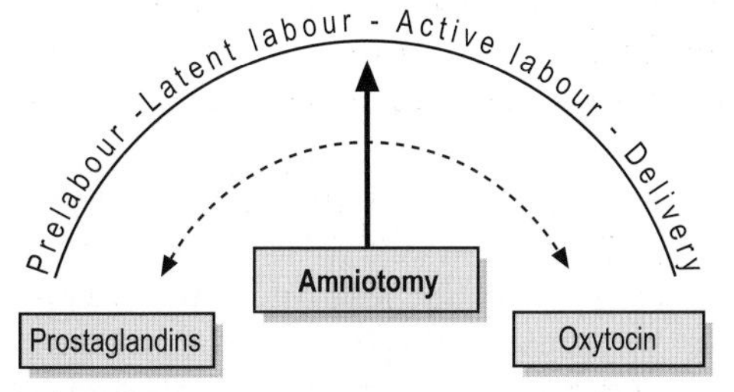

Figure 6.3 A scheme for labour induction. Prostaglandins may be used to greatest advantage in prelabour and latent labour, prior to amniotomy. Oxytocin is most effective following amniotomy. The best timing for amniotomy is after latent labour has begun.

Table 6.1 Cervical scoring systems

Cervical feature	Pelvic score			
	0	1	2	3
Bishop Score[17]				
Dilatation (cm)	0	1–2	3–4	5–6
Effacement (%)	0–30	40–60	60–70	80+
Station* (cm)	–3	–2	–1/0	+1/+2
Consistency	Firm	Medium	Soft	–
Position	Posterior	Mid-posterior	Anterior	–
Modified Bishop Score[18]				
Dilatation (cm)	< 1	1–2	2–4	> 4
Length of cervix (cm)	> 4	2–4	1–2	< 1
Station* (cm)	–3	–2	–1/0	+1/+2
Consistency	Firm	Average	Soft	–
Position	Posterior	Mid; Anterior	–	–

*In both systems, station is measured in cm relative to the ischial spines.

many women prefer what may seem a more 'natural' onset of labour from vaginal application of PGE_2.[18]

A variety of techniques have been in and out of vogue in the past 50 years. Although some of these may now seem primitive or bizarre, those which enjoyed any success had in common the provocation of those substances, especially oxytocin or prostaglandins, which participate in spontaneous labour. Thus, breast stimulation which causes release of oxytocin, and castor oil, enema, Foley catheters, Bougies and even sexual intercourse have had their advocates. All of the latter provide or provoke the release of the prostaglandins.

Oil, bath and enema

The 'OBE' much favoured in former years owed such success as it enjoyed from the stimulation of the gastrointestinal system and, presumably, the release from the gut of prostaglandin $F_{2\alpha}$, which then stimulated contractions in the adjacent uterus. This method represents an example of one that might work in women who were already on the threshold of spontaneous labour but would be unlikely to have much success otherwise.

Membrane sweeping

This technique, which by necessity is only possible once the cervix has ripened sufficiently to allow the passage of a finger, is also dependent on the release of endogenous prostaglandins but in this instance from those tissues which are normally associated with the generation of labour stimuli.[19] Its particular virtue lies in its simplicity and its comparative lack of risk and that with maintenance of the integrity of the membranes the labour may follow a more natural pattern of onset.

Transcervical Foley catheter

This has been employed both with and without the infusion of further agents with some success and once again it would seem to depend on provoking the release of those prostaglandins which soften the cervix and stimulate uterine contractility.[20,21] The pattern of cervical ripening which it appears to provoke, especially where prostaglandins are infused through the catheter, is such that the cervix dilates sufficiently to allow the Foley catheter to be expelled at 3 cm or 4 cm of dilatation (depending on the volume of fluid within the

> *'Owing to the unpredictability of the duration of labor in the nullipara, even in the presence of apparently favourable circumstances, induction of labour brings little advantage for either obstetrician or patient.'*
>
> **E H Bishop**
> *Pelvic scoring for elective induction. Obstet Gynecol 1964; 24:266.*

balloon) while the cervix may at that stage remain uneffaced. When that happens it is better to defer amniotomy until cervical effacement is more highly developed.

Amniotomy

Reference has already been made to amniotomy and its considerable success but of course it also carries additional risks. The appropriate place of amniotomy is considered later.

Oxytocin and prostaglandins

With amniotomy these form the principal agents for labour induction and the protocols of their use are given later in this chapter.

A systematic approach to induction of labour

The following stepwise approach to labour induction is considered.

Phase I

The following questions should be addressed:

- What is the state of health of the mother and what risks does she face?
- Does she have any special features in her history which require consideration? These include previous uterine surgery, precipitate delivery, difficult vaginal delivery, birth injury or stillbirth.
- What is the gestational age of the pregnancy based on the most reliable available evidence?
- What is the state of health of the fetus and the evidence of current and potential jeopardy? Assessment of liquor volume and the biophysical profile or other specific investigations may help predict how the fetus will tolerate labour.
- What is the state of the uterus and its contents?
  - are the fetal membranes ruptured or intact?
  - what is the situation of the fetus: estimated weight, presentation, and level of the presenting part?
  - is the myometrium responsive? (In practice this can really only be determined by observing its response to oxytocic drugs)
  - what is the degree of cervical ripeness? (see Table 6.1).

Phase II

Once the above information has been assembled the obstetrician should discuss matters fully with the expectant mother. The past few decades have seen a dramatic shift from a culture wherein the authoritarian clinician simply decreed the management and the mother was expected to comply. Nowadays most women expect a high level of discussion and explanation before an agreed policy is reached. Where it proves difficult to achieve such a position there may be need for compromise. A mutually satisfactory policy of clinical management can usually be reached by tactful negotiation and an honest acceptance of fallibility. There are three possible outcomes to this consultation:

1. Pregnancy should continue with appropriate surveillance.
2. Delivery should be by caesarean section.
3. Labour should be induced.

Phase III

When the decision is that labour should be induced the following approach is recommended:

Depending on the state of cervical ripeness, it may be appropriate to follow a protocol for 'priming' or 'ripening' the cervix as a prelude to labour induction *per se*. This has the important advantage of removing from both the mother and the clinical attendants the expectation that labour will be instantly established, thus reducing the likelihood that either party becomes disillusioned or disheartened by slow progress. Time taken to prepare the cervix so that the active phase of induced contractions will be effective is a worthwhile investment.

The three methods at the obstetrician's disposal to achieve successful labour and delivery are prostaglandins, amniotomy and oxytocin. The order in which these are listed here is intentional since prostaglandins are effective in ripening, effacing and dilating the cervix to the extent required for amniotomy to be appropriate, and oxytocin is largely ineffective before amniotomy. So the appropriate sequence of use is prostaglandin → amniotomy→ oxytocin (see Fig 6.3).

To emphasize the importance of this approach it should be stressed that amniotomy achieved with a struggle when the cervix is still long, firm and closed does little but condemn the woman to a long and usually unsuccessful labour[22] (Table 6.2). It is our belief that the optimal timing of membrane rupture in labour, spontaneous or induced, is when the cervix is fully effaced and ≥ 3 cm dilated. When such a policy is followed intravenous oxytocin may not be necessary, but it should be given when labour is not established or progressing following amniotomy.

Complications

Induction of labour is not an intervention to be embarked upon lightly. Indeed, the complications of induction can exceed the putative risks of the condition for which the induction was performed. The main complications are as follows:

Unsuspected fetal immaturity

A fundamental requirement before embarking on induction is confirmation of gestational age. This is not common if obsessional attention is paid to this point, particularly with the use of ultrasound in early pregnancy.

Uterine hyperstimulation

Although hypertonic uterine action can be seen in labour of spontaneous onset, it is natural to blame induction agents if their administration is followed by evidence of uterine hyperstimulation. This should be rare if protocols for administration of oxytocic agents are carefully followed but can occur within such guidelines, and may require acute tocolysis (see Chapter 26). Women of high parity (≥ 4) are at special risk and they merit particularly close monitoring.

Amniotomy

Amniotomy may lead to cord prolapse or abruptio placentae when there is polyhydramnios.

Table 6.2 Outcome of 125 consecutive labour inductions[22] by amniotomy and intravenous oxytocin titration in primigravid women at term, according to the degree of cervical ripeness (modified Bishop score[18])

Modified Bishop score	Number	Induction–delivery interval (mean)	Caesarean section rate	Depressed Apgar score
0–3: unripe	31	14.9 h	32%	23%
4–7: intermediate	69	8.9 h	4%	6%
8–11: ripe	25	6.4 h	0	0
All cases	125	9.9 h	10.4%	8.8%

It is important to take particular care to control the slow release of liquor from the uterus in these cases, otherwise the cord may be washed down and the sudden reduction in volume of the uterus may cause placental separation. With the most marked degrees of polyhydramnios it may be justified to carry out amniocentesis and reduce the liquor volume before amniotomy. Even without polyhydramnios, if the fetal head is free at the pelvic brim the risk of cord prolapse can be increased. With a normal amount of amniotic fluid and the fetal head settled into the pelvic brim, the risk of cord prolapse with amniotomy is not increased over spontaneous rupture of the membranes.

Another dreaded potential complication following amniotomy is intrauterine sepsis, in the form of chorioamnionitis.

Complications specific to oxytocin

Prolonged administration of concentrated oxytocin accompanied by large volumes of diluents carries the risk of water intoxication which has, in rare circumstances, led to maternal death. If protocols concerning dose rates and concentrations of this agent are followed this is not a risk. An association between administration of oxytocin during labour induction and an increased rate of neonatal jaundice has been proven, although this is rarely of important clinical significance.[23]

Failed induction

Although every case in which induction of labour is followed by the need for caesarean section may be considered a failed induction, some of these are in fact the result of fetal distress in labour which may have become evident during spontaneous labour. The true definition of failed induction is where the intervention is unsuccessful in leading to effective and progressive labour.[24] This is common in cases of prolonged pregnancy – which of course make up a very large proportion of those patients currently requiring induction. The constellation of failed induction, dystocia and atonic postpartum haemorrhage in women with prolonged pregnancy

Table 6.3 Protocols and dosages for the appropriate use of prostaglandins and oxytocin[27]

INTACT MEMBRANES

PGE_2 vaginal tablets 3 mg 6–8 hourly to maximum of 6 mg or PGE_2 vaginal gel – Nulliparas Bishop Score 4 or less – 2 mg

All other patients 1 mg, repeat 6 hourly to maximum 4 mg

RUPTURED MEMBRANES

(Either spontaneous or artificial) Intravenous infusion **oxytocin*** 30 international units in 500 ml normal saline = 60 milliunits per ml

∴ 1 ml per hour represents 1 mu/minute

Time (minutes)	0	30	60	90	120	150	180	210	240	270
Dose rate (mu/min)	1	2	4	8	12	16	20	24	28	32

***Oxytocin** infusion **delivered via syringe driver** or **infusion pump with non-return valve**.
12 mu/minute adequate for most women. Maximum dose 32 mu/min rarely required.
Oxytocin should not be commenced within 6 hours of last PGE_2 dose.

might lead one to speculate about a possible intrinsic myometrial dysfunction which predisposed them to failure to go into spontaneous labour, poor response to induction and postpartum uterine atony.

Special situations

Previous caesarean section

Although some clinicians regard previous caesarean as a contraindication to labour induction we do not subscribe to this view and each case must be considered on its merits. If the prospects of vaginal delivery are small and the prospects of a prolonged non-progressive labour are high, then it is prudent to recommend repeat caesarean section. That said, appropriate selection of cases will lead to safe and successful induction for a substantial proportion of such women. This topic is covered in Chapter 12.

Intrauterine fetal death

Amniotomy should be avoided in cases of intrauterine fetal death because of the increased risks of sepsis within the necrotic intrauterine tissues. Consequently prostaglandins are preferable – indeed, there may be a case for preceding prostaglandin therapy with the use of an antigestagen agent such as mifepristone. There is a school of thought who considered that amniotic fluid embolism is more likely to occur if the fetus has been long dead and the fetal membranes perhaps have begun to degenerate. While the truth of this belief remains unproven, it is prudent to be prepared to act promptly if there is any suggestion that this most serious complication may have occurred.

Interruption of pre-viable pregnancy or major fetal anomalies

The obstetrician is occasionally required to terminate a pregnancy where the fetus is pre-viable or has a lethal abnormality. This should be achieved with the minimum of distress to the mother. Although antigestagens seem to confer little or no benefit as an adjunct to labour induction at term, they are of benefit in the second trimester and in the early part of the third trimester. The reason for this is unclear. Presumably the influence of progesterone declines by term (see Chapter 1). In any event, at earlier gestations pretreatment with mifepristone 600 mg dramatically reduces the time taken to achieve delivery in response to local prostaglandins and in this circumstance vaginal misoprostol 400 µg repeated 3-hourly is highly effective.

High parity

As already mentioned, mothers of high parity have a higher risk of uterine hyperstimulation in response to induction. We therefore advocate a policy of amniotomy alone if conditions are favourable. If contractions do not become established, continuous administration of oxytocin is appropriate but this should be reduced or discontinued once contractions are established. If the cervix is unripe a preliminary single vaginal low dose of 1 mg PGE_2 in gel is appropriate.

Failure to respond

Some women resist all efforts to ripen the cervix with prostaglandins or to go into labour with prostaglandins and/or oxytocin. The reasons for this remain obscure. There may be a biological defect such as placental sulphatase deficiency[25] which prevents the sensitization of the uterus to oxytocic agents or perhaps these women lack some essential cytokine or other factor (see Chapter 1). Whatever the reason, it is never justified to continue to 'flog a dead horse' beyond the recommended protocol – to do so is often a recipe for trouble. Resort should be made to caesarean section when such cases have clearly failed to respond. This simply serves to emphasize the imperative of justifying the decision to interfere in the first place.

Prelabour rupture of the membranes

Spontaneous rupture of the membranes presents hazards to both mother and fetus, principally from intrauterine sepsis – which increases the longer delivery is delayed. Except where, for reasons of fetal immaturity, continuation of the pregnancy is proposed the need for induction of labour may arise. Since a significant proportion of such cases will go into labour within a few hours it is appropriate to anticipate this happening but we advocate stimulating contractions if this has not occurred after 12–24 hours.[26] Clearly amniotomy is not generally required but the protocols for employing prostaglandins and oxytocin are otherwise the same. Table 6.3 outlines the protocols and dosages for the appropriate use of prostaglandins and oxytocin.[27]

References

1. Barnes R. On the indications and operations for the induction of premature labour and for the acceleration of labour. Trans Obstet Soc Lond 1861; 3:132–139.
2. Champetier de Ribes CLA. De l'accouchement provoqué. Dilatation du canal genital (col de l'utérus, vagin et vulve) a l'aide de ballons introduit dans la cavité utérine pendant la grossesse. Ann Gynéc 1888; 30:401–438.
3. Voorhees JD. Dilatation of the cervix by means of a modified Champetier de Ribes balloon. Med Rec 1900; 58:361–366.
4. Dale HH. The action of extracts of the pituitary body. Biochem J 1909; 4:427–447.
5. Bell WB. The pituitary body and the therapeutic value of infundibular extract in shock, uterine atony and intestinal paresis. BMJ 1909; 2:1609–1613.
6. Kamm O, Aldrich TB, Grote IW, Rowe LW, Bugbee EP. The active principles of the posterior lobe of the pituitary gland. I. The demonstration of the presence of two active principles. II. The separation of the two principles and their concentration in the form of potent solid preparations. J Am Chem Soc 1928; 50:573–591.
7. DuVigneaud V, Ressler C, Swan JM, Roberts CW, Katsoyannis PG, Gordon S. The synthesis of an octapeptide with the hormonal activity of oxytocin. J Am Chem Soc 1953; 75:4879–4880.
8. Boissonas RA, Guttmann S, Jaquenand PA, Waller TP. A new synthesis of oxytocin. Helvetica Chimica Acta 1955; 38:1491–1495.
9. Theobald GW, Graham A, Campbell J, Gange PD, O'Driscoll WJ. The use of posterior pituitary extract in physiological amounts in obstetrics. BMJ 1948; 2:123–127.
10. Turnbull AC, Anderson AMB. Induction of labour: results with amniotomy and oxytocin titration. J Obstet Gynaecol Br Commonw 1968; 75:32–41.
11. Baskett TF. The development of prostaglandins. Best Pract Res Clin Obstet Gynaecol 2003; 17:703–706.
12. Karim SMM, Hillier K, Trussell RR, Patel RC, Tamusange S. Induction of labour with prostaglandin E_2. J Obstet Gynaecol Br Commonw 1970; 77:200–204.
13. Calder AA, Embrey MP. Prostaglandins and the unfavourable cervix. Lancet 1973; 2:1322–1324.
14. MacKenzie IZ, Embrey MP. Cervical ripening with intravaginal PGE_2 gel. BMJ 1977; 2:1369–1372.
15. Hofmeyer GJ, Gulmezoglu AM. Vaginal misoprostol for cervical ripening and labour induction in late pregnancy. Cochrane Review: Cochrane Library. Issue 4. Oxford: Update Software, 2002.
16. Hannah ME, Hannah WJ, Hellman J, Hewson S, Milner R, William A. Induction of labour as compared with serial antenatal monitoring in post-term pregnancy. A randomised controlled trial. N Engl J Med 1992; 326:1587–1592.
17. Bishop EH. Pelvic scoring for elective induction. Obstet Gynecol 1964; 24:266–269.
18. Kennedy JH, Stewart P, Barlow DH, Hillan E, Calder AA. Induction of labour: a comparison of a single prostaglandin E2 vaginal tablet with amniotomy and intravenous oxytocin. Br J Obstet Gynaecol 1982; 89:704–707.

19. Boulvain M, Stan C, Irion C. Membrane sweeping for induction of labour. Cochrane Database Syst Rev 2001; Issue 2.

20. Embrey MP, Mollison BG. The unfavourable cervix and induction of labour using a cervical balloon. J Obstet Gynaecol Br Commonw 1967; 74:44–47.

21. Calder AA, Embrey MP, Hillier K. Extra-amniotic prostaglandin E_2 for the induction of labour at term. J Obstet Gynaecol Br Commonw 1974; 81:39–46.

22. Embrey MP, Calder AA. Induction of labour. In: Proceedings of the third study group of the Royal College of Obstetricians and Gynaecologists. London: RCOG Press, 1975.

23. Calder AA, Moar VA, Ounsted MK, Turnbull AC. Increased bilirubin levels in neonates after induction of labour by intravenous prostaglandin E_2 or oxytocin. Lancet 1974; 2:1339–1340.

24. MacVicar J. Failed induction of labour. J Obstet Gynaecol Br Commonw 1971; 78:1007–1010.

25. France JT, Sneddon RJ, Liggins CG. A study of a pregnancy with low oestrogen production due to placental sulphatase deficiency. J Clin Endocrinol Metab 1973; 36:1–3.

26. Hannah ME, Ohlsson A, Farine D, et al. Induction of labor compared with expectant management for prelabour rupture of the membranes at term. TERMPROM Study Group. N Engl J Med 1996; 334:1005–1010.

27. Induction of labour. Evidence based guideline No. 9. Royal College of Obstetricians and Gynaecologists. Clinical Effectiveness Support Unit. London: RCOG Press, 2001.

7

Preterm labour

'The usual period of a woman's going with child is nine calendar months; but there is very commonly a difference of one, two or three weeks. A child may be born alive at any time from three months: but we see none born with powers of coming to manhood, or of being reared, before seven calendar months, or near that time. At six months it cannot be.'

William Hunter c. 1760
Cited by Thomas Denman. In Introduction to the Practice of Midwifery. New York: E. Bliss and E. White, 1825, p253

Although preterm deliveries constitute but a small proportion of all births their contribution to serious complications, especially those leading to perinatal death and morbidity, is hugely disproportionate. Nature has ordered that the time for delivery which offers the least risk of trouble for the fetus and newborn, and generally also for the mother, lies within what has come to be known as 'term', i.e. between 37 and 42 weeks after the last menstrual period, or 35–40 weeks after conception. Within this span the 'expected' date of delivery has been calculated to be after 40 weeks of amenorrhoea – 38 weeks after conception.

It should occasion no surprise that, as highlighted in Chapter 1, the biological changes which trigger labour are intimately linked to those which prepare and adapt the fetus for extrauterine life – notably maturation of the lungs. Thus has evolution ensured optimal survival.

Incidence

The peak incidence for spontaneous delivery, accounting for about four in every five births, is thus at term with about one in ten falling either before or after term. Historically, until the last two or three decades, 28 weeks of amenorrhoea represented another important landmark in the chronology of pregnancy. This was taken to represent, in legal terms, the lower limit of viability for the fetus. Although there had been examples of less mature infants surviving, these were exceptional and such cases as seemed to occur were often more likely due to mistaken dates.

Two comparatively recent developments have resulted in the need to rethink this definition. First, neonatal intensive care has dramatically increased the chances of survival in what were previously regarded as pre-viable infants. Second, the development of diagnostic ultrasound has enhanced our ability to determine the duration of pregnancy with a high degree of precision so that much of the former uncertainty has been dispelled. The latter facility has hitherto been relied upon as the basis on which to calculate the gestational age if the menstrual data were unreliable, but it is perhaps inevitable that, where high quality ultrasound assessment has been performed in early pregnancy, this will become the gold standard and menstrual data will become less important.

These developments have led to a lowering of the threshold of fetal viability, which in most countries is now considered to be 24 weeks. This does seem to represent an irreducible limit of viability at least for the foreseeable future and until the development of further technological advances such as would allow a less mature infant to be sustained by some sort of 'artificial placenta' until the lungs and other organs have grown and developed sufficiently. Although we are now seeing very occasional, apparently authenticated, instances of survival at 23 weeks or less, the 24-week milestone seems appropriate for the time being, not least because the prospect of intact survival is so small before that gestational age.

In defining the statistical incidence of prematurity it has always been necessary to use as the denominator the total number of births rather than the total number of pregnancies. This is because reproductive wastage – in the sense of conceptions failing to implant or those which develop and miscarry – represent a considerable and largely incalculable proportion of the whole.

On that basis the incidence of premature birth on a global scale is around one in ten births. This figure is lower in developed countries but even so the incidence varies quite widely both within and between such countries due to a variety of influences. Once again, however, such figures need to be seen in the context of the development of modern perinatal care. Just as the 25-week fetus can no longer be written off as pre-viable, neither is the 35-week fetus regarded as a source of major concern should delivery occur or become necessary. It would appear that the extent of 'viability migration' in modern obstetrics, if we might call it that, is of the order of a month. Thus as *viability* has been reduced from 28 to 24 weeks, so has the point in pregnancy where *maturity* ceases to be a major concern drifted down from 37 to around 33 weeks. After this point, all concerned, particularly the neonate, can expect to breathe more easily.

Thus, with the benefit of modern neonatal care we can now expect high levels of intact survival as early as 28 weeks. Such premature infants commonly require several weeks of intensive support and may endure a difficult sojourn in a space capsule in the neonatal unit before safe re-entry becomes possible. The nub of the problem lies not so much in prematurity as in *extreme prematurity.* The greater the degree of prematurity the greater and commoner are the hazards that are faced. Mortality and long-term handicap are inversely related to the gestational age at delivery. Although about one in ten neonates may be regarded as preterm, those in the extreme premature range of 24–30 weeks gestation account for less than 1 in 100.

Based on the assumption that survival before 24 weeks is extremely rare while, in the best of circumstances reaching 30 or even 28 weeks may give excellent prospects of survival, it will be clear that this is the stage of pregnancy when prolongation of gestation may bring the greatest benefits. In purely actuarial terms each day that the fetus remains in utero after 24 weeks should enhance its prospects of survival. In practice however, the issue is much less simple since in many instances it is not in the best interest of the fetus to remain in what may be an increasingly hostile intrauterine environment.

To place crude figures on the incidence of premature birth may thus be of limited value. Suffice it to say that most populations will see around one in ten of their offspring delivering before the traditional definition of term. Of these, a greater or lesser proportion will face significant perils depending on the stage of gestation at delivery and the obstetric and paediatric facilities available. Unhappily, the greater the degree of immaturity the greater is the likelihood of long-term handicap among the surviving children. It is therefore imperative that if preterm delivery is inescapable, the child should be delivered in the best condition possible.

Table 7.1 shows recent survival rates according to gestational age at delivery in one neonatal unit. During the period in question overall survival rates continued to improve. The rate of survival at less than 28 weeks gestation rose from 56% in 1995 to 71% in 2002–2004. Against these increasingly optimistic figures it must be emphasized that the handicap rates in extremely preterm babies remain depressingly high. The Epicure Study[1–3] of babies born at less than 26 weeks gestation showed a handicap rate of 50% at 30 months of age and in half of these the handicap was assessed as severe.[1–3] Even at 26–28 weeks about one surviving infant in six is likely to be handicapped.

Table 7.1 Survival rates by gestational age at delivery of infants liveborn in the Simpson Maternity Unit of Edinburgh Royal Infirmary (1994–2004)

Gestational age (weeks)	Survival (%)
< 24	18
24	57
25	75
26	80
27	80
28	85
29	92
30	98

Aetiology

When considering the reasons why most pregnancies progress happily to term while others fail to do so, account must be taken of the current state of knowledge concerning the biological control of parturition. This has been briefly reviewed in Chapter 1. An underlying assumption must be that if labour begins before term this must be the result of the influence of one or more factors which distort the normal mechanism. Since we believe that normal mechanism to consist of a cascade of biological changes which ultimately have the effect of causing myometrial contractility and cervical dilatation, we might reasonably expect that this may happen either as a result of premature triggering of the whole biological process, or alternatively that some event or influence may have resulted in a short-circuiting of the normal sequence of events. The most obvious example of the latter is where significant intrauterine infection causes

> *'But sometimes it happens, that women bring forth their young before the time; or to preserve their lives, the fetus is taken from them before their time, whether this happens by some remarkable foregoing accident, viz. by a fall, a blow, a concussion or hurt, or by some violent passion of the mind, by a fright, by fear or great sorrow or whether it happens of its own accord, without such remarkable accident.'*
>
> **Hendrick van Deventer**
> *The Art of Midwifery Improved. London: E. Curll, 1716, p87*

Table 7.2 Aetiology of preterm labour

Direct causes	Associated factors	Idiopathic (cause unknown)
Infection Antepartum haemorrhage Premature rupture of the membranes Structural abnormalities of uterine corpus (congenital malformations, fibromyomata, etc) Incompetence of the uterine cervix Trauma Multiple pregnancy Polyhydramnios Clinical induction of labour	Socioeconomic deprivation Marital status Substance abuse, including tobacco Extremes of maternal age Short maternal stature Extremes of maternal weight Extremes of haemoglobin concentration Previous history of preterm delivery	?

the release of inflammatory mediators such as prostaglandins and cytokines with the direct effect of provoking cervical softening and myometrial contractility.

In drawing up a catalogue of aetiological factors we may list them under three principal categories (Table 7.2). The first consists of specific events or conditions which can be identified as the *direct cause* of preterm labour in the individual case. The second category concerns *associated factors* which may put an individual pregnancy at greater risk of preterm delivery. The third are *idiopathic*, in which no explanation can be found.

Complications

Although the mother who experiences premature labour may thereby incur greater risks to herself as a result of either the cause or the need for obstetric intervention, the principal risks are to the fetus. These may be considered under three main headings:

- The first is simply the catalogue of risks which surround immaturity of the neonate as a result of preterm delivery. The most prominent of these is respiratory distress from incomplete pulmonary development and the absence of pulmonary surfactant. There may be problems which result from the immaturity of organs such as the liver, inadequacy of temperature control, and others resulting from metabolic considerations such as mineral and electrolyte balance and glucose homeostasis.
- The second category derives from the risks, principally of trauma, which are increased as a result of labour and delivery. The most important of these is intracranial haemorrhage.
- The third threat is the direct deleterious effects on the neonate from the underlying cause of the premature delivery. Notable among these are infection and hypoxia associated with complications such as abruptio placentae. It is now recognized that infectious processes provoke the release of inflammatory cytokines which may have a directly damaging effect on delicate structures, especially in the fetal brain.[4] In essence the main aim of management is to avoid the three major hazards to the fetus/neonate – infection/hypoxia/trauma.

From all the above it will be clear that the challenge to the preterm infant is not simply one of survival but rather survival without permanent damage to vital organs and systems.

Prediction

Because of our inability to influence the course of events once labour has become clearly established, a situation akin to trying to lock the stable door after the horse has bolted, attempts have been made to improve the prediction of preterm labour. It may seem surprising, faced with such an array of factors which may cause or contribute to the onset of preterm labour, that it has proved so difficult to predict this complication. It may be precisely because the condition has such a multifactorial aetiology that this remains one of the largest sources of frustration in clinical obstetric practice. Among all these factors the one with the single largest relative risk is history of a previous preterm birth, but this is clearly of no help in predicting preterm labour in first pregnancies – and even given a history of two previous preterm births the incidence of recurrence is less than 30%.[5]

Although normal parturition at term is known to be preceded by a significant period of prelabour, characterized by cervical softening, effacement and increasing uterine contractility over several weeks (see Chapter 1), it is still not clear whether any or all preterm labours demonstrate a similar preterm prelabour phenomenon. Attempts to recognize such a pattern by regular digital examination of the cervix or observing its condition with ultrasound have so far yielded inconsistent results. Similarly, risk-scoring systems based on assessment of a wide range of factors have been developed with the object of directing a tailored programme of antenatal surveillance to those women whose scores suggest that they are at particularly increased risk. While these are attractive on theoretical grounds they have not yet produced any measurable dividends.[6]

Diagnosis

The over-riding obstacle to progress in seeking to reduce the impact of premature labour lies in the difficulty of precise diagnosis. On the one hand it may be obvious that a woman is in established preterm labour because she has regular painful uterine contractions, with or without rupture of the membranes or a 'show', and the cervix is undergoing progressive dilatation. In these circumstances it is inevitable that delivery will follow in spite of the most determined efforts to arrest or delay it. On the other hand it has become increasingly clear in recent years that where such obstetric interventions have appeared to be effective it is probable that many of the patients concerned were never in established labour in the first place.

It is clearly unsatisfactory to rely solely on observation of myometrial contractility. Even where this is supported by a continuous tocographic record showing regular contractions, these may be very misleading. The definitive evidence that labour is established lies in observing progressive cervical dilatation. This however brings further difficulties, since in most circumstances this depends on at least two vaginal examinations separated by a significant period of time. The very performance of such examinations may provoke the local release of prostaglandins in the genital tract or introduce infection.

In practice if a woman suspects that she might be in preterm labour, by the time medical or midwifery staff have attended her if the cervix then remains closed and uneffaced it may reasonably be assumed that she is not in preterm labour despite apparent myometrial contractility. Although diagnostic ultrasound has made an enormous impact on obstetric practice its contribution in this area of care is limited. There was excitement some 20 years ago when it was demonstrated that if fetal breathing movements could be recognized this effectively ruled out the possibility of established preterm labour.[7] On the other hand where breathing movements are absent this *may* equate with preterm labour, but because this phenomenon is sporadic it could equally be due to a period of fetal 'sleep' and not evidence of established labour. Although the theoretical basis for this approach has been demonstrated it has never reached the point of practical utility.

Where diagnostic ultrasound may be of some value is in observing changes in the uterine cervix without the need for digital examination. The value of this is probably restricted to following women considered to be at risk of preterm delivery, particularly from cervical incompetence and in multiple pregnancy.[8]

A variety of biochemical factors have been suggested as potential diagnostic indicators but the only one to have achieved widespread application is the detection of fetal fibronectin. This substance may be released from intrauterine tissues such as the decidua and fetal membranes if these are disturbed by the onset of preterm labour and may be detected in vaginal secretions. Again in practice it is often found that where this test is positive the reality of labour is clinically very obvious and as a result the principal value of this test lies in the exclusion of the diagnosis of preterm labour where the test is negative – this is of considerable value in limiting the use of tocolytics and hospital admission.[9] There may be value in combining ultrasound assessment of the cervix with fetal fibronectin testing.

As indicated above, where the clinical situation is unclear a digital vaginal examination may not be in the patient's best interests, particularly where there is a possibility of premature rupture of the membranes. On the other hand a careful speculum examination may be very useful in clarifying the situation. It affords the option of testing for fetal fibronectin and also obtaining specimens for bacteriological investigation, such as culture for group B Streptococcus.

Management

Treatment with the object of reducing the incidence, risks and complications of preterm labour falls into three principal categories:

- Measures aimed at preventing preterm labour including early recognition and treatment of infection, cervical cerclage where the cervix is considered to be incompetent and, however unrealistically optimistic, encouragement to modify high-risk practices such as drug abuse and smoking.
- Tocolysis to try to abolish or arrest preterm labour.
- Obstetric interventions aimed at minimizing the complications of preterm delivery, including the administration of glucocorticoids to accelerate fetal lung maturation and decisions concerning the safest and least traumatic mode of delivery for the baby.

Tocolytic treatment

The use of drugs to suppress or inhibit the onset of myometrial contractility may reasonably be described as one of the most outstanding examples of clinical self-delusion. For decades clinicians continued to administer drugs which appeared to produce effective suppression of preterm labour. It was only when placebo controlled trials were properly conducted that they were shown to be of very limited efficacy for this purpose.[10,11] Many of these agents are now seen to carry risks to either the mother or the fetus, or both, which hardly justifies their use. The catalogue of therapeutic agents which have come into and out of vogue as tocolytics is extremely long. Agents such as progesterone and ethyl alcohol had their advocates but have long since fallen out of favour – although there may be some resurgent enthusiasm for progesterone therapy which would seem to have a logical basis in our understanding of myometrial contractility. Although ethyl alcohol may have a direct inhibitory effect on the myometrium its principal role was thought to lie in its inhibition of oxytocin secretion. While this may well be its effect, the clinical reality is that any impact it may have had was generally at best short lived before the myometrium escaped inhibition.

Worldwide the most extensively used group of tocolytics has been the β-sympathomimetics.[12] These agents have been used with great enthusiasm but with little persuasive evidence of benefit. Add to that the very real danger to which they expose some mothers, notably from complications such as pulmonary oedema, and it is hardly surprising that they have fallen out of favour in the past few years. Although they appear to be capable of delaying delivery in the short term there is little to suggest that they can produce any long-term postponement and their greatest virtue lies in their use to delay labour long enough to allow maternal transfer and glucocorticoids to take effect.

Other agents which appear to act at the myometrial level include magnesium sulphate, which may act as a calcium channel blocker.[13] Specific agents designed for that purpose, such as nifedipine, have also been used.[14]

The therapeutic approach which perhaps has the firmest basis in the physiology of parturition is the use of prostaglandin synthesis inhibitors. The one which has been most widely used for this purpose is indometacin. Its use however has been largely eschewed because of serious concerns that it may cause dangerous complications to the fetus, notably pulmonary hypertension as a result of closure or partial closure of the fetal ductus arteriosus.[15] The risks of necrotizing enterocolitis and intraventricular haemorrhage may also be increased. Because it is now recognized that there are two separate cyclo-oxygenase enzymes and that selective inhibition of COX-2 might avoid some of the above complications, agents developed with this degree of specificity are currently under evaluation, although the early results do not appear to be encouraging.[16]

Most recently a specific oxytocin receptor blocker (atosiban) has been marketed. It would not appear to be more effective than any of these other agents but it may have the advantage of fewer serious complications, especially on the mother.[17]

On the assumption that infection may underlie many cases of preterm labour, the routine use of antibiotics to try to avert it when it seems to threaten has proved disappointing.[18] The assumption must be that although it may be possible to eradicate the infective organisms, they will already have provoked the inflammatory cascade which triggers preterm labour.

All agents aimed at achieving tocolysis should be used with caution since they are capable of causing adverse effects on the mother, the fetus, or both. A suggested regime for attempting to suppress preterm labour in selected pregnancies is as follows:

Betamimetic agents

Ritodrine hydrochloride: intravenous infusion of 100 µg/min stepped up by an additional 50 µg/min at 15-minute intervals until suppression of contractions is achieved or the maternal pulse rate exceeds 120 bpm. The maximum dose range should not exceed 350 µg (i.e. 5 increments). Careful monitoring of the maternal condition is essential.

Oxytocin receptor blockers

Atosiban: Bolus intravenous injection of 6.75 mg followed by 300 µg for 3 hours. Thereafter maintenance dose of 100 µg/min for 48 hours.[17]

Calcium channel blockers

Nifedipine: 10–20 mg by mouth every 4–6 hours. The maternal blood pressure should be measured regularly and evidence of hypotension calls for interruption of therapy.[14]

Cyclo-oxygenase inhibitors

Indometacin: 25–50 mg orally 4–6-hourly or 100 mg by rectal suppository every 12 hours. This agent is often favoured as prophylactic therapy in conditions or during procedures considered to carry an increased risk of preterm labour. Examples of these are polyhydramnios, multiple pregnancy, uterine malformations and cervical suture insertion. It should be avoided after 32 weeks gestation because of the increased risk of premature closure of the fetal ductus arteriosus. If exposure is continued beyond a few days the amniotic fluid volume and the condition of the fetus should be carefully monitored.

Nitric oxide donors

Glyceryl trinitrate facilitates smooth muscle relaxation including that of the uterus. It is under study using a slow-release transdermal patch.

Antimicrobial agents

Apart from treatment of specifically diagnosed infections such as group B Streptococcus, empirical use of antibiotics should be limited to cases where the membranes are ruptured.[18] The appropriate agent is erythromycin 250–500 mg every 6 hours.

Glucocorticoids

Glucocorticoids should be given on one occasion before 34 weeks gestation. The usual routine is betamethasone 12 mg IM on two occasions 12 hours apart. If at all possible delivery should be postponed for 24 hours after giving the last dose. Glucocorticoids given before 34 weeks gestation are associated with a significant reduction in rates of respiratory distress syndrome, neonatal death and intraventricular haemorrhage.

Premature prelabour rupture of membranes

The terminology surrounding rupture of the fetal membranes before the onset of labour at term has suffered from considerable confusion. The phrase 'premature rupture of the membranes' has been applied by some to mean that the membranes have ruptured but the mother is not in labour regardless of the gestational age. The modern terminology is 'prelabour rupture of the membranes' when the mother is not in labour – when this occurs before 37 weeks, it should be prefixed with 'preterm'. Where there is preterm prelabour rupture of the membranes there are two principal sources of anxiety:

- The potential for chorioamnionitis is very considerable and, at least in some cases, the initiating cause is intrauterine infection. In this circumstance a decision requires to be made as to whether conservative management is or is not appropriate. Our ability to diagnose chorioamnionitis is limited but careful observation of the maternal temperature, the white blood cell count and specific markers such as C-reactive protein (CRP) may be helpful.[19]
- The second anxiety arises from the increased likelihood that, although it may be desirable to continue the pregnancy longer, rupture of the membranes may be followed by the onset of uterine contractility. If this does happen the use of tocolytic drugs is neither likely to succeed nor clinically sensible.

Diagnosis

Although there may have been an apparent convincing loss of amniotic fluid from the vagina, it is not uncommon for this to be confused with sudden loss of bladder control. Sterile speculum examination may confirm the presence of a pool of liquor within the vagina and such an observation may be supported by the use of a variety of tests – the simplest and most specific of which is ferning. Ultrasound examination may suggest that the amount of fluid within the uterus is reduced, but this could be for obstetric reasons other than rupture of the membranes. Conversely, a seemingly adequate volume of amniotic fluid does not preclude rupture of the membranes.

Management

In some circumstances it may be plain that the best approach is to secure delivery. This will be best accomplished by induction of labour with oxytocin, unless caesarean section is warranted. The principal indication for delivery is convincing evidence of chorioamnionitis – in these circumstances appropriate antibiotic therapy should be administered. Corticosteroids should also be given if the gestation is less than 34 weeks.

If it is felt prudent to manage the case conservatively, careful surveillance should be conducted for evidence of infection. If a conservative policy is adopted it must be accepted that, especially if the membranes have ruptured at a very early gestation, there is an increased risk of impaired fetal lung development and of limb deformities from pressure effects within the uterus ('fetal crush syndrome'). It is our view that once the gestational age has reached 35 weeks there is little to be gained from continuing a policy of conservative management and induction of labour becomes appropriate.

Although the impact of antimicrobial therapy on preventing and suppressing preterm labour or improving its outcome has been disappointing, the one area in which benefit has been demonstrated is preterm prelabour rupture of the membranes.[18]

Mode of delivery

Controversy continues to surround the appropriate mode of delivery of the premature baby. Caesarean section is indicated in many circumstances in which the mother is not in labour. For instance if there is severe maternal disease and/or fetal compromise – either impaired fetal growth or direct evidence of intrauterine hypoxia – caesarean delivery is appropriate.

In the absence of such problems, however, it may be better to allow vaginal delivery to take place, although most would favour caesarean section where there is a breech presentation, which is more common at earlier gestations.

The second controversy surrounds a policy of elective use of forceps. This has been advocated on the basis that the forceps act as a protective cage for the delicate fetal skull, thereby perhaps reducing the incidence of intracranial haemorrhage. An alternative school of thought holds that the forceps might actually increase trauma, particularly as forceps are designed for the term-size fetal head. However, if assisted delivery is required this should be by the use of forceps as the vacuum extractor should not be used before 34 weeks gestation. Thus, the best principle is to allow a carefully controlled spontaneous delivery and avoid compression forces on the fetal head, if necessary by use of episiotomy. As indicated above, the over-riding objective in dealing with preterm labour and delivery is to minimize the damaging trio of complications to the infant from infection, asphyxia and trauma. If this can be accomplished, much of the financial and emotional cost associated with perinatal death and permanent handicap may be avoided.

References

1. Wood NS, Marlow N, Costeloe K, Gibson AT, Wilkinson AR. Neurologic and developmental disability after extremely preterm birth. EPICure Study Group. N Engl J Med 2000; 343:378–384.
2. Costeloe K, Hennessy E, Gibson AT, Marlow N, Wilkinson AR. The EPICure study: outcomes to discharge from hospital for infants born at the threshold of viability. Pediatrics. 2000; 106:659–671.
3. Wood NS, Costeloe K, Gibson AT, Hennessy EM, Marlow N, Wilkinson AR. EPICure Study Group. The EPICure study: associations and antecedents of neurological and developmental disability at 30 months of age following extremely preterm birth. Arch Dis Child Fetal Neonatal Ed 2005; 90:F134–140.
4. Dammann O, Leviton A. Maternal intrauterine infection, cytokines, and brain damage in the preterm newborn. Pediatr Res 1997; 42:1–8.
5. Bakketeig LS, Hoffman HJ. Epidemiology of preterm birth: results from a longitudinal study of births in Norway. In: Elder MG, Hendricks CH, eds. Preterm labor. London and Boston: Butterworths, 1981:17–46.
6. Papiernik E, Kaminski M. Multifactorial study of the risk of prematurity at 32 weeks of gestation. I. Study of 30 predictive characteristics. J Perinat Med 1974; 2:30–36.
7. Castle BM, Turnbull AC. The presence or absence of fetal breathing movements predicts the outcome of preterm labour. Lancet 1983; 2:471–473.
8. Iams JD, Paraskos J, Landon MB, Teteris JN, Johnson FF. Cervical sonography in preterm labour. Obstet Gynecol 1994; 84:40–46.
9. Honest H, Bachmann LM, Gupta JK, Kleinjnen J, Khan KS. Accuracy of cervicovaginal fetal fibronectin test in predicting risk of spontaneous preterm birth: systematic review. BMJ 2002; 325:301.
10. The Canadian Preterm Investigators Group. Treatment of preterm labor with the beta adrenergic agonist ritodrine. N Engl J Med 1992; 327:308–312.
11. Gyetvai K, Hannah ME, Hodnett ED, Ohlsson A. Tocolytics for preterm labor: a systematic review. Obstet Gynecol 1999; 94:869–877.

12. King JF, Grant A, Keirse MJ, Chalmers I. Beta-mimetics in preterm labour: an overview of the randomised controlled trials. Br J Obstet Gynecol 1988; 95:211–222.

13. Crowther CA, Hiller JE, Doyle LW. Magnesium sulphate for preventing preterm birth in threatened preterm labour. Cochrane Database Syst Rev 2002; (4):CD001060.

14. King JF, Flenady VJ, Papatsonis DN, Dekker GA, Carbonne B. Calcium channel blockers for inhibiting preterm labour. Cochrane Database Syst Rev 2003; (1):CD002255.

15. Norton ME, Merrill J, Cooper BA, Kuller JA, Clyman RI. Neonatal complications after the administration of indomethacin for preterm labor. N Engl J Med 1993; 329:1602–1607.

16. Sawdy RJ, Lye S, Fisk NM, Bennett PR. A double-blind randomised study of fetal side effects after short-term maternal administration of indomethacin, sulindac, and nimesulide for the treatment of preterm labor. Am J Obstet Gynecol 2003; 188:1046–1051.

17. Worldwide Atosiban versus Beta-agonists Study Group. Effectiveness and safety of the oxytocin antagonist atosiban versus beta-adrenergic agonists in the treatment of preterm labour. Br J Obstet Gynaecol 2001; 108:133–142.

18. Kenyon S, Taylor DJ, Tarnow-Mordi WO; ORACLE Collaborative Group. ORACLE – antibiotics for preterm prelabour rupture of the membranes: short-term and long-term outcomes. Acta Paediatr (Suppl) 2002; 91:12–15.

19. Hvilsom GB, Thorsen P, Jeune B, Bakketeig LS. C-reactive protein: a serological marker for preterm delivery? Acta Obstet Gynecol Scand 2002; 81:424–429.

8

Assisted vaginal delivery

There is no chapter in the history of obstetrics that is more central to the development of the clinical art of obstetrics than the invention and evolution of the obstetric forceps. Indeed, there are few surgical instruments that remain in use, albeit modified, more than three centuries after their introduction. In contrast, the other instrument used to assist vaginal delivery, the vacuum extractor, while having its origins some 150 years ago, has really only been developed in practical clinical terms over the past half century. Because assisted vaginal delivery was and remains an essential clinical obstetrical skill its history and evolution over almost four centuries will be recorded here. Indeed, to a large extent it was the development of the obstetric forceps in the hands of the 'man-midwife' that allowed the physician access to the birth chamber, formerly almost the sole purview of the midwife.

Historical Background

Four important events mark the evolution of the obstetric forceps: (1) the invention, (2) the introduction of the pelvic curve, (3) the introduction of axis-traction devices, (4) the return to a modified 'straight' forceps for application to the low, transversely placed head.

THE INVENTION OF THE FORCEPS

On 3 July 1569 there disembarked at Southampton a Huguenot refugee family by the name of Chamberlen (Chamberlayne, Chamberlaine and Chamberlin are other spellings). The family consisted of William

Historical Background

the father (whether he ever practiced medicine or was qualified to do so has not been determined), his wife and three children. Two other sons were born a year and 3 years, respectively, after the family had settled in England. The eldest and the youngest son were both named Peter and are referred to by obstetric historians as 'Peter the older' and 'Peter the younger'. To add to the confusion there was a third Peter, a son of Peter the younger, known under the designation 'Dr Peter Chamberlen' because he was Doctor of Medicine at Padua (1619), Oxford (1620), and Cambridge (1621) and a Fellow of the College of Physicians (1628); while the father and uncle were of the Barber Surgeons Company (date of admission round about the years 1596–8). Further reference to these three Peters will be under the respective numbers I, II, and III which some historians have very wisely adopted for the purpose of distinguishing them.

For many years the invention was attributed to Peter III (Dr Peter Chamberlen), who was born in 1601 and died in 1683. This impression, however, is almost certainly refuted by his own statement:[1] 'My Fame begot me envie and secret enemies which mightily increased when my Father added to me the knowledge of "Deliveries and the Cures of Women".' There is therefore every justification for concluding that the inventor of the obstetric forceps was either Peter I or Peter II, or possibly both.

Peter I (1560?–1631) attained the greater distinction and his rise to fame was as dramatic as it was rapid. He attended Anne of Denmark, Queen Consort of James I, and other notable women in society in their confinements. And for so doing as a Barber Surgeon he was arraigned before the College of Physicians in 1612 and incarcerated in Newgate Prison. By the intervention of the Queen and the Archbishop of Canterbury, the President and Censors of the College were prevailed upon to permit his release.

Peter II (1572–1626), the brother, some 10 or 12 years younger, was also interested in midwifery and he was the first to suggest the creation of an Incorporation of Midwives, a project with which Peter III, his son, was more particularly identified.

The probability is that Peter I was the inventor and that the date of the invention was shortly before or shortly after 1600. There is of course the other remote possibility that if 'Old Father William' did practice medicine, as some historians thought was the case, he may have been the actual inventor of the instrument.[2]

The secret was kept in the family for 100 years or more. But many attempts were made – presumably the secret was beginning to leak out – to trade the instrument in Paris and Amsterdam by Hugh Chamberlen Senior (son of Peter III), who possessed all his father's combativeness and business instincts, coupled with his ability to retain a position at Court and amongst numerous clients in the highest social scale. Historical was his encounter with the great obstetrician Francois Mauriceau (1637–1709) in Paris in 1670 when, to test the value of the forceps, Mauriceau gave him a rachitic dwarf (who had been many days in labour) to deliver. Of course, Chamberlen failed and Mauriceau chuckled! Yet, like all commercial travellers, so little was he abashed by his failure that within 6 months we find him again in Paris, on this occasion attempting to sell the invention to the French Government.[3,4]

It was not until the 18th century was well advanced that the secret of the forceps became known. It was first announced by Edmund Chapman (1680?–1756), the obstetrician of Essex and London, who publicly made known the forceps used by the Chamberlens.[5]

Space does not permit, nor is the occasion suitable, to pursue here the story of this most remarkable family and its doings; nor to describe the schemes – medical, political and commercial – which they sponsored. Fortunately in Aveling's historic volume[1] *we possess a complete record of all these details and of what perhaps was the crowning event in the romance of the forceps, the discovery in 1818 of a number of the Chamberlens' instruments (Fig 8.1) in a well-concealed chest in Woodham Mortimer Hall, Essex, which had been purchased by Peter III round about 1630 and continued in the possession of the family until 1715.*

On the death in 1728 of Hugh (Junior), son of Hugh (Senior) and grandson of Peter III, the male line of the Chamberlens became extinct. He too was a popular obstetrician and physician and carried on a most successful practice amongst the highest classes of society of London. As far as can be judged, he shed the aggressive enthusiasm, commercial instincts and timely sanctimoniousness of his forebears. He mellowed, was popular with the fellows and was three times elected a Censor of the College of Physicians. His memory is commemorated in the cenotaph in the north aisle of the choir in Westminster Abbey erected by the son of his patron the Duke of Buckingham, no doubt at the instigation of the Duchess, with whom he lived on intimate terms following the death of the Duke. Thus is the story of the family rounded off by these events!

The forceps of the Chamberlens – admittedly those illustrated here were early patterns – was simple in design and possessed only a cephalic curve, and in this form they remained for well over 100 years (1600?–1747).

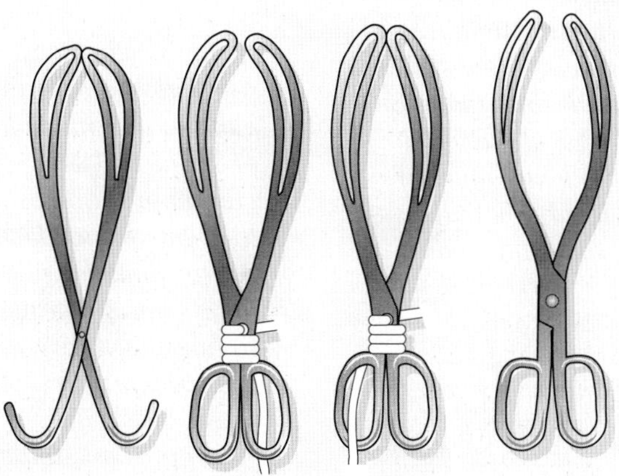

Figure 8.1 Chamberlen's forceps.

THE INTRODUCTION OF THE PELVIC CURVE

To André Levret (1703–1780) is attributed this improvement, which he brought to the notice of the Paris Academy in 1747. As is often the case other individuals came up with the same idea at about the same time. Benjamin Pugh (1715–1798), an obstetrician in Chelmsford, Essex, claimed, in the preface of his 1754 Treatise of Midwifery, 'The curved forceps I invented upwards of 14 years ago…'[6] It is likely that about the same time William Smellie (1697–1763) independently conceived the same modification, but in respect of the design of the forceps it is mainly for the simplification of the lock ('English lock') that we are indebted to him. The lock Chapman designed was simply a slot in each blade and not nearly so secure as Smellie's lock.

Incidentally we would mention here that Smellie was the first to recommend forceps for the delivery of the after-coming head in breech extractions and it was largely because he found the straight forceps unsuitable that he invented a long double-curved forceps.[7]

With the addition of this new pelvic curve the instrument was obviously more suitable for extracting a fetal head arrested high in the pelvis, but it still suffered from one of the chief faults of the long straight forceps: namely that when applied to a high head much of the traction force (a third to a half) was expended by pulling the head against the pubes.

THE INTRODUCTION OF AXIS-TRACTION DEVICES

Etienne Stéphane Tarnier (1828–1897) will ever be honoured as the inventor of axis-traction forceps.[8] But long before Tarnier described his instrument in 1877 it had been fully appreciated that, even with the long double-curved forcep, traction in the axis of the pelvis was impossible and that a great deal of the force exerted by the operator was lost by the head being pulled against the anterior pelvic wall. Levret, Smellie and Baudelocque, for example, in order to obviate this, gave directions how traction was to be made as far back as possible. Charles Pajot (1816–1896) of Paris popularized the manoeuvre to assist this posteriorly directed traction (Fig 8.2). Although known as Pajot's manoeuvre it was first described by the Danish obstetrician Mathias Saxtorph (1740–1800).[9]

With the object of obtaining traction in the axis of the pelvis, many alterations and additions to the ordinary double-curved forceps were suggested in times past. One of the earliest – that of Saxtorph – was the use of bands through the fenestrae of the blades. A century later this suggestion reappeared in the recommendation of Poullet to pass cords through holes made immediately below the fenestrae of the blades; in more recent times Haig Ferguson once again recommended this primitive device.[10]

As far as can be ascertained, the suggestion of having special traction handles was made first by Hermann of Berne in 1844.[11] But the rods in Hermann's forceps were employed on the same principle as that by which Saxtorph and Pajot effected their manoeuvres. Hermann's device seems to have been forgotten, if, indeed, it ever became very generally known.

An important step in the evolution of the instrument was Hubert's traction

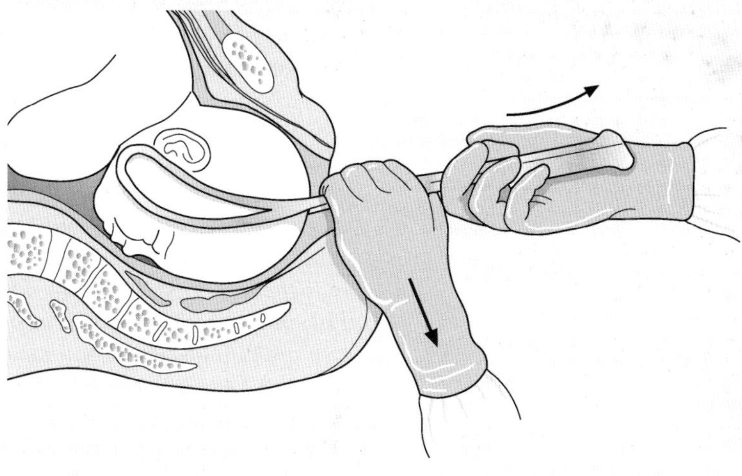

Figure 8.2 Pajot's manoeuvre.

bar, described in 1860, for by it traction could undoubtedly still be exerted in the axis of the pelvis. Still later, the ends of the handles were bent backwards in a wide perineal curve. Alternatively, a detachable traction handle incorporating a perineal curve was applied to either the upper or the lower ends of the handles – some patterns recently employed (Neville-Barnes, Haig Ferguson) have the latter arrangement. It is perfectly evident to everyone that, in employing the ordinary forceps with the head at the brim, a large amount of force is dissipated against the anterior pelvic wall: Tarnier estimated that nearly half the traction force was lost. With axis-traction forceps this is avoided in greater part. The mechanics of axis-traction forceps were very carefully considered by Tarnier[8] and by Milne Murray.[12] To those interested in this now historical subject we would commend the writings of those two authorities.

THE INTRODUCTION OF STRAIGHT FORCEPS FOR ROTATION OF THE FETAL HEAD

The Norwegian obstetrician, Christian Kielland (1871–1941), designed straight forceps without a pelvic curve to facilitate delivery from the mid-pelvis in cases of malrotation with occipito-transverse and occipito-posterior positions of the fetal head.[13] In fact, William Smellie had used the same principles of rotation almost two centuries before.[14] Kielland laid down very precise rules for the use of his forceps which could be more correctly applied than forceps with a pelvic curve to the incompletely rotated fetal head in the mid or upper pelvis.[15] In 1928, Lyman Barton (1866–1944), a rural general practitioner in New York State, developed straight forceps with a hinged anterior blade to facilitate application to the fetal head arrested in the transverse position at the pelvic brim.[16] *Arvind Moolgaoker later modified the Kielland forceps to incorporate a distance-spacing wedge between the handles to maintain the parallel positions of the forcep blades around the fetal head.*[17] *Kielland's forceps enjoyed considerable use in the middle part of the 20th century and continue to be applied in some hospitals for arrested occipito-posterior and occipito-transverse positions in the low–mid-pelvis.*

THE VACUUM EXTRACTOR

The history of the vacuum extractor is much shorter but its use is increasing, so that a majority of assisted vaginal deliveries are now performed using this instrument as opposed to the obstetric forceps. The vacuum principle was probably first applied in medicine with a cupping-glass to treat depressed skull fractures in infants and adults.[18] *The first attempted obstetrical application was in 1705 by James Yonge, surgeon to the Naval Hospital in Plymouth, England. He unsuccessfully attempted to deliver a fetus 'by a cupping-glass fixt to the scalp with an air pump'.*[19] *Neil Arnott (1788–1874), a Scot who received his education in Aberdeen and London, practiced medicine in London and outlined the principles of a pneumatic tractor.*[20] *There is no evidence that Arnott used his tractor for clinical purposes but he did propose its application in obstetrics: 'Now it seems peculiarly adapted to the purpose of obstetric surgery, viz, as a substitute for the steel forceps in the hands of men who are deficient in manual dexterity, whether from inexperience or natural inaptitude'.*[20]

Some 20 years later James Young Simpson of Edinburgh (1811–1870), acknowledging the work of Arnott, developed a practical suction-tractor[21] *(Fig 8.3). After his initial publications Simpson wrote no more on the subject and in the same year developed the obstetric forceps that bear his name and continue in use 150 years later.*

The next century saw a number of attempts to apply the vacuum principle to assist vaginal delivery, but none achieved clinical utility.[18] *Tage Malmström of Sweden (1911–1995) was the father of the modern extractor. His unique contribution was a metal cup with an in-curved rounded margin. Thus, the peripheral margin of the cup attached to the fetal scalp had a narrower diameter than the upper margin, thereby producing a 'chignon' and effectively increasing the total surface area of application and reducing the risk of cup detachment during traction. Malmström introduced his prototype in 1953 with refinements culminating in 1957.*[22,23] *Malmström's cup had the suction and traction portions attached by one port in*

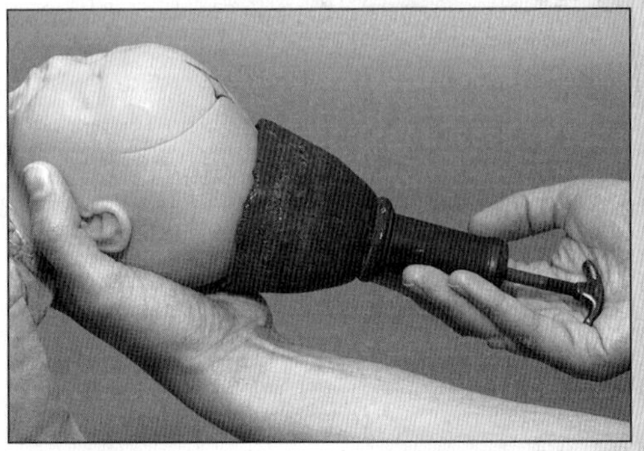

Figure 8.3 Simpson's air tractor. This early attempt to develop an instrument was hampered by an inability to produce sufficient negative pressure. The piston was of metal, the cup of wood and the rim was lined with leather which when wet allowed an air tight seal with the presenting part of the fetus. (Property of the Department of Obstetrics and Gynaecology, University of Edinburgh).

HISTORICAL BACKGROUND

the centre of the cup. The English obstetrician Geoffrey Bird (1922–2001), who worked in Kenya, Australia and Papua New Guinea, made the next significant contribution to development of the vacuum extractor. He separated the traction and suction ports and emphasized the importance of accurate cup placement over the flexion point of the fetal head to minimize the presenting diameter.[24] In order to facilitate placement of the cup over the flexion point in deflexed occipito-transverse and occipito-posterior positions Bird further modified the cup so that the suction port originated from the lateral margin. This so-called 'posterior cup' facilitated placement over the flexion point in the deflexed fetal head.[25]

In the 1970s, in an attempt to reduce scalp trauma attributed to the metal cups, vacuum cups were manufactured with soft material. These softer cups did reduce the superficial scalp trauma but were associated with a much higher failure rate of achieving delivery, up to 25%, compared to a failure rate of < 5% with the metal cups.[18] By the end of the 20th century, due to this high failure rate, vacuum cups were manufactured with harder plastic, and these continue in widespread use.[26]

General considerations

Assisted vaginal delivery of cephalic presentations involves the use of either forceps or vacuum to achieve delivery of the fetal head. These instruments allow the operator to apply extraction forces along the pelvic curve. In the case of the vacuum this is achieved by applying suction and traction to the fetal scalp, while the forceps cradle the parietal and malar bones of the fetal skull and, in addition to applying traction, laterally displace maternal tissue. The second stage of labour is one of the most dramatic occasions in a woman's life and the decision to intervene and use instrumental delivery of the fetal head is a significant one. From the obstetrician's point of view assisted vaginal delivery is the application of the art of obstetrics in stressful circumstances. The spectre of litigation looms and the level of expectation is high. In an increasing number of areas in obstetrics evidence-based data are available, but for assisted vaginal delivery this is very limited and the outcome depends more on the judgement, training and experience of the obstetrician.

The rates of assisted vaginal delivery vary from country to country and within countries from hospital to hospital. In broad terms the range varies between 5 and 25% and it is commonly about 10–12% of all deliveries.[27] Similarly, there are variations in obstetric practice worldwide which influence the choice of forceps and vacuum for assisted vaginal delivery. These variations depend on operator choice, clinical indications, local policies and, occasionally, maternal choice. However, the last 10–15 years have seen an almost universal increase in the frequency of use of vacuum extraction and a decline in the use of forceps assisted delivery.[28] There is no evidence to support improved safety of either instrument over the other. A Cochrane systematic review[29] showed that compared with forceps the vacuum extractor is:

- more likely to fail to achieve vaginal delivery
- more likely to be associated with cephalhaematoma and retinal haemorrhage
- more likely to be associated with maternal worries about the baby
- less likely to be associated with significant maternal perineal and vaginal trauma
- no more likely to be associated with low 5-minute Apgar scores or the need for phototherapy.

The vacuum extractor has been favoured by many because of the reduction in maternal pelvic floor injury compared with forceps delivery. Although this is the case in the short-term, a 5-year follow-up of women in one randomized controlled trial showed no difference in long-term maternal pelvic floor function between the two instruments.[30] A potential drawback to the use of the vacuum extractor is the higher rate of failed delivery compared with forceps. This then raises the dilemma of the sequential use of forceps following failed vacuum with potentially increased risk to mother and infant. We will not further debate in detail the comparative merits of the two instruments as the well-trained obstetrician should be adept with both and should select the one best suited to the woman's individual circumstances.

Utero-fetal-pelvic relationships

A number of these principles have been reviewed in Chapter 3 but the main elements will be emphasized here. The interaction between uterine work, descent of the fetal head and the pelvic architecture should be viewed as a dynamic relationship rather than a set of mathematical measurements. Factors to be assessed are: uterine work; maternal effort; fetal head, including: presentation, position, attitude (flexed/deflexed), synclitism, station, caput and moulding; and the bony pelvis.

Uterine work

Before considering operative vaginal delivery one should ensure that there has been adequate uterine action to provide maximum descent of the fetal head by propulsion before resorting to traction. This is particularly important in the nulliparous woman and in those with epidural analgesia. It is important to recognize that in normal spontaneous labour there is an increase in the endogenous production of oxytocin in the second stage. Thus, nature actively manages the second stage of labour with increased oxytocin production to augment uterine action and aid descent of the presenting part.[31] Epidural analgesia blocks Ferguson's reflex so that this normal endogenous surge of oxytocin in the second stage of labour does not occur.[32] This is particularly evident in the nulliparous woman in whom the addition of oxytocin in the second stage of labour will, to some extent, offset the increased need for operative vaginal delivery associated with epidural analgesia.[33] This is much less often required in the multiparous woman but, occasionally, and after careful appraisal to rule out cephalopelvic disproportion, oxytocin augmentation may be necessary for the multiparous woman with epidural analgesia in the second stage of labour.

Maternal effort

It is essential that the resource of maternal effort should be guided appropriately. During the second stage of labour the fetal head descends, flexes and rotates anteriorly. These cardinal movements are accomplished by effective uterine action and maternal expulsive efforts. From the aspect of maternal effort there are two phases to the second stage of labour. In the first, *passive phase*, uterine action causes descent of the fetal head to the pelvic floor. At this point maternal effort will be productive and should be added as the *active phase*. In the multiparous woman the passive phase may be very brief as the head often descends rapidly to the pelvic floor after full cervical dilatation. In the nulliparous woman, however, the fetal head is often only at the level of the ischial spines at full dilatation and time, aided by effective uterine action, is required to allow descent to the pelvic floor before enlisting maternal effort and entering the active phase of the second stage.

As with the first stage of labour the progressive nature of the second stage is more important than a fixed time limit. A working definition of arrest of progress in the second stage is no descent after 30 minutes in the multiparous woman and 60 minutes in the nulliparous woman. Protracted progress is < 2 cm/hour descent in multipara and < 1 cm in nullipara. Protracted progress in the second stage of labour is much more common in the nulliparous woman than in multipara. In the nulliparous woman it is reasonable to encourage no maternal effort for 1 hour after full cervical dilatation. In about half of nulliparous women the descent of the fetal head will be quite rapid during this time and descent to the pelvic floor will be obvious – productive maternal effort can then be encouraged. In the remaining half, however, progress is protracted and after 1 hour oxytocin augmentation should be started. This can be administered for another hour, after which maternal effort is encouraged as the oxytocin augmentation is continued. The virtue of this approach is that it reduces the likelihood of exhausting the mother in achieving fetal descent through the mid-pelvis, which is more appropriately accomplished by uterine contractions. Although individual women's stamina varies considerably, 1 hour of full maternal effort is usually the most productive. Thus, with the above guiding principles, by 3 hours of the second stage one should be in a position to decide whether vaginal delivery is imminent with continued maternal effort, or whether assisted vaginal delivery may be necessary. If there is continued arrest of descent in the mid-pelvis then caesarean section may be more appropriate (Fig 8.4).

Fetal head

There are a number of characteristics of the fetal head that can be assessed to evaluate its accommodation by the bony pelvis and pelvic floor.

Position

The position may be occipito-anterior, occipito-transverse or occipito-posterior. Usually the head descends to the mid-pelvis in the transverse position. The normal progression is for the head to rotate anteriorly as it descends to the pelvic floor. Such rotation is favoured by the available space and the tone of the pelvic floor musculature, a benefit which may be lost with regional anaesthesia. If the pelvic floor muscle tone is not maintained the forward and medial sloping nature of the pelvic floor is lost, favouring deflexion and malrotation of the fetal head. Posterior rotation is less advantageous as it presents a larger diameter to the pelvis.

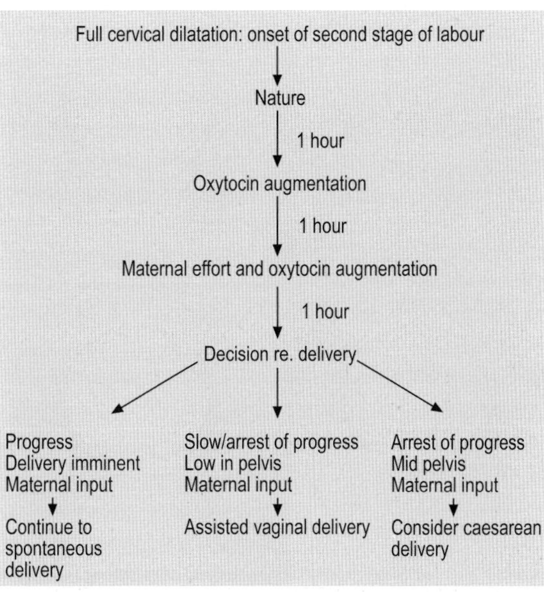

Figure 8.4 Guideline for arrest/protraction of second stage of labour in nullipara.

Attitude

The attitude of the fetal head may be flexed (smaller diameter) or deflexed (larger diameter).

Synclitism

Synclitism is the parallel relationship between the planes of the fetal head and of the pelvis. This is assessed by feeling the sagittal suture of the fetal head and its relationship to the transverse plane of the pelvic cavity. Anterior asynclitism, which is normal, occurs when the anterior parietal bone is felt more easily because the sagittal suture is further back in the transverse plane of the pelvis. In posterior asynclitism, a sign of cephalopelvic disproportion, the posterior parietal bone occupies more of the transverse plane and the sagittal suture is more anterior (Fig 8.5).

Station

The station of the fetal head is the relationship of the foremost bony part of the fetal head to the ischial spines. When this is at the level of the ischial spines the station is zero, levels above and below the ischial spines are designated −1 cm to −5 cm and +1 cm to +5 cm respectively.

Caput succedaneum

Caput succedaneum is the oedematous swelling formed on the presenting portion of the fetal scalp during labour. This is a serous effusion which overlies the aponeurosis. The assessment of caput is rather subjective but is expressed as none, +, ++, or +++. One+ or two+ is quite compatible with normal spontaneous delivery. Three+ may also be compatible with normal or easy assisted vaginal delivery, but in general is more indicative of a tighter fit between the fetal head and the pelvis.

Moulding

Moulding is the change in shape of the fetal head as it adapts to the pelvic canal. This is associated with compression of the bones of the skull and the relationship of the edges of these bones to each other is how moulding is classified. Depending on accessibility to the examining finger, this is usually assessed by the relationship of the two parietal bones at the sagittal suture or the occipital and parietal bones in the area of the posterior fontanelle. In this regard the parietal bones always override the occipital bone. This point is a guide to identification of the posterior fontanelle.

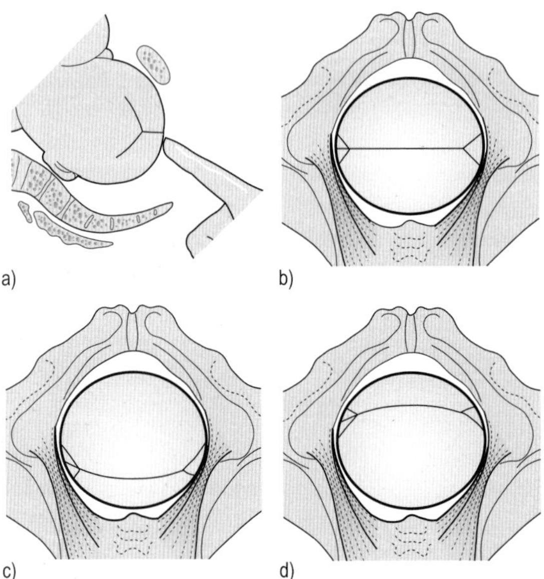

Figure 8.5 Synclitism and asynclitism. (a) Detection of asynclitism, estimating how far from the symphysis the sagittal suture lies. (b) LOT normal synclitism, both parietal bones present equally. (c) LOT anterior asynclitism, anterior parietal presentation. (d) LOT posterior asynclitism, posterior parietal presentation.

The classification of moulding is as follows: none = bones normally separated; + = bones touching; ++ = bones overlapping but easily separated with digital pressure; +++ = bones overlapping and not separable with digital pressure (Fig 8.6). The + and ++ degrees of moulding are compatible with normal vaginal delivery. Three+, however, is more likely to denote relative cephalopelvic disproportion, particularly if it exists at both the sagittal suture and the posterior fontanelle.

Bony pelvis

X-ray pelvimetry has a limited, if any, role in modern labour management. Ultrasound has been used as an aid to documenting the position and station of the fetal head and the extent of overlap of the fetal cranial bones.[34] This application of ultrasound has not found widespread clinical application on the labour floor.

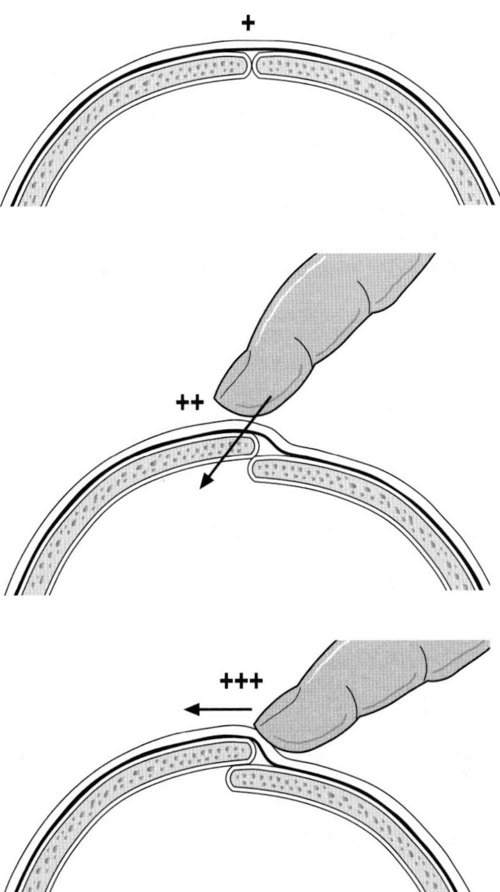

Figure 8.6 Degrees of moulding. + Parietal bones together but not overlapped. ++ Parietal bones overlap but reduced by digital pressure. +++ Parietal bones overlap but not reducible by digital pressure.

Description of the pelvic diagonal conjugate

'With the tip of my finger I could hardly reach the jutting forward of the last vertebra of the loins and upper part of the sacrum; from which circumstances I understood the pelvis at that part was not above half or three-quarters of an inch narrower than those that are well formed.'

William Smellie
A Treatise on the Theory and Practice of Midwifery. London: D. Wilson, 1752

Clinical pelvimetry has limitations but is still a worthwhile endeavour. If one carries this out in every patient managed during labour a useful bank of clinical experience will be obtained. By measurement of your own fingers and fist you should be able to assess the following points:

- diagonal conjugate – at least 12 cm (Fig 8.7)
- curve of the sacrum – should be curved and the lower end should not be inclined anteriorly

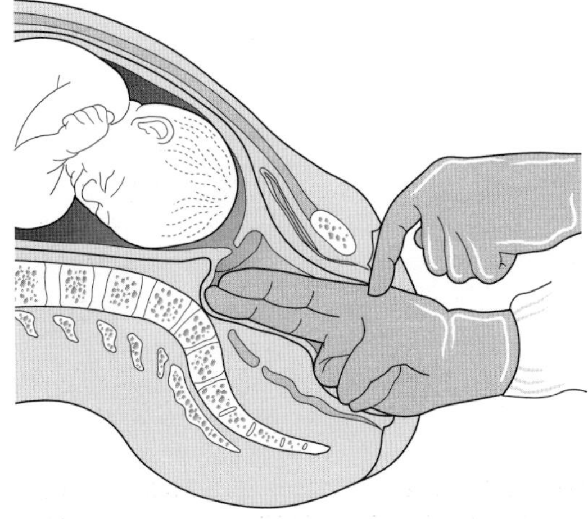

Figure 8.7 Measurement of the diagonal conjugate.

- pelvic sidewalls – should be parallel and not converge
- ischial spines – blunt and not prominent
- sacrospinous ligaments – should accept two finger-breadths (> 4 cm)
- subpubic arch – not narrowed, should accommodate two fingers
- inter-tuberous diameter – should hold the closed fist (at least 10 cm).

Assessment for assisted vaginal delivery

In assessing suitability for assisted vaginal delivery, it is essential that a combined abdominal and vaginal examination be performed to accurately establish the level of descent of the fetal head. In this context vaginal examination can be misleading because of the difficulty in assessing the contribution of caput and moulding to the true level of descent (Fig 8.8). It is here that careful abdominal palpation following the principles laid down by Crichton are most helpful.[35] He proposed a clinical estimation of descent of the fetal head in fifths, as palpable above the pelvic brim (Fig 8.9). The occiput and sinciput should be carefully palpated. In general, if only the sinciput is palpable the head is one-fifth above the pelvic brim and this corresponds to the lowest part of the fetal bony skull being at the level of the ischial spines. With vaginal examination alone and a moderate or major degree of moulding the bony part of the fetal skull may appear to be much lower. If none of the fetal head can be palpated above the pelvic brim then it has descended to at least spines +1 to +2 cm. In modern obstetrics it is rarely indicated to assist vaginal delivery at a level higher than this. Thus, abdominal palpation is in many ways the critical and decisive component of the combined abdominal–vaginal assessment. As Chassar Moir (1964) noted in a previous edition of this book:

> *'It is a good working rule never to apply the forceps if the sinciput can still be felt per abdomen. This should be remembered when examining the patient that has been long in labour, for the extreme moulding of the head and the considerable size of the caput succedenaum may give a false impression to the examining vaginal fingers to the degree of descent already achieved.'*

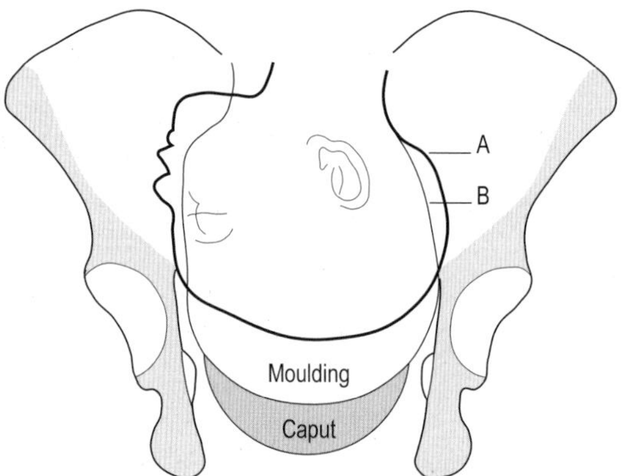

Figure 8.8 Caput and moulding may give a false sense of fetal descent. (a) Fetal head before descent without caput and moulding. (b) Fetal head after descent with caput and moulding.

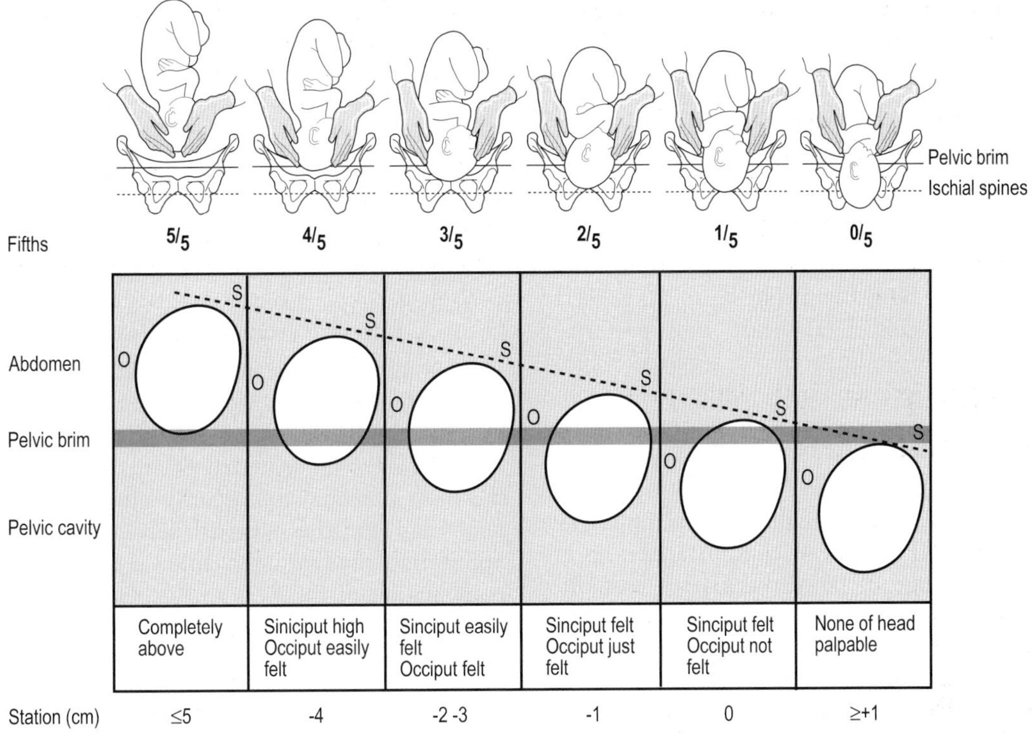

Figure 8.9 Clinical estimation of the fetal head in fifths palpable above the pelvic brim, and the relationship to station.

In addition to accurately determining the level of descent of the fetal head, the position and attitude of the fetal head are very important. These can be ascertained by identifying the sagittal suture and the anterior and posterior fontanelles. In this context the occipital and frontal bones always ride under the parietal bones with moulding. By identifying the posterior fontanelle of the fetal head the position (OA, OT, OP) can be readily identified. If the posterior fontanelle is easily palpable the head must be well flexed which presents the smallest diameter to the pelvis.

If, however, the posterior fontanelle cannot be felt, move in the opposite direction along the sagittal suture to see if the anterior fontanelle is palpable. Normally, with a well-flexed fetal head the anterior fontanelle is difficult to feel as it is much deeper in the pelvis towards the sinciput. If it is easily palpable the head is usually considerably deflexed which presents a larger diameter to the pelvis. If, due to caput, there is difficulty in identifying the sutures one should feel anteriorly for the fetal ear. Feel for the pinna and canal, as the ear can be folded forward to give a false impression of the true position. The ear as a landmark can be useful in assessing the level of the head as it is just below the maximum biparietal diameter. Thus, if it is easily felt during maternal bearing-down effort, there is unlikely to be significant disproportion.[36] The acquisition of these clinical skills requires the proverbial 'long apprenticeship at the bedside of women in labour'.

Indications for operative vaginal delivery

Most indications for assisted vaginal delivery are relative and fall into three categories: maternal, fetal and non-progressive labour/dystocia.[37,38]

Maternal

The mother's medical condition may limit the desirability or ability for maternal effort, e.g.

cerebrovascular disease, severe pre-eclampsia/ eclampsia, cardiac disease. Maternal fatigue and exhaustion may lead to unproductive, non-progressive and demoralizing effort. This may culminate in maternal request for assisted vaginal delivery.

Fetal

Presumed fetal compromise as manifest by non-reassuring fetal heart rate pattern is a common indication for assisted vaginal delivery. Here again, the indication is often relative and dependent upon the interpretation of the fetal heart rate abnormality, the presence or absence of meconium, and the availability of fetal scalp blood sampling (see Chapter 4). In these circumstances, in the second stage of labour, the fetus can often be delivered more rapidly by assisted vaginal delivery than by caesarean section. However, it is essential to be sure that assistance with either forceps or vacuum is straightforward as the combination of hypoxia and trauma is potentially damaging to the fetal brain.

Non-progressive labour/dystocia

In a prolonged, non-progressive second stage of labour the indication to assist delivery is usually based on a combination of maternal and fetal reasons. The mother may be exhausted and demoralized that her efforts are not productive. Prolonged second stage of labour may damage the maternal pelvic floor.[39] The fetal contribution to a non-progressive second stage of labour may be due to macrosomia or an unfavourable position and attitude of the fetal head presenting a wider diameter to the pelvis. Most commonly this occurs with a deflexed occipito-transverse or occipito-posterior position of the fetal head, with the larger diameter resulting in relative cephalopelvic disproportion. Skillfully performed, assisted vaginal delivery can correct the unfavourable position and flex the fetal head allowing safe and easy vaginal delivery. A prolonged, non-progressive second stage of labour may cause the potentially lethal combination of trauma and hypoxia to the brain, noted above. The following guidelines have been suggested for time limits in the second stage of labour, at which point consideration should be given to assisted delivery:[40]

- nullipara: 2 hours without regional anaesthesia and 3 hours with regional anaesthesia
- multipara: 1 hour without regional anaesthesia and 2 hours with regional anaesthesia.

Although these are reasonable guidelines it is emphasized that no rigid time limits should be applied. Of relevance is the duration of the active phase with maternal effort, as this has the most potential for negative effects on the fetal head and the maternal pelvic floor. The appropriate time for intervention is based upon combination of the fetal and maternal factors noted above, a careful appraisal of the feto-pelvic relationships, and the mother's wishes.

Classification of assisted vaginal delivery

The American College of Obstetricians and Gynecologists has been the organization that has most consistently defined the types of operative vaginal delivery.[40] Other speciality organizations have adopted this classification[37,38] (Table 8.1).

Prerequisites for assisted vaginal delivery

Indication and assessment

The indication should be clearly established and documented. The essentials of the feto-pelvic relationship should be confirmed and these include, full cervical dilatation and membranes ruptured; vertex presentation; the exact position and attitude of the head should be known; the head should be ≤ one-fifth palpable per abdomen and the pelvis should be deemed adequate. As mentioned previously, it should be rare that operative vaginal delivery

Table 8.1 Types of operative vaginal delivery[40]

Mid	Fetal head is ≤ one-fifth palpable per abdomen Leading point of the skull is above station + 2 cm (0 ⇒ +1 cm) but not above the ischial spines Two subdivisions: (a) rotation ≤ 45° (b) rotation >45°
Low	Leading point of the skull (not caput) is at station ≥ + 2 cm and not on the pelvic floor Two subdivisions: (a) rotation of ≤ 45° (b) rotation > 45°
Outlet	Fetal scalp visible without separating the labia Fetal skull has reached the pelvic floor Sagittal suture is in the antero-posterior diameter, or right or left occiput anterior, or occiput posterior position (rotation ≤ 45°) Fetal head is at or on the perineum

is undertaken with the head even one-fifth palpable above the pelvic brim. The bladder should be emptied by straight catheterization and if an indwelling catheter is in place, the bulb should be deflated and the catheter removed just before the procedure to reduce the risk of urethral or bladder damage.

Informed consent

Genuinely informed consent can be difficult to obtain in the stressful environment surrounding the second stage of labour. However, the options generally include waiting, assisted vaginal delivery or caesarean section – and these should be discussed with the woman and her partner. In some circumstances the course of action is quite clear, e.g. acute fetal bradycardia with the head at the pelvic outlet requiring only easy assistance with forceps or vacuum. On other occasions the head may be arrested in the low–mid-pelvis and a more detailed outline of the options and answers to the woman's questions is more appropriate.

Analgesia

If the assistance required is in the low or outlet portion of the pelvis, infiltration of the perineum with local anaesthetic may be all that is required. Alternatively, pudendal block is effective for most low assisted deliveries. In general, more analgesia is required for forceps than for vacuum assisted deliveries. If the fetal head is in the low–mid-pelvis, and particularly if rotation is required, then epidural or spinal anaesthesia is optimum.

Training

The potential for maternal and fetal trauma with assisted vaginal delivery performed by inexperienced operators is considerable. Obstetricians in training should have adequate supervised experience with spontaneous vaginal delivery and low and outlet assisted vacuum and forceps delivery. The judgement and technical skills required for assisted vaginal delivery in the low–mid pelvis, particularly with rotation, is considerable and more senior obstetrical staff with experience should directly supervise juniors in the acquisition of these skills.[41] This is an area of obstetrics fraught with risks of poor clinical outcome and litigation. The two go hand-in-hand and it is not acceptable for inadequately trained staff to be unsupervised in the performance of these procedures.

Trial of assisted vaginal delivery

To the experienced obstetrician it is usually clear that the head is in the low or outlet pelvis and that assisted vaginal delivery can be accomplished with ease in the delivery room. However, in cases where the fetal head is arrested in the low-mid pelvis, particularly at spines +1 cm to + 2 cm, the potential for difficulty is greater and it is usually prudent to declare a trial of forceps or trial of vacuum. This is a long-established principle in obstetrics, well articulated on both sides of the Atlantic ocean, and remains relevant.[15,42,43]

It entails moving the woman to the operating theatre so that either an assisted vaginal delivery or caesarean section can be undertaken. This is explained to the woman and her partner, as well as to the anaesthetist and nursing staff, and they are told that if the forceps or vacuum delivery proceeds smoothly then vaginal delivery will be accomplished with safety. However, if there are any difficulties then the attempt at vaginal delivery will not be sustained and the obstetrician can immediately back off and proceed to caesarean section. In this way any pressure on the obstetrician to persist with attempted vaginal delivery when difficulty is encountered is removed. In most instances vaginal delivery is achieved with ease and safety, but on other occasions difficulty is encountered and caesarean section can be promptly undertaken with minimal risk of damage to mother or fetus. This was nicely summarized by Chassar Moir (1964) in a previous edition of this book:

> *'Although seemingly simple, the conception of trial forceps is a most important advance in policy, and is the logical outcome of the increased safety of the modern caesarean operation … I have on several occasions deliberately pursued this policy and believe that by so doing I have acted in the best interest of both the mother and child, avoiding an unnecessary caesarean section in some cases, and a mutilating vaginal delivery in others'.*

and by Ian Donald in his emphasis of the difference between a failed forceps delivery, undertaken without preparations for immediate caesarean section if necessary, and a failed trial of forceps:

> *'Trial of forceps, advisedly undertaken, however comes into a completely different class. Here, one recognizes all the difficulties in advance and has made due preparations for them … The decision to abandon forceps and to proceed to caesarean section must not be regarded as a matter of "failed forceps" but as an enlightened step in recognition of the hazards, particularly to the baby of persisting with vaginal delivery.'*
>
> Practical obstetric problems. 5th ed. London: Lloyd-Luke, 1979, p654

Forceps assisted delivery

The ambivalent attitude of the medical profession towards obstetrics forceps is exemplified by the different viewpoints expressed by two of the great obstetricians of the 18th century, Edmund Chapman and William Hunter:

> *'I can, from my own experience, affirm it to be a most excellent instrument, and so far from hurting or destroying, that it frequently saves the mother's life, and that of the child … All I can say in praise of this noble instrument, must necessarily fall short of what it justly demands'.*
>
> Edmund Chapman. A Treatise on the Improvement of Midwifery. Chiefly with Regard to the Operation. 2nd ed. London: Brindley Clarke and Corbett, 1735.

> *'To a poor woman that is quite exhausted, forceps may be of considerable service – but I wish to God they had never been contrived …*

I am convinced the forceps has killed three, I may say ten women to one that it has saved, and therefore we should never use it on any occasion but where it is absolutely necessary.'

William Hunter, c1760

Almost three centuries later medical and lay opinion remains divided about the role of forceps in modern obstetric practice, although not quite to the extreme views expressed above. Nevertheless, if assisted vaginal delivery was to be abandoned the some 5–25% of women currently delivered by this method would only have two options: either delivery by caesarean section or a return to days before forceps when some women would labour for many hours and even days in the second stage of labour, with disastrous consequences for them and their infant.

The construction and anatomy of the forceps is shown in Figure 8.10. Over three centuries more than 700 types of forceps have been invented and new ones continue to be produced. In clinical terms there are the classical forceps exemplified by Simpson's and similar types such as Neville–Barnes, Haig Ferguson and Tucker–MacLean, which has solid blades. The two right and left branches are composed of blades, shanks and handles. The cephalic curve of the blade relates to the fetal head and the pelvic curve to the maternal pelvis. The blades are usually locked at the junction of the shanks and handles. Forceps designed for rotation, most commonly Kielland's forceps, have a cephalic curve but minimal pelvic curve of the blades. This allows rotation within the pelvis and helps avoid trauma to the maternal soft tissues by narrowing the rotational arc of the toes of the blades. When using rotation forceps it is common to

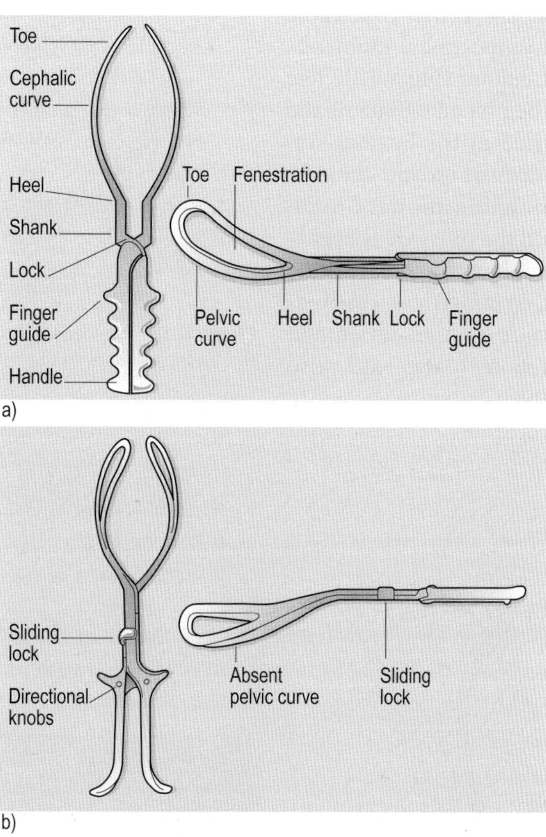

Figure 8.10 Anatomy of the forceps. (a) Simpson's classical forceps. (b) Kielland's rotation forceps.

encounter asynclitICism so these forceps have a sliding lock which allows for its correction. Individual obstetricians have their favourite make of forceps, usually depending on their training and familiarity. In clinical terms one needs to be familiar with a pair of classical forceps such as Simpson's, and a rotational forceps, such as Kielland's. Those interested in details of the various types of forceps available should consult the bibliography at the end of this chapter.

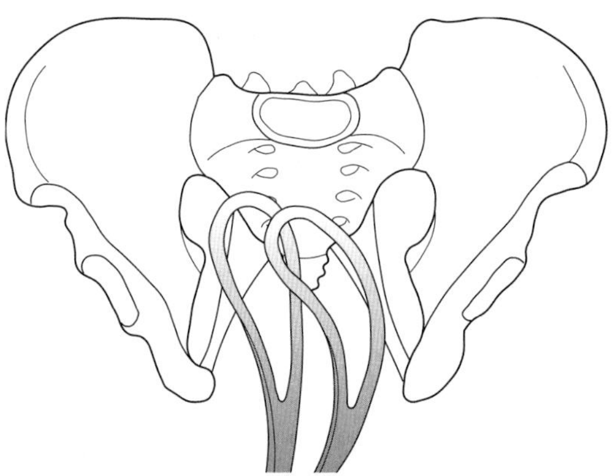

Figure 8.12 The range of safe movement of the forceps blades relative to the pelvis.

Classical forceps

Once the indications for assisted forceps delivery has been established and the prerequisites mentioned have been fulfilled the woman is placed in the lithotomy position with appropriate leg supports. The blades of classical forceps are so constructed that they are in perfect position transversely in the pelvis (Fig 8.11) with a safe range of movement of approximately 45° on either side from the transverse: these limits are between the iliopectineal eminence and the sacroiliac joint behind (Fig 8.12). The forceps blades should be placed as a cephalic application along the side of the head covering the space between the orbits and the ears (Fig 8.13). This cephalic application is biparietal and bimalar. As such the pressure is evenly distributed to the least vulnerable areas. If the cephalic application is asymmetrical – such as a brow-mastoid application – the subsequent compression and traction forces are also

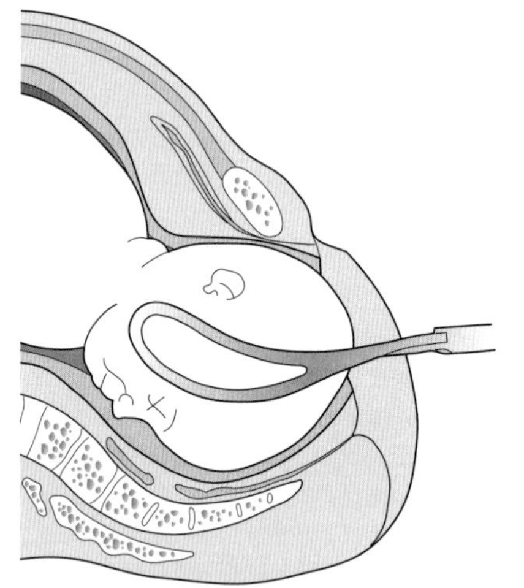

Figure 8.13 The ideal biparietal bimalar application of the forceps blades to the fetal head.

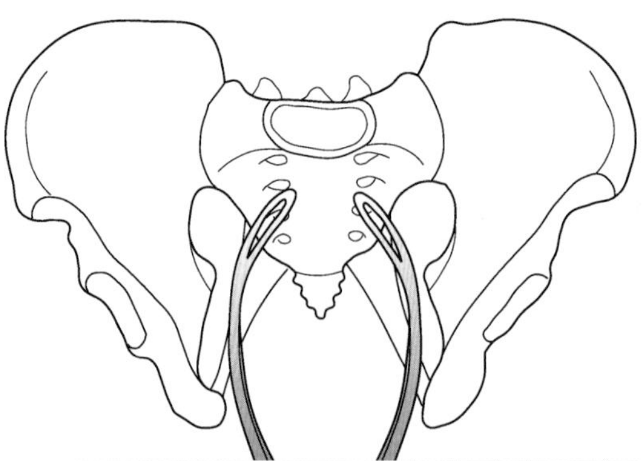

Figure 8.11 The ideal position of the forceps blades relative to the maternal pelvis.

'Branche gauche à la main gauche, à gauche la première: tout doit être gauche, sauf l'accoucheur ...'

'Left blade in the left hand, to the left at first; all is gauche, except the skill of the obstetrician ...'

Charles Pajot
Travaux d'obstetrique et de Gynécologue Précédés d'Elements de practique Obstetricale. Paris: H. Lauwereyns, 1882

asymmetrically applied to the underlying falx cerebri and tentorium, risking intracranial haemorrhage.

Once the precise position of the fetal head has been ascertained – either direct occipito-anterior (OA) or left or right occipito-anterior (LOA, ROA) – the forceps are placed together and lined up as a ghost or phantom application holding the forceps in front of the perineum in the same orientation as they will be applied to the fetal head. The left blade is held in the left hand and inserted to the left side of the pelvis just in front of the left ear of the fetus. In doing this the fingers of the right hand are placed just inside the vagina and the thumb of the right hand against the heel of the blade. The left hand holding the handle is then rotated down in an arc while the fingers and thumb of the right hand guide the blade into correct position (Fig 8.14a). Changing hands the same procedure is used to insert the right blade (Fig 8.14b). Most forceps have the 'English lock' in which the right handle fits into the lock on the left shank. Thus, there is

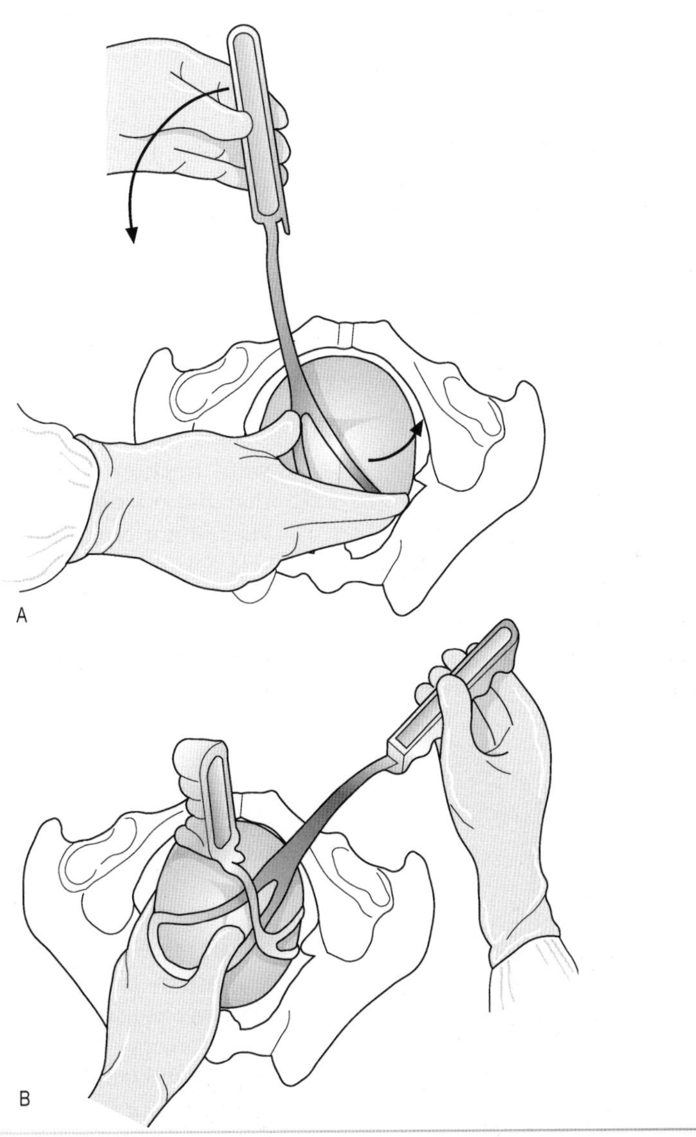

Figure 8.14 (a) Insertion of left blade. The fingers and thumb of the right hand guide the blade into correct position while the left hand rotates the handle in a downward arc. (b) The same procedure is carried out for insertion of the right blade using the opposite hands.

no need to manipulate one handle above the other as they just lock in naturally. The above description is for the direct OA position. For LOA and ROA positions the procedure is the same, taking care to line up the blades and their application to the oblique orientation of the fetal head. No force should be required to apply or lock the blades of the forceps. Unless they can be applied and locked easily one should stop and recheck the position of the fetal head. One of the more common reasons for difficulty is an unsuspected occipito-posterior position.

Once the handles have locked satisfactorily check that the application is correct by the following:

- The posterior fontanelle should be located midway between the sides of the blades with the lambdoidal suture lines equidistant from the forcep blades.
- The posterior fontanelle should be one finger-breadth above the plane of the shanks. If the fontanelle is more than one finger-breadth above this plane, traction will tend to deflex the head, presenting a larger diameter to the pelvis.

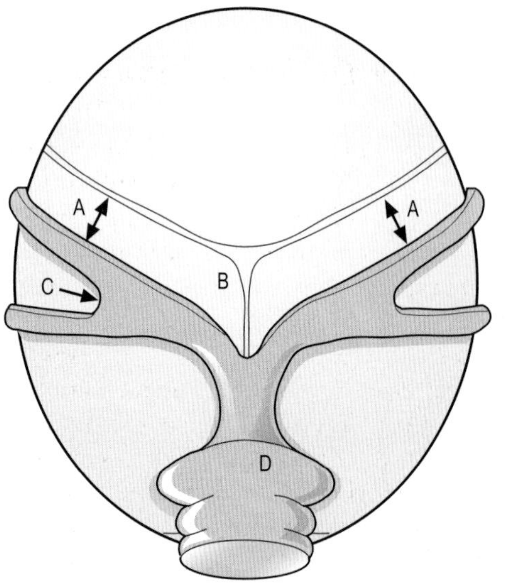

Figure 8.15 Checks for correct position of forceps relative to the head. (A) Blades equidistant from lambdoidal sutures. (B) Posterior fontanelle one finger-breadth above plane of shanks. (C) At most one finger-breadth between fenestra and head. (D) Shanks perpendicular to sagittal suture.

- The sagittal suture should be perpendicular to the plane of the shanks throughout their length. If the shanks run obliquely to the sagittal suture the application is asymmetrical – towards a brow–mastoid orientation.
- The amount of palpable fenestration of each of the blades should be equal on each side. In fact, there should be barely any fenestration felt and at most one finger should be able to be inserted between it and the head (Fig 8.15).

Unless all the above checks are fulfilled the forceps will need to be manipulated or reapplied.

The compression forces of the forceps are the least desirable aspect. These can be kept to a minimum if the operator grasps and applies traction via the finger guards which are placed close to the lock so that the least compression force is applied, as opposed to squeezing the handles at their end. This is best achieved using an underhand grip with the index and middle fingers on the finger guards while the other hand is placed on the shanks of the forceps to help apply downward traction (Pajot's manoeuvre) to ensure that the traction is in the curve of the pelvis and not dissipated against the pubic arch (Fig 8.16).

Traction is applied during a uterine contraction and, aided by maternal effort, should be carefully directed along the pelvic curve – the curve of Carus. During traction the obstetrician can be seated or standing and the arms should be flexed at the elbows. It is difficult to teach how much traction is appropriate – obviously the least required is the best. A recent study using an isometric strength testing unit shows that junior obstetricians can be trained to reproduce and not exceed the 'ideal' traction forces of 30–45 lb.[44] Muscular obstetricians, of both sexes, are capable of applying considerable and undesirable force with forceps. The guiding principle is that mild to moderate traction, which admittedly is in the eye of the beholder, should cause progressive descent when co-ordinated with each uterine contraction. Generally it is clear whether there is descent of the fetal head or

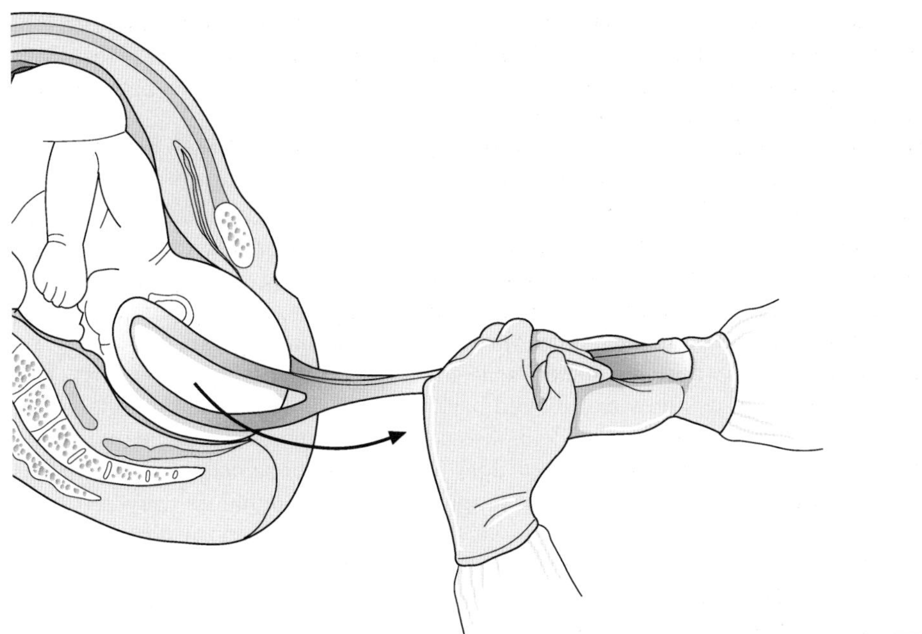

Figure 8.16 Appropriate grip for traction which should be directed along the pelvic curve.

not with the first pull. There is an unyielding feel to obstructed cases that dictates that the trial of forceps should be abandoned. Strong traction should not be applied or necessary for safe assisted vaginal delivery.

As the head descends to the perineum and the occiput passes under the symphysis the direction of traction is gradually changed forwards and upwards to end up about 45° above the horizontal. As the head extends over the perineum the handles are elevated to about 75° above the horizontal, and one hand is removed from the forceps to guard the perineum or perform episiotomy if necessary. Once the head is almost delivered the forceps blades can be removed by reversing the manoeuvres used for their insertion. Usually the right blade is removed first. If too much force is required to remove the blades then the head can be gently eased out with the blades in position.

When the head is LOA or ROA, after the blades have been appropriately placed and checked, rotation through the 45° towards the midline should be performed in a gradual and gentle manner without traction. This is carried out by slightly elevating the handles and rotating slowly through an arc, allowing the maternal tissues and fetal head to adapt to the changing position. Once the rotation is completed the position of the blades should be checked again to make sure that they have not slipped during rotation.

Occipito-posterior delivery

If the fetal head has descended and arrested low in the pelvis ***(spines ≥ +3 cm)*** with the head in the direct occipito-posterior position, or a few degrees to either side of direct OP, it may be best to assist delivery in this position, 'face-to-pubes', rather than attempt rotation. In most of these cases it seems that the fetal head fits the pelvis best in the direct OP position. This is more likely in the anthropoid type of pelvis with a longer anteroposterior diameter compared with the transverse dimensions. In these cases the head descends low in the pelvis and, if the pelvis is large and the fetus small, delivery will be spontaneous in the face-to-pubes position. In those cases in which arrest occurs low in the pelvis it may be necessary to assist the delivery with forceps, although this entails a greater risk of perineal trauma compared with the OA position.

The technique for insertion and application of the forceps is the same as for the OA position, but the pelvic curve of the blades is reversed in its relationship to the sides of the fetal head. The toes of the blades, rather than facing towards the ears as in the OA application, curve toward the mouth (Fig 8.17). In checking the application of the forceps to the landmarks of the skull, the shanks should be parallel to the sagittal suture but the posterior fontanelle will be one finger-breadth below, rather than above the shanks as in the OA check. Traction is downwards and backwards initially but the occiput will distend the perineum more than the sinciput does in the OA position. Thus, a mediolateral episiotomy is usually required. As the occiput distends the perineum, traction is progressively directed upwards to flex the occiput over the perineum. Excessive downward traction in the initial phase will tend to deflex the fetal head and increase the diameter presenting to the perineum.

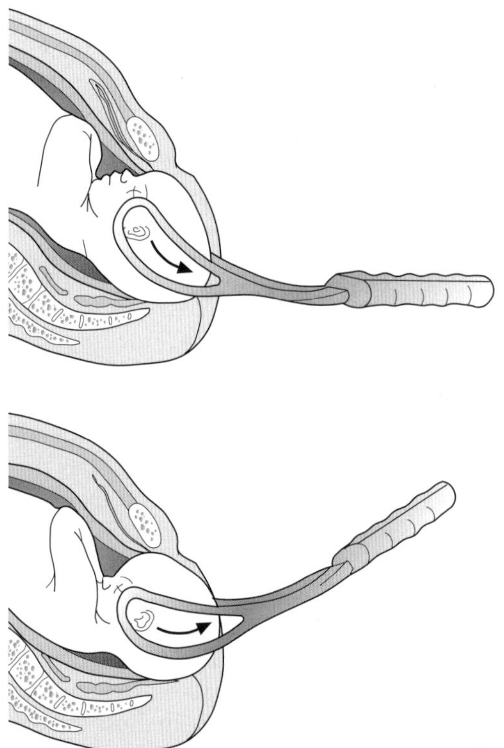

Figure 8.17 Relationship of forceps blades to the fetal head in occipito-posterior position.

Delivery with rotation

Assisted vaginal delivery involving rotation of occipito-transverse and occipito-posterior positions of the fetal head requires some of the finest clinical judgment in obstetrics. For it is in these situations that the risk of maternal trauma and, particularly, fetal trauma is highest. The reader is referred again to the earlier parts of this chapter and the prerequisites for assisted vaginal delivery. For any assisted vaginal delivery involving rotation it is sensible to encapsulate these considerations by asking oneself the question 'why am I not doing a caesarean section?'. Having said that, in many instances of malrotation of the fetal head, deflexion is involved, presenting a larger diameter of the fetal head to the pelvis. If rotation and flexion of the fetal head can be safely and successfully achieved the diameter of the fetal head is reduced, and often light traction is all that is required to effect delivery. In contrast, the arrested fetal head in the occipito-anterior position already has the narrowest diameter presenting so that more traction may be required to effect delivery.

In addition to the risks of intracranial trauma, rotation procedures carry the extremely rare but potentially catastrophic risk of cervical spinal cord trauma – at its worst producing quadriplegia. This risk is probably due to a combination of reasons. Usually there has been a prolonged labour, the amniotic fluid has drained, and the uterus 'hugs' the fetus. Under these circumstances, if the fetal head is rotated the shoulders (which are grasped by the uterus) may not rotate, making the cervical spine vulnerable. If, in addition, there is a degree of fetal hypotonia associated with hypoxia there may be no protection of the cervical spinal column from the hypotonic fetal neck and shoulder muscles. Thus, rotation procedures should be avoided in the presence of fetal hypoxia. It is also logical that any rotational manoeuvre of the fetal head should be accompanied by concomitant rotation of the fetal shoulders.

Digital rotation

In some cases of left and right occipito-transverse positions (LOT, ROT) it is possible to rotate the occiput anterior with digital pressure alone. This will allow the use of the classical occipito-anterior forceps to aid delivery. For the LOT position, the tips of the index and middle fingers of the right hand are placed against the elevated edge of the anterior parietal bone along the lamboidal suture and close to where it joins the posterior fontanelle (Fig 8.18). Using counterclockwise and downward pressure during a uterine contraction, with or without maternal bearing-down effort, the head can often be rotated to LOA or even direct OA. This obviates the need to use rotational forceps. Once the head has been rotated the fingers of the right hand remain against the left parietal bone to counteract any tendency for the occiput to rotate back to LOT. With the head thus held in the OA position the right blade of the forceps can be applied. The fingers can then be withdrawn and while the right blade steadies the position of the head in the OA position the left blade can be applied. For ROT positions the left hand is used and the manoeuvres are carried out in the opposite direction.

Manual rotation

If digital rotation is unsuccessful the manual technique can be used. However, if the head is deeply impacted in the pelvis it may be difficult to get a good enough grasp of the head to achieve manual rotation. The hand is inserted into the vagina fully supinated – the left hand for ROP and the right hand for LOP positions. The head is grasped with the fingers high and widespread on one side of the head, and the thumb high on the other; the occipital region should now be well in the palm of the hand. The head is elevated only enough to allow flexion and rotation such that the sinciput comes round to the position previously occupied by the occiput (Fig 8.19). Thus, one tends to overcorrect the rotation. Simultaneously with this rotation the other hand is placed on the maternal abdomen behind the shoulder pulling it toward the midline. In some cases, if the vaginal hand can reach high enough to the posterior shoulder this is also dislodged from one side of the sacral promontory to the other, again while the external hand on the maternal abdomen puts concomitant rotational pressure on the anterior shoulder. This is sometimes known as Pomeroy's manoeuvre (Fig 8.20).[45]

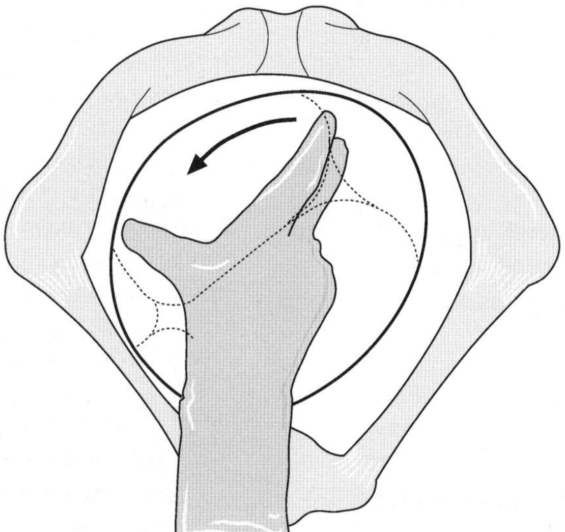

Figure 8.18 Digital rotation.

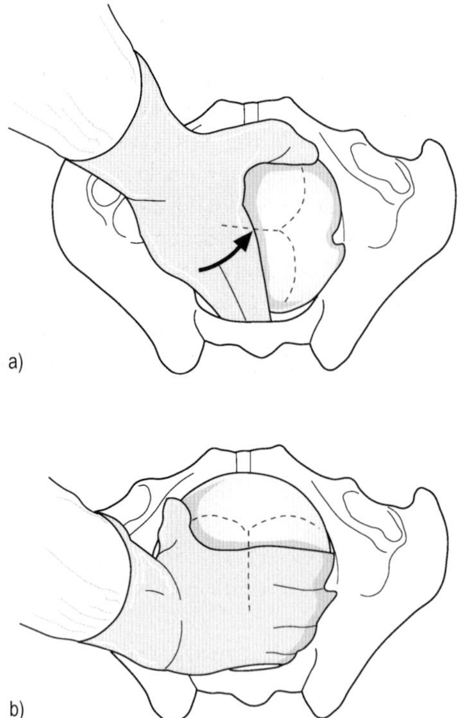

Figure 8.19 Manual rotation. (a) LOT head grasped with right hand. (b) LOT rotated to OA.

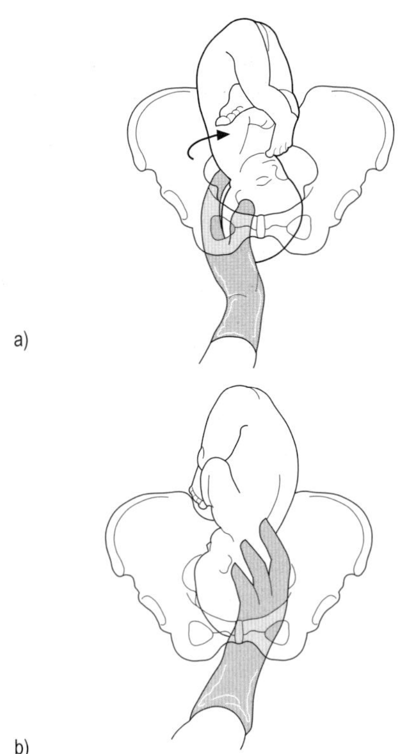

Figure 8.20 Manual head and shoulder rotation: Pomeroy's manoeuvre. (a) ROP left hand grasps head with fingers behind the anterior shoulder. (b) Head and shoulders rotated from ROP to LOA.

In some cases, provided the head remains occipito-anterior after the rotation, oxytocin augmentation may help bring the head down to spontaneous delivery. In most instances, however, forceps delivery from the OA position will be required following the manual rotation.

Regional anaesthesia and an adequately relaxed uterus are necessary for satisfactory manual rotation. Epidural and spinal anaesthesia provide good pain relief but, if the uterus is firmly contracted around the fetus, tocolysis with intravenous nitroglycerine may have to be given. Most of the large series with successful manual rotation were carried out in the days when general anaesthesia with profound uterine relaxation was used.

Forceps rotation

If digital or manual rotation of the head is not feasible, forceps rotation can be considered. Although a number of forceps have been used for this purpose there is greatest experience with those devised by Kielland in 1915. He designed his forceps without a pelvic curve so that rotation of the fetal head arrested in the transverse position could be achieved without the trauma to maternal tissues that is incurred by the wide excursion of the

> *'If the head is in the pelvic cavity, rotation can be completed with the forceps ... the head is rotated 90° from the transverse into the exact anteroposterior diameter before its extraction through the pelvic narrows is begun. In such a case rotation is carried out* without *simultaneous traction. The forceps, held tightly closed, are turned about the axis of the handles.'*
>
> **Christian Kielland**
> *Eine neue form und einführungsweise der geburtszange, stets biparietal an den kindlichlen schädel gelagt. Munchen Med Wchnscr 1915; 62:923*

toes of forceps that have a pelvic curve. In many hospitals, forceps rotation has been abandoned but there are still units where the skill with this instrument has been retained. The main indication is the deflexed fetal head arrested in the transverse or posterior position. In modern obstetrics this is often associated with epidural analgesia and, while the head may be low *(≥ +2 cm)*, the deflexed and malrotated head presents a larger diameter. If the head can be safely rotated and flexed the presenting diameter is reduced and often mild traction will safely effect delivery.

In order to allow for correct application and manoeuvre of Kielland's forceps the woman's perineum should protrude slightly over the edge of the delivery table. Before application the Kielland forceps are assembled and held outside the pelvis in the position to which they will be applied to the fetal head (Fig 8.21a). The directional knobs on the shanks should be toward the fetal occiput. The obstetrician then takes the anterior blade and there are three techniques by which this can be applied – classical, wandering and direct.

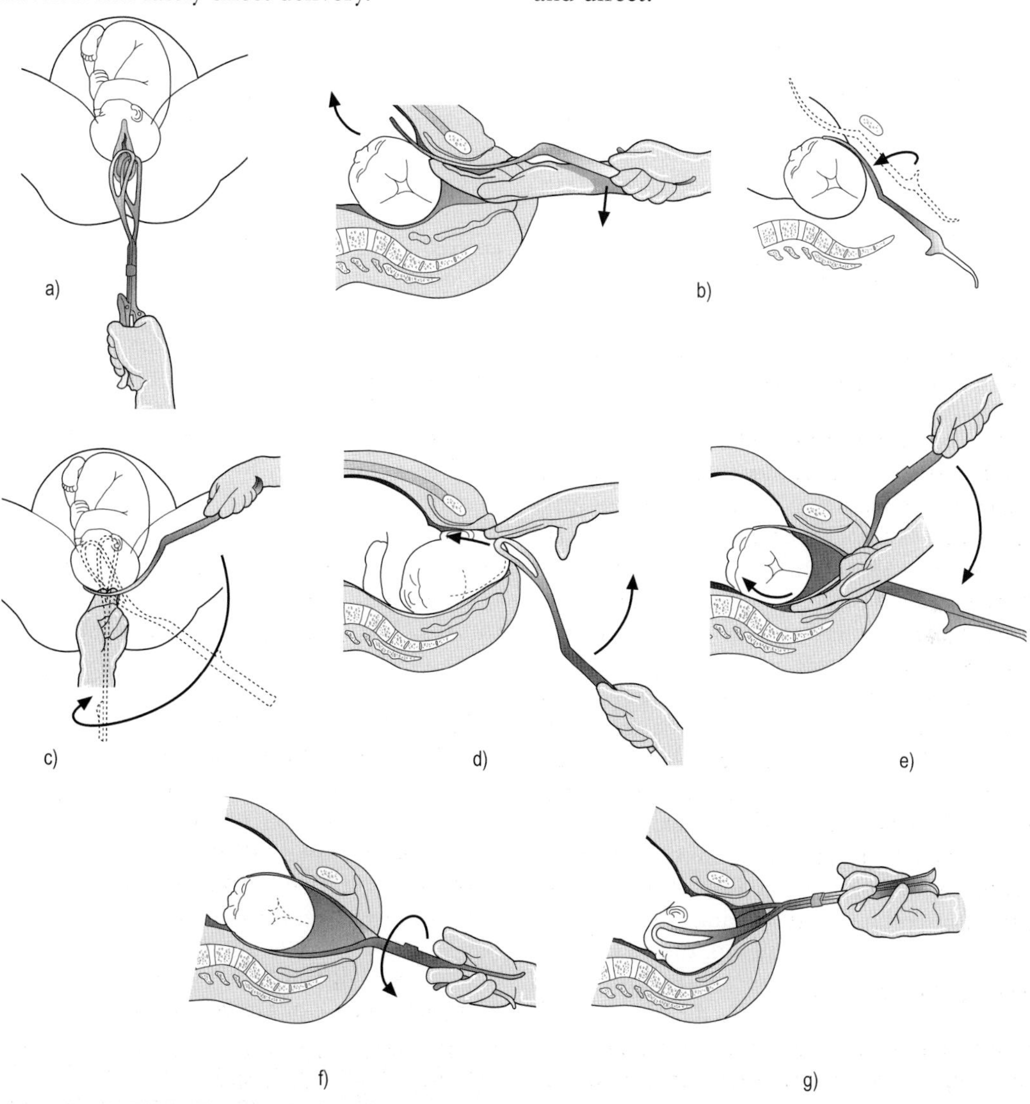

Figure 8.21 Kielland's forceps: left occipito-transverse. (a) Orientation of forceps, directional buttons towards occiput. (b) Classical (inversion) application of anterior blade. (c) Wandering technique of applying anterior blade. (d) Direct application of anterior blade. (e) Introduction of posterior blade. (f) Gentle rotation from LOT to OA. (g) Traction with Kielland's forceps.

The *classical* or inversion technique was that originally described by Kielland for use when the fetal head was higher in the pelvis than would be acceptable for forceps delivery today. It will be described here, largely for historical interest, as it is associated with a small risk of perforation of the lower uterine segment and entanglement of the fetal hand, forearm or umbilical cord. The middle and index fingers of one hand are inserted under the symphysis with the palmer surface up. The anterior blade is held in the other hand at an angle of about 45° above the horizontal with the cephalic surface up (Fig 8.21b). The toe of the blade is guided over the finger tips and the handle is pressed down and the blade passed up until it occupies the space in the lower uterine segment between the anterior shoulder and the side of the fetal head. The shank is now lying over the anterior parietal bone. The blade is then rotated through 180° and fits down over the parietal bone (Fig 8.21b). Throughout these manoeuvres extreme gentleness should be exercised. If there is any resistance the technique should be abandoned.

The *wandering* technique has less potential for trauma to the maternal tissues than the classical technique. Nonetheless, great care has to be exercised or trauma to the vaginal vault can occur with the toe of the blade. The anterior blade is inserted posteriorly into the vagina and the fingers guide the blade around the sinciput and face of the fetus while the other hand rotates the blade in a downward arc. Once again this move must be gentle and no force should be necessary (Fig 8.21c). If the head is very deflexed the face may present an obstruction to this manoeuvre. In this case it may be best to use the reverse wandering technique over the occiput.

If the fetal head is low, and particularly if there is anterior asynclitism, the *direct* technique can be used. The middle and index fingers of one hand are inserted palmer surface down between the anterior parietal bone and the maternal symphysis. The other hand guides the blade directly over the parietal bone to the correct cephalic application (Fig 8.21d).

The posterior blade is inserted into the hollow of the sacrum. A protective hand is placed as high as possible posteriorly and the blade guided between that and the posterior parietal bone of the fetal head. The tips of the fingers should guide the toe of the blade around the fetal head and away from the vaginal tissues overlying the sacrum and sacral promontory. This is aided by depression on the handle with the other hand (Fig 8.21e). Most junior obstetricians are surprised at how much depression of the handle is required to guide the toe of the blade around the fetal head. Once both blades have been appropriately placed the operator often finds that there is more of the shank of the anterior blade protruding then there is of the posterior blade. This may be due to incorrect application but is usually due to anterior asynclitism. Thus, provided the obstetrician is secure in the parietal application of each blade, they are locked. The sliding lock allows one to, at least partially, correct the asynclitism. However, much of the asynclitism will not be corrected until rotation has occurred. The relationship of the blades to the sagittal suture and posterior fontanelle should be checked. Before rotation it is helpful to try and flex the fetal head. This can be achieved, after the correct application has been confirmed, by moving the handles towards the sinciput.

Rotation should be gentle and easy. If it is not then one should check the application very carefully and consider again whether forceps delivery is safely feasible. With the hand in the supine position the index and middle fingers and the thumb grasp the finger guides and the handles are depressed posteriorly. Rotation should occur slowly and gently with pronation of the hand (Fig 8.21f). At the same time the other hand, or that of an assistant, applied to the abdomen should guide the anterior shoulder around in the same direction as the occiput. Provided one has an assistant to manipulate the shoulder it is useful for the obstetrician to use the other hand to retract the vaginal wall so that the rotation of the fetal head can be observed directly. This ensures that the forceps remain properly applied, rather than just rotating around the surface of the head. Once rotation is achieved the correct application of the forceps is checked again.

Traction with Kielland's forceps should take account of the reduced pelvic curve. Thus, the appropriate position for the obstetrician is on one knee. One hand with the index and middle fingers below the finger grips applies traction and the heel of the other hand applies downward traction on the shanks (Pajot's manoeuvre). The head is guided downwards and backwards and as the occiput appears below the symphysis the handles are slowly elevated to the horizontal position (Fig 8.21g). There are some obstetricians who will use the Kielland's only to rotate the fetal head and then remove the blades and apply a pair of classical forceps with a pelvic curve for traction and final delivery of the head. There is no doubt that safe use of Kielland's forceps requires considerable training and supervision. In many training programmes this is not now available.

Vacuum assisted delivery

In recent years obstetricians have moved from using forceps to the vacuum for the majority of assisted vaginal deliveries. There are those who feel that the training and experience required to perform safe forceps delivery is more than that for vacuum assisted delivery. There is an element of truth in this supposition, but it is a potentially dangerous assumption. The 'suck-it-and-see' school of vacuum assisted delivery assumes that placing the vacuum device on the fetal head and applying traction is a safe and simple option to overcome dystocia. Nothing could be further from the truth and the potential for fetal damage with the vacuum is as great as it is with the forceps. The predelivery assessment and prerequisites discussed earlier in this chapter should be just as stringent for vacuum assisted as for forceps assisted deliveries.

Vacuum assisted delivery does have a lower risk of maternal vaginal and perineal trauma compared with forceps. In addition, it can often be performed with less profound anaesthesia: local infiltration or pudendal block, compared to epidural or spinal.

There are many different varieties of vacuum cups and devices, but they fall into two main categories – rigid cup and soft cup. The original rigid cups were metal and usually the Malmström or the Bird modification of the Malmström. More recently, rigid plastic cups have been manufactured.[26,46] In the 1970s cups were developed with softer material in an attempt to reduce scalp trauma attributed to the hard cups. The first of these was the Kobayashi Silastic cup[47] and there have been many other soft cups developed since that time. In general the soft cups do reduce superficial scalp trauma but have a higher failure-to-deliver rate than the hard cups. The principles of use with all of the cups, however, is the same and will be reviewed here.

The first and most essential piece of information is the identification of the *flexion point*.[25] This is situated approximately 3 cm in front of the posterior fontanelle. If traction is directed from this point the fetal head is flexed to the narrowest suboccipito-bregmatic diameter (9.5 cm). Most of the vacuum cups are 5 or 6 cm in diameter. Thus, if the cup is applied so that the rear edge is just at the posterior fontanelle it should be over the flexion point. The other way of assessing this is to gauge the relationship of the leading edge of the cup to the anterior fontanelle. The distance between the anterior fontanelle and the flexion point is approximately 6 cm. Thus, when the cup is correctly placed there should

FLEXION AND VACUUM ASSISTED DELIVERY

'The large amount of force apparently required in some cases is because it is misdirected. The head is not properly flexed, and traction is exerted in a direction that would tend to pull the occiput through the pubic symphysis, instead of under the pubic arch.'

Peter McCahey
Atmospheric tractor: a new instrument and some new theories in obstetrics. Med Surg Rep (Philadelphia) 1890; 43:619–623

be about 3 cm (two finger-breadths) between the leading edge and the anterior fontanelle (Fig 8.22). In addition to correct flexion of the head one wants to avoid asynclitism, which will also increase the diameter of the fetal head presenting to the pelvis. The biparietal diameter is 9.5 cm and this assumes no asynclitism. If the cup is applied off the central sagittal suture, this paramedian application will cause asynclitism during traction and increase the presenting diameter of the fetal head. Thus, there are four possible applications of the vacuum cup (Fig 8.23):

- flexing median – which provides the optimum and narrowest suboccipito-bregmatic and biparietal diameters
- deflexing median – which produces the wider occipito-frontal diameter
- flexing paramedian – which produces a wider paramedian diameter
- deflexing paramedian – which provides the worst combination of wider diameters with the occipito-frontal and paramedian diameters.

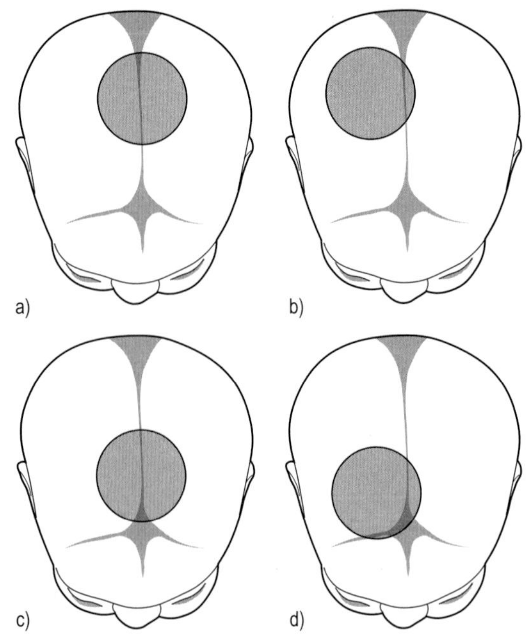

Figure 8.23 The four potential vacuum cup applications. (a) Flexing median. (b) Flexing paramedian. (c) Deflexing median. (d) Deflexing paramedian.

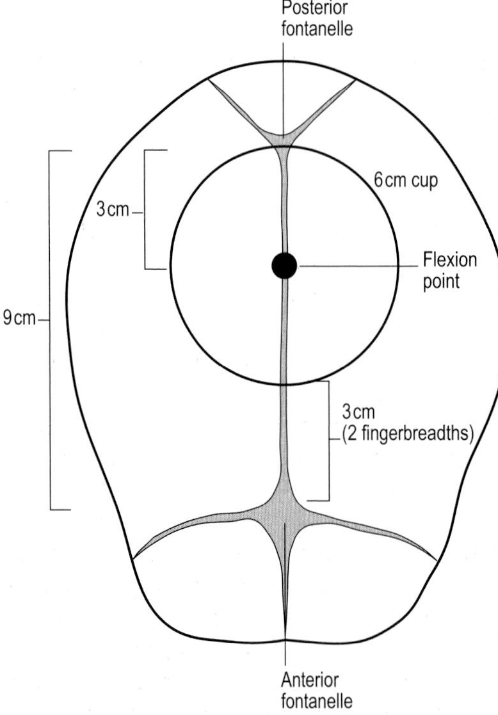

Figure 8.22 Relationship of the vacuum cup to the flexion point.

It has been shown that the amount of fetal scalp trauma is least with the correct flexing-median cup application.[48]

The above rationale dictates the correct placement of the vacuum cup in a median position over the flexion point. Once the cup has been applied the vacuum is created to about 0.2 kg/cm^2 and the index finger carefully run around the periphery of the cup to ensure that no maternal tissue has been included. If all is clear the vacuum is increased to 0.8 kg/cm^2 (600 mmHg). There is no need to increase the vacuum in increments and, other than a delay of a minute or two while one carefully checks its application and the exclusion of maternal tissues, there is no need to wait several minutes for the 'chignon' to develop.

Both the metal and rigid plastic cups have an in-curved margin. Thus, the peripheral margin of the cup attached to the fetal scalp has a narrower diameter than the upper curved margin and it is this that produces the chignon. In addition to the atmospheric pressure on the cup against the vacuum created,

Table 8.2 Force needed to detach the vacuum cup

Cup diameter	Vacuum		Traction force (lb)
	mmHg	kg/cm²	
5 cm	500	0.65	29
	600	0.80	35
	700	0.96	41
	760	Atmospheric	45
6 cm	500	0.65	42
	600	0.80	51
	700	0.95	59
	760	Atmospheric	64

this has the effect of reducing the risk of cup detachment and also adds to the effective diameter of the cup, such that a 5 cm cup effectively becomes a 6 cm cup.

The traction force needed to detach the vacuum cup will depend on the diameter of the cup and the vacuum created. The calculation of the force needed to detach the cup ('pop-off') when the cup is pulled in a perpendicular direction is given in Table 8.2.

Traction force is the maximum theoretical force possible based on the vacuum holding over the given cross-sectional area of the cup and pulling at right angles to the cup surface seal. There is additional force added from the trapping of the tissue that wedges itself into the cup. One can use 760 mmHg vacuum as the upper limit as that is as close to pure vacuum as one can get at sea level. The force calculation assumes a perpendicular traction force pulling out from the back surface of the cup ignoring frictional effects. Traction angled off the perpendicular will be modified by the vector angle.

Clinically, traction is carried out in conjunction with the uterine contractions and maternal effort. If the traction is carried out an angle off the perpendicular the force required to pull off the edge of the cup can be quite low (Fig 8.24). It is essential that the axis of traction be perpendicular to the cup – the best guiding rule is that the direction of pull should never go outside the circumference of the cup. Traction should be with the index and middle fingers on the traction bar and the thumb of the other hand should be placed on the surface of the cup with the forefinger placed against the scalp and underlying bone. This allows one to detect what Bird called 'negative traction', in which the scalp is drawn away from the skull but the bony skull does not descend.[25]

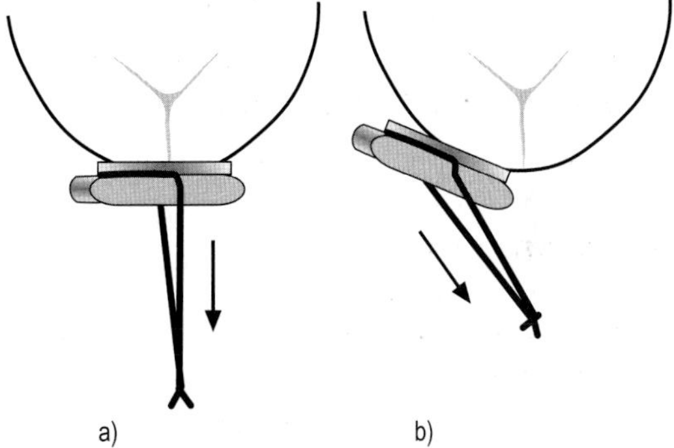

Figure 8.24 Cup placement and traction. (a) Correct perpendicular traction within the circumference of the cup diameter. (b) Oblique traction and/or paramedian application predispose to cup detachment.

Repeated negative traction may result in fluctuations of pressure within the cranium and increase the risk of scalp and intracranial haemorrhage. Therefore, the thumb applies counter-traction to reduce the chance of cup detachment and the index finger assesses whether the scalp is just being pulled off the bone or the bone is descending appropriately. Thus, the two hands work in combination with the finger and thumb of the left hand, keeping the cup pressed to the surface of the scalp and the index finger assessing descent, while

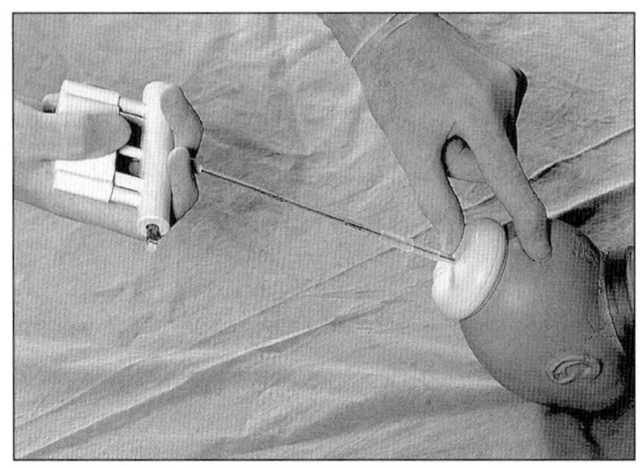

Figure 8.25 Technique of vacuum extraction.

the right hand ensures that the traction is in the perpendicular plane to the cup (Fig 8.25). This co-ordinated effort between the two hands and fingers should be practiced on manikins.

Some of the vacuum delivery devices, such as the commonly used OmniCup, have traction force indicators.[49] In clinical use most vacuum deliveries are achieved using ≈9 kg (20 lb) traction force, although up to 14 kg (30 lb) may be necessary.[26,48]

The advantage of the rigid cups, in addition to their lower risk of pop-off, is that the vacuum port is placed laterally or recessed – which allows placement of the cup over the flexion point in cases of deflexed occipito-transverse and occipito-posterior positions. The problem with the soft cups that have a central stem is that it is not possible, due to this stem, to place the cup over the flexion point in many of these deflexed positions. Another disadvantage of the soft cup is that it is not possible to use the finger and thumb placement as easily as with the hard cup. However, using the fingers and thumb spread around the periphery of the soft cup the same principles can be applied.

No attempt should be made to encourage rotation of the fetal head by applying shearing tangential pressure to the cup. Provided the cup has been placed with a correct flexing median application the head will undergo autorotation during traction at the level in the pelvis most suitable for that particular head in that pelvis. In some cases of occipito-posterior position the head does not rotate but is delivered OP.

If the head has descended to the perineum with traction but further progress is slow check posteriorly between the fetal head and the sacrum. Vacca has described entrapment of the fetal hand between the sacrum and the fetal head – which he calls the 'sacral hand wedge' and which can delay final delivery of the head over the perineum.[50] Thus, if there is delay in descent check posteriorly and, if present, grasp the fetal wrist with the fingers and deliver the posterior arm.

If the vacuum cup detaches during traction the situation should be carefully reappraised. If everything still seems suitable for vacuum assisted delivery the cup can be reapplied and traction carried out. If the cup detaches for a second time then further reappraisal will have to be undertaken to determine whether vaginal delivery is safe or whether one should move to caesarean section – which would be necessary if there is inadequate descent and rotation. If the head has rotated and descended to the perineum delivery can be assisted with forceps. This needs especially careful evaluation as it is associated with a higher risk of fetal trauma. At times the chignon can prevent accurate re-application of the vacuum cup.

It is useful to regard vacuum assisted delivery as having two phases. The *descent phase* is from the time of cup application until the head is at the pelvic outlet, at which level the vacuum cup will be completely visible at the introitus. The *outlet phase* is the time from when the cup is completely visible until delivery of the head.[50]

Traction during one uterine contraction is regarded as one 'pull'. One should expect that during three pulls delivery will occur or the head will have progressively descended to the perineum (with the cup completely visible) so that vaginal delivery is clearly safe and feasible. Sometimes it takes two to four more pulls to gently assist delivery of the fetal head over the perineum. When there is progressive descent with traction the pull on the scalp is less compared with no descent. Hence the three pulls during three contractions should have produced enough descent and rotation to signify that additional pulls will achieve safe delivery without trauma to the fetus. Thus, the vast majority of vacuum assisted deliveries should be carried out within 20 minutes from the initial application of the cup. Just as with forceps delivery certain vacuum assisted deliveries should be carried out as a trial of vacuum with the obstetrician prepared to back off in the face of any difficulty and move straight to caesarean section.

Once delivered, the vacuum is released and the cup removed. The chignon should be explained to the parents and that the majority of this swelling will disappear within hours and usually completely within 48 hours. Although subgaleal haemorrhage is rare its potential should be considered in all infants delivered by vacuum and the appropriate nursing observation in the postnatal ward instituted.

In the postpartum period the events leading to assisted vaginal delivery, either by forceps or vacuum, and its implications should be explained to the woman. She can be reassured that in the vast majority of cases (> 80%) spontaneous delivery will occur in a subsequent delivery.[51,52]

Complications of assisted vaginal delivery

Maternal

Instrumental vaginal delivery is associated with a higher incidence of maternal injuries compared with spontaneous vaginal delivery. These include perineal, vaginal, labial, periurethral and cervical lacerations. There is often significant haemorrhage of an insidious nature associated with these lacerations. Assisted delivery of the head with an emphasis on posteriorly directed traction risks trauma to the perineum and anal sphincter complex, while traction that is directed more anteriorly will result in anterior labial and periurethral lacerations.

In general, vaginal and perineal trauma is less with vacuum assisted delivery than with forceps delivery. The management of lower genital tract trauma is covered in Chapter 21.

Fetal

Scalp and facial skin trauma

Superficial bruising, blistering and even minor lacerations can occur at the site of the vacuum cup on the fetal scalp. These are usually trivial and of no lasting significance. Similarly, with forceps assisted delivery, bruising can occur over the fetal cheeks, which is equally benign. These features should be explained to the parents immediately after delivery along with appropriate reassurance.

Caput succedaneum

Caput succedaneum is a serosanguinous, subcutaneous and extraperiosteal fluid collection with poorly defined margins. It extends across suture lines – in contrast to cephalhaematoma (Fig 8.26a). Caput succedaneum is found normally in spontaneous vaginal delivery and is

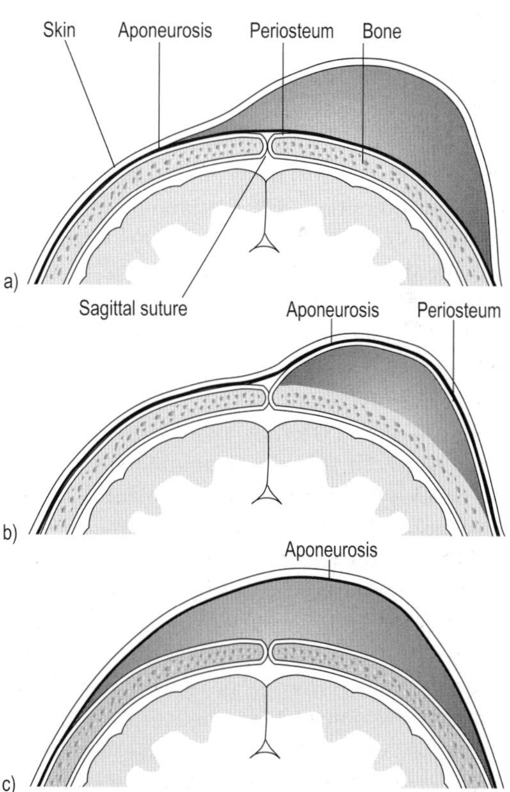

Figure 8.26 Fetal scalp trauma. (a) Caput succedaneum. (b) Cephalhaematoma. (c) Subgaleal haemorrhage.

associated with pressure on the presenting part by the dilating cervix and pelvis. It is often more marked in assisted vaginal deliveries, due to the dystocia present in many of these cases. The vacuum cup produces a well-defined caput succedaneum which is known as a 'chignon'. Both the chignon and the physiological caput succedaneum usually resolve within 24–48 hours and have no long-term significance.

Cephalhaematoma

Cephalhaemtoma is a subperiosteal collection of serosanguinous fluid secondary to rupture of small blood vessels between the bony skull and the periosteum. The swelling does not cross the suture line; in contrast to both caput succedaneum and subgaleal haemorrhage (Fig 8.26b). Cephalhaematoma is more common following vacuum delivery compared with forceps delivery. Other than the disfigurement, which should be explained to the parents, most cephalhaematomas are benign and resolve within a few weeks. Occasionally there may be residual calcification leading to a hard swelling for several months.

Subgaleal haemorrhage

Subgaleal haemorrhage is one of the most serious and potentially life threatening complications of vaginal delivery. It is also known as subaponeurotic haemorrhage, as the bleeding develops in the space between the periosteum and the galea aponeurotica (Fig 8.26c). This aponeurosis is a sheet of fibrous tissue that extends from the orbital margins anteriorly, the temporal fascia laterally and the nuchal ridges posteriorly. In the loose subaponeurotic area lie emissary veins connecting the dural sinuses and the scalp veins. In term infants the subaponeurotic space has a capacity of about 250 ml and this therefore can lead to life threatening hypovolaemia in the newborn.

A recent review reported the incidence of subgaleal haemorrhage as approximately 1 in 2000–3000 spontaneous deliveries and 1 in 150–200 vacuum assisted deliveries.[53] One observational study found a rate as high as 21% of vacuum assisted deliveries.[54] The rate with forceps assisted delivery is higher than spontaneous vaginal delivery, but about one-third that of vacuum assisted delivery. The occurrence is the same for vacuum assisted delivery with both rigid and soft cups and is likely to be increased with improper placement of the cup and with failed vacuum delivery.

Subgaleal haemorrhage presents as a diffuse, firm but fluctuant mass that crosses suture lines and will shift as the infant's head is repositioned. It is usually observed within the first 12 hours of delivery but may progress insidiously over the next 48–72 hours. Anaemia and hypovolaemic shock are the presenting signs. The treatment is early detection and correction with transfusion of blood products if necessary.

Eye injuries

Minor injuries such as periorbital oedema, subconjunctival haemorrhages and retinal haemorrhages can occur after spontaneous and assisted vaginal delivery. These are usually trivial and of no long-term significance. Retinal haemorrhage is more common with vacuum assisted delivery compared with spontaneous and forceps delivery.

Facial palsy

The facial nerve is vulnerable to compression as it exits the stylomastoid foramen or as it passes over the ramus of the mandible. The nerve may be compressed by forceps or by pressure against the bony pelvis, usually the sacral promontory. Facial nerve palsy occurs in about 1 in 2000 spontaneous deliveries, 1 in 1000 vacuum assisted deliveries and 1 in 200 forceps deliveries. The injury is virtually always a neuropraxia and recovery is complete.

Brachial plexus injury

Brachial plexus injury is increased with assisted vaginal delivery, probably due to the fact that the indication for assistance is dystocia and often associated with fetal macrosomnia. In most reviews there is a slightly increased risk of shoulder dystocia with vacuum assisted delivery rather than forceps, although this association is by no means consistent.[55]

Skull fracture

Skull fracture can occur with spontaneous and assisted vaginal delivery. Most fractures are linear, of no clinical significance and require no treatment. Depressed skull fractures are rare and, if greater than 2 cm in width and accompanied by neurological symptoms, require neurosurgical elevation. The fracture may be associated with forceps or vacuum delivery or due to pressure of the skull against the maternal bony pelvis.

Intracranial haemorrhage

Symptomatic intracranial haemorrhage occurs in about 1 in 2000 deliveries. The risk for assisted vaginal delivery is approximately twice that of spontaneous delivery. The risk seems about equal between vacuum (both rigid and soft cups) and forceps delivery. The highest risk is with failed vacuum followed by forceps assisted delivery.

Spinal cord injury

Cervical spine cord injury is very rare, about 1 in 80 000 deliveries. It is more likely to be associated with delivery by rotation, particularly with forceps. The possible pathogenesis and safeguards against this injury have been outlined in the section on forceps rotation earlier in this chapter.

Perhaps the evolution of assisted vaginal delivery is best shown by the attitude expressed by Sir Anthony Carlisle in 1834, when he addressed the select committee on medical education in the British Parliament:[56]

> *'I consider it derogatory to any liberal man to assume the office of a nurse, of an old woman: it is an imposture to pretend that a medical man is required at labour. The craft therefore involves imposture, mischievous interference and gross indecency. Not only is it beneath our dignity, but it is not within our province. I do not consider the delivery of a woman as a surgical operation: it is a natural operation. The man-midwives have recourse to surgical operations, to make themselves in request, and to make it believed that parturition is a surgical act, which it ought not to be. All interference in my opinion is injurious, particularly premature interference, or a meddling with the process of nature.'*

References

1. Aveling JH. The Chamberlens and the midwifery forceps. London: J & A Churchill, 1882.
2. Spencer HR. The history of British midwifery from 1650 to 1800. London: John Bale, Sons and Danielsson, 1927.
3. RadcliffeW. A secret instrument. London: William Heinemann, 1947.
4. Radcliffe W. Milestones in midwifery. Bristol: John Wright & Sons, 1967.
5. Chapman E. A treatise on the improvement of midwifery; chiefly with regard to the operation. 3rd ed. London: L. Davis and C. Reymers, 1759.
6. Pugh B. A treatise of midwifery, chiefly with regards to the operation. London: J. Buckland, 1754.
7. Smellie W. A treatise on the theory and practice of midwifery. London: E. Wilson, 1752.
8. Tarnier ES. Descriptions des deux nouveaux forceps. Paris: Martinet, 1877.
9. Saxtorph M. Theoria de diverso partu. Copenhagen: A. H. Godiche, 1772.
10. Ferguson JH. A simple and improved modification of the midwifery forceps. Trans Edinb Obstet Soc 1925–26; 46:78–92.
11. Das K. Obstetric forceps: its history and evolution. Calcutta: The Art Press, 1929.
12. Murray RM. The axis traction forceps: their mechanical principles, construction and scope. Trans Edinb Obstet Soc 1891; 16:58–89.
13. Kielland C. Eine neue form und einfuhrungsweise der geburtszange, stets biparietal an den kindlichen schadel gelegt. Munchen Med Wscher 1915; 62:923.
14. Baskett TF. On the shoulders of giants: eponyms and names in obstetrics and gynaecology. London: RCOG Press, 1996:110–111,134–135.
15. Jones EP. Kielland's forceps. London: Butterworth and Co., 1952.
16. Barton LG, Caldwell WE, Studdiford WE. A new obstetric forceps. Am J Obstet Gynecol 1928; 1516–1526.

17. Moolgaoker A. A new design of obstetric forceps. J Obstet Gynaecol Br Commonw 1962; 69:450–457.

18. Baskett TF. The history of vacuum extraction. In: Vacca A. Handbook of vacuum delivery in obstetric practice. 2nd ed. Brisbane: Vacca Research, 2003:11–23.

19. Yonge J. An account of balls of hair taken from the uterus and ovaria of several women. Phil Trans R Soc Lond 1706; 725–6:2387–2392.

20. Arnott N. Elements of physics or natural philosophy. 4th ed. London: T&G Underwood, 1829, Vol. 1:650–652.

21. Simpson JY. On a suction-tractor; or new mechanical power as a substitute for the forceps in tedious labours. Monthly J Med 1849; 9:556–559.

22. Malmström T. The vacuum extractor: an obstetrical instrument and the parturiometer: a tokographic device. Acta Obstet Gynecol Scand 1957; 36:(Suppl 3) 7–50.

23. Chalmers JA. The ventouse. The obstetric vacuum extractor. Chicago: Yearbook Medical Publisher, 1971.

24. Bird GC. Modification of Malmström's vacuum extractor. BMJ 1969; 2:52–56.

25. Bird GC. The importance of flexion in vacuum delivery. Br J Obstet Gynaecol 1976; 83:194–200.

26. Vacca A. Operative vaginal delivery: clinical appraisal of a new vacuum extraction device. Aust NZ J Obstet Gynaecol 2001; 41:156–160.

27. Drife JO. Choice and instrumental delivery. Br J Obstet Gynaecol 1996; 103:608–611.

28. O'Grady JP, Pope CS, Hoffman DE. Forceps delivery. Best Pract Res Clin Obstet Gynaecol 2002; 16:1–16.

29. Johanson RB, Mennon V. Vacuum extraction versus forceps for assisted vaginal delivery. Cochrane Database Syst Rev 2004; (2).

30. Johanson RB, Heycook E, Carteer J, Sultan AH, Walklate K, Jones PW. Maternal and child health after assisted vaginal delivery: five-year follow up of a randomised controlled study comparing forceps and ventouse. Br J Obstet Gynaecol 1999; 106:544–549.

31. Baskett TF. Non-progressive labour: dystocia. In: Essential management of obstetric emergencies. 4th ed. Bristol: Clinical Press Ltd, 2004:119–133.

32. Goodfellow CF, Howell MGR, Swaab DF. Oxytocin deficiency at delivery with epidural analgesia. Br J Obstet Gynaecol 1983; 90:214–219.

33. Saunders NJ, Spiby H, Gilbert L, et al. Oxytocin infusion during second stage of labour in primiparous women using epidural analgesia: a randomised double-blind placebo-controlled trial. BMJ 1989; 299:1423–1426.

34. Sherer DM, Onyje CI, Bernstein PS. Utilization of real-time ultrasound on labor and delivery in an active academic teaching hospital. Am J Perinatol 1989; 16:303–307.

35. Crichton D. A reliable method of establishing the level of the fetal head in obstetrics. South Afr Med J 1974; 48:784–787.

36. Baskett TF, Arulkumaran S. Assisted vaginal delivery. In: Intrapartum care. London: RCOG Press, 2002:63–74.

37. Royal College of Obstetricians and Gynaecologists. Instrumental vaginal delivery. Guideline No. 26. London: RCOG, 2005.

38. Society of Obstetricians and Gynaecologists of Canada. Guidelines for vaginal birth. Clinical practice guideline No. 148. J Obstet Gynaecol Can 2004; 26:747–753.

39. Cheung YW, Hopkins LM, Caughey AB. How long is too long? Does a prolonged second stage of labor in nulliparous women affect maternal and neonatal morbidity? Am J Obstet Gynecol 2004; 191:933–938.

40. American College of Obstetricians and Gynecologists. Practice Bulletin No. 17. Operative vaginal delivery. Washington, DC: ACOG, 2000 (Obstet Gynecol 2000; 95:6).

41. Cheong YC, Abdullahi H, Lashen H, Fairlie FM. Can formal education and training improve the outcome of instrumental delivery? Eur J Obstet Gynecol Reprod Biol 2004; 113:139–144.

42. Douglass LH, Kaltreider DF. Trial forceps. Am J Obstet Gynecol 1953; 65:889–896.

43. Jeffcoate TNA. The place of forceps in present-day obstetrics. BMJ 1953; 2:951–957.

44. Leslie KK, Lehnerz PD, Smith M. Obstetric forceps training using visual feedback and the isometric strength testing unit. Obstet Gynecol 2005; 105:377–382.

45. Pomeroy RH. The treatment of occipito-posterior positions. Am J Obstet Dis Wom 1914; 69:354–356.

46. Hayman R, Gilby J, Arulkumaran S. Clinical evaluation of a 'hand-pump' vacuum delivery device. Obstet Gynecol 2002; 100:1190–1195.

47. Maryniak GM, Frank JB. Clinical assessment of the Kobayashi vacuum extractor. Obstet Gynecol 1984; 64:431–435.

48. Baskett TF, Fanning CA, Young DC. A prospective observational study of vacuum-assisted delivery with the OmniCup device. J Obstet Gynaecol Can (Suppl) 2003; S23.

49. Whitlow BJ, Tamizian O, Ashworth J, Kerry S, Penna LK, Arulkumaran S. Validation of traction force indicator in ventouse devices. Int J Gynecol Obstet 2005; 90:35–38.

50. Vacca A. The 'sacral hand wedge': a cause of arrest of descent of the fetal head during vacuum assisted delivery. Br J Obstet Gynaecol 2002; 109:1063–1065.

51. Mawdsley SD, Baskett TF. Outcome of the next labour in women who had a vaginal delivery in their first pregnancy. Br J Obstet Gynaecol 2000; 107:932–934.

52. Bahl R, Strachan BK. Mode of delivery in the next pregnancy in women who had a vaginal delivery in their first pregnancy. J Obstet Gynaecol 2004; 24:272–273.

53. Uchil D, Arulkumaran S. Neonatal subgaleal hemorrhage and its relationship to delivery by vacuum extraction. Obstet Gynecol Surv 2003; 58:687–693.

54. Boo NY, Foong KW, Mahdy ZA, Yang SC, Jaafar R. Risk factors associated with subaponeurotic haemorrhage in full-term infants exposed to vacuum extraction. Br J Obstet Gynaecol 2005; 112:1516–1521.

55. Caughey AB, Sandberg PL, Zlatnik MG, Thiet MP, Parer JT, Laros RK. Forceps compared with vacuum: rates of neonatal and maternal morbidity. Obstet Gynecol 2005; 106:908–912.

56. Arulkumaran S, Gibb DMF, Tamby Raja RL, Heng SH, Ratnam SS. Rising caesarean section rates in Singapore. Singapore J Obstet Gynaecol 1985; 16:5–14.

Bibliography

Chalmers JA. The ventouse – the obstetric vacuum extractor. London: Lloyd-Luke, 1971.

Dennen PC. Dennen's forceps deliveries. 4th ed. Washington, DC: American College of Obstetricians and Gynecologists, 2001.

Dill LV. The obstetrical forceps. Springfield, Illinois: Charles C. Thomas, 1953.

Groom KM, Jones BM, Miller N, Paterson-Brown S. A prospective randomised controlled trial of the Kiwi OmniCup versus conventional ventouse cups for vacuum-assisted vaginal delivery. Br J Obstet Gynaecol 2006; 113:183–189.

Hankins JD, Rowe TF. Operative vaginal delivery – Year 2000. Am J Obstet Gynecol 1996; 175:275–282.

Laufe LE, Berkus MD. Assisted vaginal delivery: obstetric forceps and vacuum extraction techniques. New York: McGraw-Hill, 1992.

O'Grady JP. Modern instrumental delivery. Baltimore: Williams and Wilkins, 1988.

O'Grady JP, Gimovsky ML, McIlhargie CJ. Vacuum extraction in modern obstetric practice. New York: Parthenon Publishing Group, 1995.

O'Mahony F, Settatree R, Platt C, Johanson R. Review of singleton fetal and neonatal deaths associated with cranial trauma and cephalic delivery during a national intrapartum-related confidential enquiry. Br J Obstet Gynaecol 2005; 112:619–626.

Patel RP, Murphy DJ. Forceps review in modern obstetric practice. BMJ 2004; 328:1302–1305.

Robson S, Pridmore B. Have Kielland forceps reached their use-by date? Aust NZ J Obstet Gynaecol 1989; 39:301–304.

Vacca A. Handbook of vacuum delivery in obstetric practice. 2nd ed. Brisbane: Vacca Research, 2003.

Vacca A. Vacuum assisted delivery. Best Pract Res Clin Obstet Gynecol 2002; 16:17–30.

Vacca A, Grant A, Wyatt G, Chalmers I. Portsmouth operative delivery trial. A comparison of vacuum extraction and forceps delivery. Br J Obstet Gynaecol 1983; 90:1107–1112.

Whitby EH, Griffiths PD, Rutter S, et al. Frequency and natural history of subdural haemorrhages in babies and relation to obstetric factors. Lancet 2004; 363:846–851.

9

Malpresentations

Fetal malpresentation exists when the presenting part is other than the normal vertex of the fetal head. This includes two malpresentations that are covered in other chapters: breech (Chapter 14) and cord presentation (Chapter 16). The remaining malpresentations which will be covered in this chapter are face, brow, transverse lie with shoulder or arm presentation, and compound presentations. In modern obstetrics, particularly in the developed world, the incidence of malpresentations has fallen. This is due to the association of many malpresentations with high parity and the fact that women are having fewer children.

The various anteroposterior diameters (Fig 9.1) of the term fetal head vary depending upon the position: normal flexed vertex (9.5 cm), deflexed occipito-posterior position (11–12 cm), and malpresentation: face presentation, submento-bregmatic (9.5 cm) and brow, mento-vertical (13.5 cm). These are illustrated in Figure 9.2.

Face presentation

In face presentation the attitude of the fetal head is one of complete extension with the chin as the denominator and leading pole. The presenting diameter is the submento-bregmatic, which in the term fetus is about 9.5 cm. This is the same as the favourable flexed vertex presentation, but the facial bones do not mould to the same extent as the cranial vault does in vertex presentation. The incidence of face presentation is about 1 in 500 births.

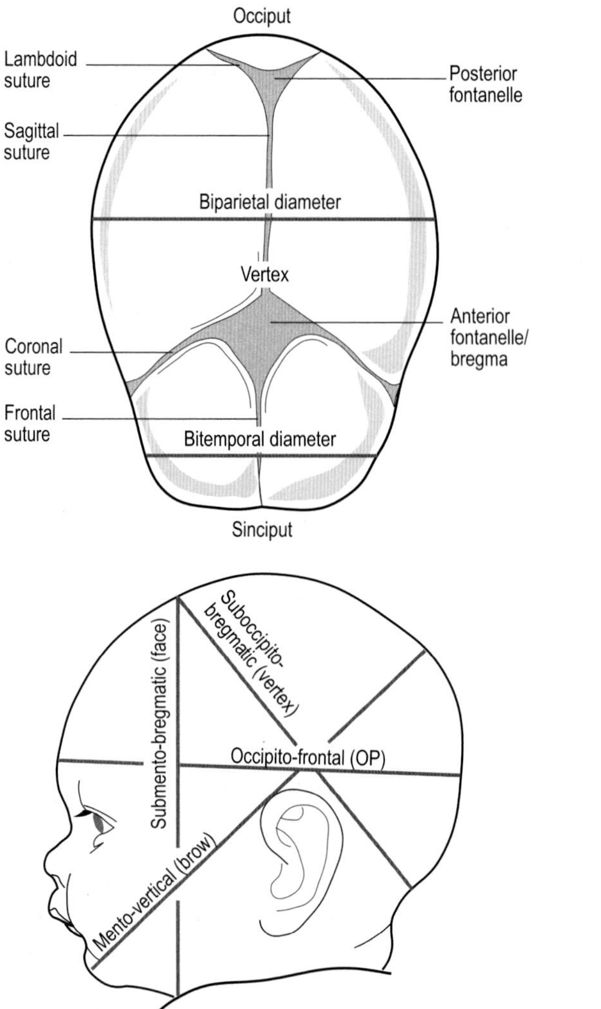

Figure 9.1 Diameters and landmarks of the fetal skull.

Causes

- Fetal anomalies are found in about 15% of face presentations. The commonest are major CNS anomalies such as anencephaly and meningomyelecoele. Tumours of the neck may also cause extension and face presentation.
- Prematurity.
- Mild cephalopelvic disproportion has been incriminated. It is probable that in some cases of deflexed occipito-posterior position with relative disproportion the fetal head may extend completely to a face presentation.
- It has been postulated that excessive tone in the extensor muscles may predispose to face presentation. This theory has been used to explain cases of primary face presentation which occur before the onset of labour. The development of face presentation during labour is called secondary face presentation.
- High parity is associated in the majority of cases.
- In most cases, other than parity, no obvious cause is found.

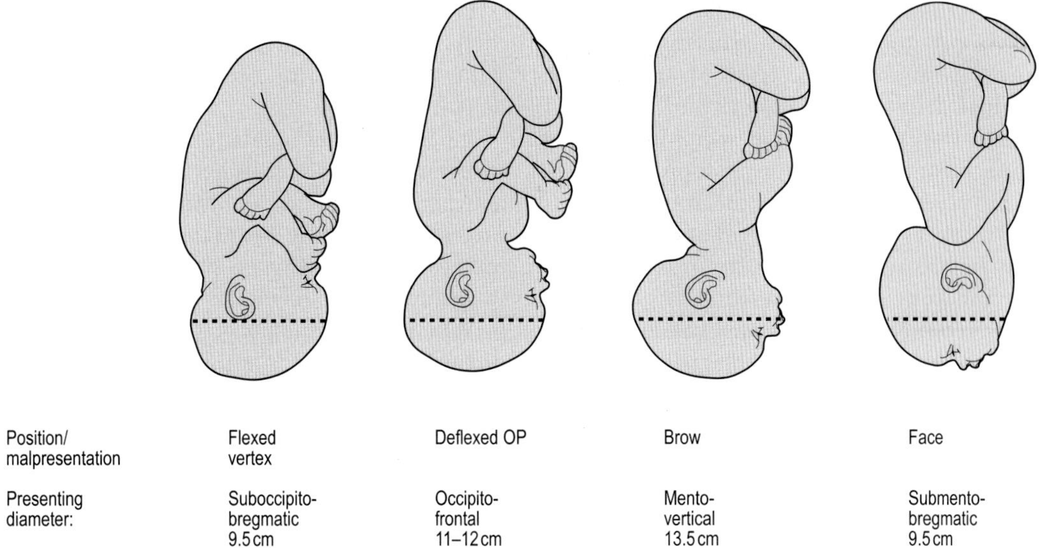

Figure 9.2 Positions and malpresentations of the fetal head.

Diagnosis

The presenting part of the face is between the chin and supraorbital ridges. Usually the characteristic landmarks of the eyes, nose, mouth and chin can be felt with the examining finger during labour. Considerable oedema often develops which may, to a degree, obscure these landmarks. Although the distinction is usually obvious there may be confusion in distinguishing between the mouth and the anus. If this is so, the finger is inserted into the orifice and the gum ridges can easily be felt as a distinguishing landmark.

Diagnosis before labour is rare but may be suspected if on abdominal examination the fetus is easily palpated and its back is lying dorsoanterior. In cases with a normally flexed vertex, palpation of the back and head will reveal only a slight depression at the neck between the back and occiput. In face presentations on the other hand, with the head extended, there is a marked depression between the back and occiput. If there is clinical suspicion, ultrasound will establish or refute the diagnosis.

The position of a face presentation is defined with the chin as the denominator and is therefore recorded as mento-anterior, mento-posterior or mento-transverse, left or right accordingly. The majority of cases are mento-anterior.

Management

On the rare occasions that face presentation is diagnosed before labour a careful ultrasound examination should be made to exclude structural fetal anomalies. One can make the case for observation until the onset of labour or full term, on the grounds that a number of these cases will revert spontaneously to a normal flexed vertex position. However, if face presentation persists and the fetus is normal, it should be delivered by elective caesarean section.

When the diagnosis is made in labour a gross fetal anomaly should be excluded and clinical pelvimetry should rule out obvious pelvic contraction or deformity. The position of the face presentation is then assessed. Depending upon the estimated fetal weight, the position, station, clinical assessment of pelvic capacity and the progress of labour the following guidelines may be used:

If the fetus has an anomaly incompatible with life then progress to vaginal delivery should be followed.

If the position is mento-anterior, which presents the same diameters as a flexed vertex, if the fetus is normal or small in size and the pelvis is of good capacity, progress can be followed with the expectation of spontaneous vaginal delivery. The majority of cases with mento-transverse position will rotate to the more favourable anterior position.

Fifty years ago, when the morbidity and mortality associated with caesarean section was high, vaginal manipulation was used to try and convert face presentations to a vertex presentation. This was carried out at advanced or full cervical dilatation and usually done under deep general anaesthesia with uterine relaxation. In a previous edition of this book Chassar Moir (1964) described his technique:

> *'In cases discovered early in labour (mentolateral) positions, I succeeded in five consecutive cases in correcting the position to a vertex position by the simple intrauterine manipulation of hooking down the occiput with the fingers and simultaneously pressing up the chin and brow with the thumb, labour then proceeded normally in each case.'*

Nowadays, we would not advise such manipulation, except perhaps a tentative attempt which is most likely to succeed with a small fetus and a large pelvis. One would only continue with such a manoeuvre if it proved easy and atraumatic.

> *'When the chin is turned towards the pubis, at the lower part of that bone, the woman must be laid on her back, the forceps introduced ... and when the chin is brought out from under the pubis, the head must be pulled half round upwards; by which means, the fore and hind head will be raised from the perineum.'*
>
> **William Smellie**
> *A Treatise on the Theory and Practice of Midwifery. London: D. Wilson, 1752, p281*

Provided labour continues normally and there is good progress in the second stage with mento-anterior positions, spontaneous delivery is likely.

If progress is inadequate with mento-anterior positions consideration of forceps delivery is appropriate. One has to be very careful that there is adequate descent for safe forceps assisted delivery. Even when the face is visible at the vulva the cranium may not be fully through the pelvic brim. The guiding dictum is 'the head is higher than you think'. If forceps delivery is to be considered there should be no head palpable at the pelvic brim and the sacral hollow should be filled with the cranium. Either classical or Kielland's forceps can be used and in face presentations the chin replaces the occiput for orientation. If Kielland's forceps are used the directional buttons on the shanks should point toward the chin. With both types of forceps the blades are applied as for classical forceps to the occiput anterior positions (see Chapter 8). The orientation is along the mento-occipital diameter of the head. With the pelvic curve of the classical forceps the chin is between the heels of the blades and the face is beneath the level of the shanks (Fig 9.3). With Kielland's forceps the upper part of the blades is at the level of the supraorbital ridges with the face above the level of the shanks (Fig 9.4).

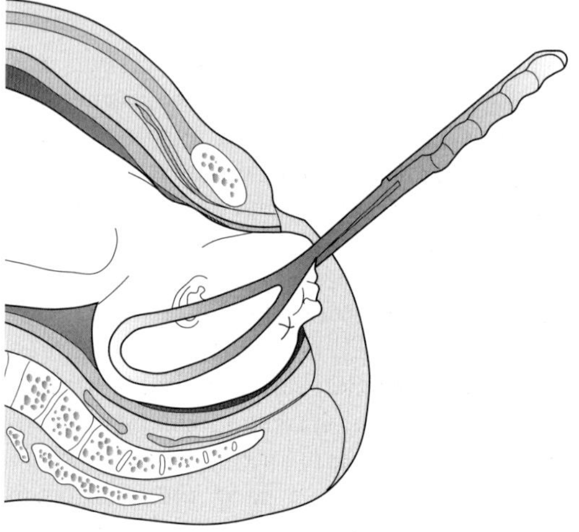

Figure 9.3 Face presentation, mento-anterior. Delivery with classical forceps.

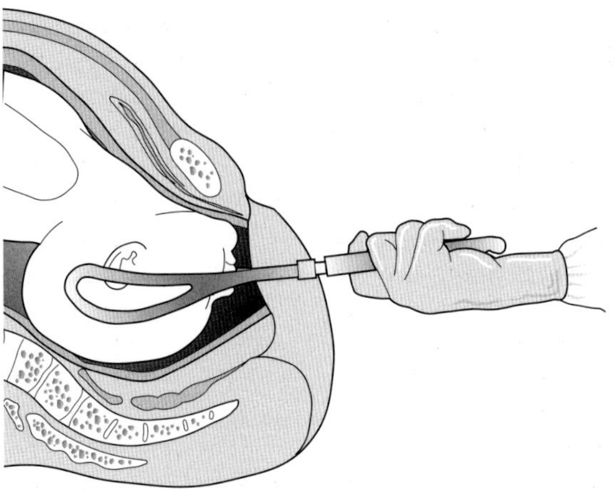

Figure 9.4 Face presentation, mento-anterior. Delivery with Kielland's forceps.

Once locked in position the handles of both types of forceps should be slightly lowered to give maximum extension of the head, which presents the narrowest diameter. With both types of forceps a slight downward traction is applied during a uterine contraction and with maternal effort until the chin is delivered beneath the symphysis. With the classical forceps the handles are gradually elevated up to about 45° to allow flexion of the occiput over the perineum. Using Kielland's forceps, with their lack of pelvic curve, the handles should only be elevated up to the horizontal level to achieve flexion and delivery of the occiput.

In cases of mento-posterior position which do not rotate to anterior during labour, vaginal delivery is impossible (Fig 9.5). In the past Kielland's forceps were sometimes used to rotate mento-posterior and mento-transverse cases to mento-anterior. However, the risks associated with this are considered excessive in modern obstetrics. Thus, these cases should be delivered by caesarean section.

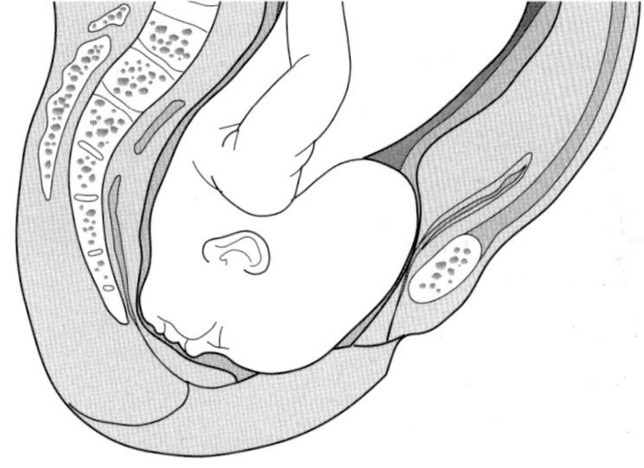

Figure 9.5 Face presentation, impacted mento-posterior position.

Brow presentation

In brow presentation the attitude of the fetal head is midway between the flexed vertex and face presentation. It is the most unfavourable of all cephalic presentations with its mento-vertical diameter of 13 cm in the term fetus. The incidence is approximately 1 in 1000–2000 births.

The potential causes are the same as those for face presentation, although the prevalence of lethal fetal anomalies is less with brow presentation than with face presentation. In a number of cases the cause is cephalopelvic disproportion, in which the fetal head deflexes progressively from vertex, to occipito-posterior, to brow.

Diagnosis

It is rare to diagnose brow presentation before the onset of labour. During labour the landmarks for the examining fingers are the root of the nose, the supraorbital ridges, and the anterior fontanelle. Over this presenting area, in neglected cases, considerable moulding and caput can occur, making the identification of these landmarks difficult. Usually, however, the supraorbital ridges and root of the nose can be identified.

> *'The child appearing in a very unnatural posture ... with the arm and the shoulder foremost. I then endeavoured with all the strength I had to bring back the arm and shoulder, but to no purpose, this being one of the most troublesome cases that can happen to a man-midwife ... I got my hand into the womb as well as I could ... At last I got hold of one foot, which whilst I was pulling toward me the arm that was before in the passage drew back within the womb of course, and the other foot following the first to the orifice of the womb, I joined them close together, and delivered the child, which proved a daughter and alive ...'*
>
> **Paul Portal**
> *The Compleat Practice of Men and Women Midwives. London: J. Johnson, 1763, p178–179*

Management

In a small number of cases brow presentation is associated with a small fetus in a capacious pelvis. In such cases labour may progress normally to spontaneous delivery. In the normally grown term fetus the wide presenting diameter, unless there is an exceptionally capacious pelvis, is incompatible with vaginal delivery. Attempts have been described with digital manipulation to try and flex the head to a vertex presentation – these are usually fruitless. The other alternative is to manually encourage deflexion to a face presentation. In modern obstetrics neither of these options is usually feasible or desirable. Thus, in the vast majority of cases with brow presentation, caesarean section should be performed.

Transverse lie

Transverse lie is the most unfavourable lie which the fetus can assume. At term the incidence is about 1 in 500 births. The fetus may be either dorso-anterior or dorso-posterior. In many cases the lie is oblique rather than transverse with either the head or breech occupying one iliac fossa. With a transverse or oblique lie in labour the most common presentation is the shoulder and sometimes the arm prolapses through the cervix (Fig 9.6).

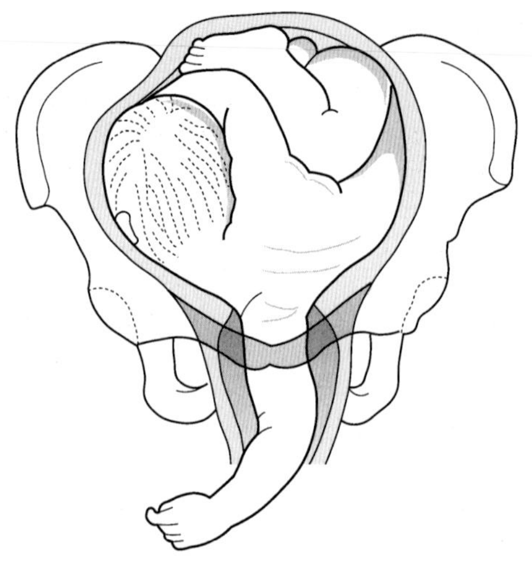

Figure 9.6 Shoulder presentation with prolapsed arm.

Causes

- Placenta praevia, which should be considered in all cases.
- Uterine anomaly – most often a septate or subseptate uterus. When this is the cause the fetus is usually relatively fixed in its position and not amenable to version.
- Polyhydramnios.
- Fetal anomaly – abnormal babies do abnormal things, including lying abnormally within the uterus. A dead, toneless fetus may also lie transversely.
- Fibroid in the lower uterine segment. On rare occasions an ovarian tumour may have the same effect by preventing the presenting part from entering the lower uterine segment.
- Gross prematurity.
- High parity. Both the uterine and abdominal musculature will lack tone, which may facilitate transverse or oblique lie of the fetus.
- Full bladder can on rare occasions prevent descent of either fetal pole into the lower uterine segment.

Diagnosis

Diagnosis may be suspected by simply inspecting the abdomen, where the uterus is enlarged transversely and shortened vertically. With palpation the emptiness of the lower pole of the uterus is obvious and the head and breech can usually be felt at each side connected by the transverse or obliquely lying fetal back. Only in cases of considerable maternal obesity should it be necessary to resort to ultrasound to confirm the diagnosis. However, ultrasound is usually advisable to rule out placenta praevia or structural fetal anomaly.

In labour the presentation can be confirmed by vaginal examination and it is usually the shoulder that comes to present. This is felt as a small rounded body and the palpable landmarks are the clavicle and the ribs. In a neglected labour after the membranes have ruptured one or more limbs may prolapse through the cervix. The most common is for an arm to prolapse but both a foot and an arm can prolapse together. The prolapsed hand, which may be quite oedematous, can be distinguished from a foot by the absence of the projecting heel (see Chapter 14).

Course of labour

There are four possible outcomes for a transverse/oblique lie in labour:

- As uterine tone increases in early labour while the membranes remain intact the fetus may convert to a longitudinal lie. This is most likely to happen when the aetiology is lax uterine musculature associated with high parity.
- The shoulder presents and is pushed down into the pelvis. This results in total obstruction and the uterus may become exhausted or rupture.
- Spontaneous delivery of the fetus with the body doubled-up (*partus conduplicato corpore*). This only occurs when the fetus is unusually small or macerated. The head and thorax or pelvis are pressed together and deliver doubled-up.
- Spontaneous evolution, in which the shoulder becomes impacted behind the symphysis and the trunk, the breech and limbs are driven past, followed by the shoulders and head (Fig 9.7). This is exceptionally rare and only occurs with a small premature or macerated fetus with a capacious maternal pelvis.

Management

There are three circumstances to consider in the management of transverse lie and shoulder presentation: late pregnancy before the onset of labour, during labour with the fetus alive and during labour with the fetus dead.

Late pregnancy before the onset of labour

When transverse or oblique lie is diagnosed ≥*36* weeks gestation, the common associated causes should be sought. This involves the use of ultrasound to rule out placenta praevia, fetal anomaly and multiple pregnancy. It is also essential to ensure that the gestational age is correct. If these causes are ruled out then external cephalic version should be carried out as outlined in Chapter 26. If this is successful and the fetus remains stable as a cephalic

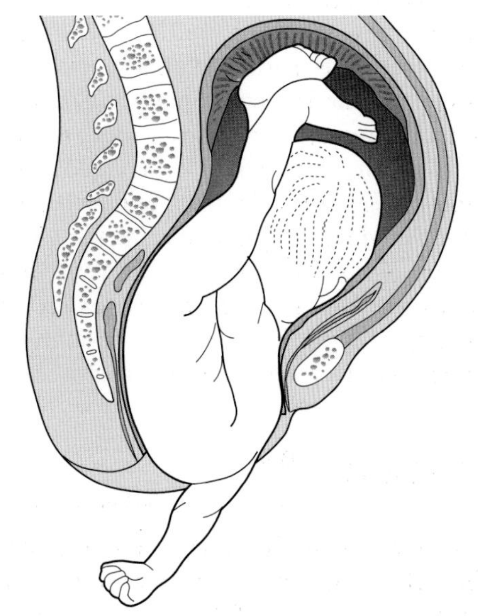

Figure 9.7 Spontaneous evolution.

Spontaneous evolution

'In the year 1772, I was called to a poor woman in Oxford Street ... I found the arm much swelled and pushed through the external parts in such a manner, that the shoulder nearly reached the perineum. The woman struggled vehemently with her pains, and during her continuance, I received the shoulder of the child to descend ... I remained at the bed-side til the child was expelled and I was very much surprised to find, that the breech and inferior extremities were expelled before the head, as if the case had originally been a presentation of the inferior extremities.'

Thomas Denman

Observations to prove that in cases where the upper extremities present, at the time of birth, the delivery may be affected by the spontaneous evolution of the child. Lond Med J 1784; 564–570

presentation, the rest of the antenatal care can be normal. The problem arises, and this is most often in cases of higher parity, when the lie remains unstable changing from day to day, or even hour to hour between transverse, oblique, cephalic, and breech. In such cases, close to term the risk of labour or spontaneous rupture of membranes occurring with the fetus transverse or oblique could result in umbilical cord prolapse or obstructed labour. In these cases it is best to admit the woman to the antenatal ward so that at the earliest signs of labour external cephalic version can be performed, or immediate caesarean section be carried out should there be spontaneous rupture of the membranes and prolapse of the umbilical cord or of an arm.

In many of these cases uterine tone increases in the days before labour and either spontaneous version or external cephalic version successfully stabilizes the fetus to a favourable presentation. In these cases, provided gestational age is a secure ≥38 weeks, a stabilizing induction can be considered. For a stabilizing induction the patient is taken to the labour ward, the lie is corrected to vertex presentation if necessary, and intravenous oxytocin is started as per the normal induction protocol (see Chapter 6). Once uterine contractions have become established a pelvic examination is performed and amniotomy carried out, after excluding cord presentation. The fetal head is carefully controlled with the other abdominal hand during this procedure and amniotic fluid slowly drained off until the head is well settled in the lower uterine segment on to the cervix.

If the transverse lie is not amenable to version then elective caesarean section should be carried out at 39 weeks gestation.

During labour with the fetus alive

In early spontaneous labour it is sometimes possible to carry out external cephalic version in between the uterine contractions. The mother's bladder should be emptied before version. This is most likely to be successful in patients with high parity as the cause of the transverse lie. Unless this is simple and in cases where labour is well established, caesarean section should be performed immediately.

Caesarean section for transverse and oblique lie requires careful appraisal of the lower uterine segment once the abdomen has been entered. Unless the membranes are intact and a broad well-developed lower uterine segment is present, which is not likely in these circumstances, a vertical incision should be made starting in the lower uterine segment. This incision will usually have to be extended into the upper uterine segment to allow adequate room to manoeuvre the fetus into position for delivery. If accessible it is usually better to deliver the feet first, unless the head is much lower.

During labour with the fetus dead

This is a situation which should rarely, if ever, be encountered in well developed health services. However, it still has to be confronted in areas of developing countries with limited hospital resources. In these circumstances decapitation with the Blond–Heidler saw is the most appropriate treatment if the skill exists to carry this out. The rationale and technique of this procedure is covered in Chapter 26. In regions where there is less experience with such procedures, or where the mother may not accept this management, caesarean section may be preferable.

Compound presentation

By definition, compound presentation is prolapse of part or all of one or more limbs in association with cephalic presentation and of prolapse of a hand or arm in association with breech presentation. In practical clinical terms, compound presentation is usually confined to cephalic presentations.

Any condition which interferes with the engagement of the fetal head may predispose to the prolapse of a limb or limbs along with the head. These include contracted pelvis, pelvic tumours and polyhydramnios. Prematurity and a dead macerated fetus are additional causes. It is very unusual for a foot to be alongside or below the fetal head, and if it is the fetus is usually so premature as to be pre-viable or it is macerated.

The commonest situation is a small fetus with a roomy pelvis and a hand and forearm beside and just below the head. Having ruled out any of the other serious causes it is usually a simple matter to push the hand and forearm back beside and above the fetal head. Retaining one's fingers in this position, subsequent uterine contractions will usually cause the fetal head to descend and the hand and arm to remain above. If the arm prolapses beside and in front of the head it obstructs labour and if it cannot be replaced delivery will have to be by caesarean section.

Bibliography

Breen JL, Weismeier E. Compound presentation: a survey of 131 patients. Obstet Gynecol 1968; 32:419–422.

Cruikshank DP, Cruikshank JE. Face and brow presentation: a review. Clin Obstet Gynecol 1981; 24:333–350.

Edwards RL, Nicholson HO. The management of the unstable lie in late pregnancy. J Obstet Gynaecol Br Commonw 1969; 76:713–715.

Kawatheker P, Kasturilal MS, Srinivis P, Sudda G. Etiology and trends in the management of transverse lie. Am J Obstet Gynecol 1973; 117:39–44.

Kovacs SG. Brow presentation. Med J Aust 1972; 280–284.

Laufe LE, Berkus MD. Assisted vaginal delivery: obstetric forceps and vacuum extraction techniques. New York: McGraw-Hill, 1992.

Moore EJT, Dennen EH. Management of persistent brow presentation. Obstet Gynecol 1955; 6:186–189.

O'Grady JP. Modern instrumental delivery. Baltimore: Williams and Wilkins, 1988:150–152.

Posner AC, Friedman S, Posner LB. Modern trends in the management of the face and brow presentations. Surg Gynecol Obstet 1957; 104:485–490.

Posner LB, Ruben EJ, Posner AC. Face and brow presentations: a continuing study. Obstet Gynecol 1963; 21:745–749.

Vacca A. The 'sacral hand wedge', a cause of arrest of descent of the fetal head during vacuum assisted delivery. Br J Obstet Gynaecol 2002; 109:1063–1065.

Weissberg SM, O'Leary JA. Compound presentation of the fetus. Obstet Gynecol 1973; 41:60–62.

10

Shoulder dystocia

'The delivery of the head with or without forceps may have been quite easy ... time passes. The child's face becomes suffused. It endeavours unsuccessfully to breathe. Abdominal efforts by the mother or by her attendants produce no advance, gentle head traction is equally unavailing. Usually equanimity forsakes the attendants. They push, they pull. Alarm increases. Eventually "by greater strength of muscles or by some infernal juggle" the difficulty appears to be overcome, and the shoulders and trunk of a goodly child are delivered. The pallor of its body contrasts with the plum coloured cyanosis of the face and the small quantity of freshly expelled meconium about the buttocks. It dawns upon the attendants that their anxiety was not ill-founded. The baby lies limp and voiceless, and only too often remains so despite all efforts and resuscitation.'

J Morris
Obstet Gynaecol Br Emp 1955; 62:302

It is a measure of the increasing clinical and medicolegal importance of shoulder dystocia that we devote a whole chapter to the topic which was covered in only one and a half pages in the last edition.

Shoulder dystocia occurs when the fetal head has delivered but the shoulders do not deliver spontaneously or with the normal amount of gentle downward traction. This is because one, or rarely both, shoulders remain trapped above the pelvic brim. The clinical diagnosis is confirmed when the head delivers but external rotation does not occur and the head recoils tightly against the perineum – the so-called 'turtle sign'. The fetal neck is neither visible nor palpable. The diagnosis may be based on the opinion of the accoucheur or, more objectively, by a head-to-completion-of-delivery interval of more than 60 seconds, or the need to use additional manoeuvres to deliver the shoulders.[1] The diagnosis is, however, to a large extent in the eye of the beholder, which, along with the varying prevalence of predisposing factors, accounts for the widely reported range of the condition from 1 in 50 to 1 in 500 cephalic deliveries. Perinatal death is rare but trauma and asphyxia are not uncommon and of increasing clinical and medicolegal relevance.

Pathophysiology

It is important to recognize the anatomical relationship between the fetus and pelvis so that the mechanism of shoulder dystocia and the rationale for its management can be understood. In addition, the potential reduction of fetal oxygenation during delivery of the head and shoulders is relevant.

Feto-pelvic relationships

Of the three diameters of the pelvic brim the anteroposterior is the narrowest, the oblique is larger and the transverse is the widest diameter. In spontaneous delivery the fetal head passes through the pelvic brim in the occipito-transverse position and the posterior shoulder descends via the sciatic notch or sacral bay. The anterior shoulder descends to the retropubic space and is accommodated by the obturator foramen. In the term fetus the bisacromial diameter is larger than the biparietal diameter and thus some flexibility and rotation of the shoulders is required to ensure their unobstructed descent through the pelvis. If the bisacromial diameter is large and the shoulders confront the pelvic brim in the narrow anteroposterior diameter the conditions are set for shoulder dystocia. In these cases the posterior shoulder almost always descends below the sacral promontory and it is the anterior shoulder that becomes impacted behind the pubic symphysis. On extremely rare occasions both shoulders may remain above the pelvic brim – bilateral shoulder dystocia – which requires considerable extension of the fetal neck and is usually associated with assisted mid-pelvic forceps or vacuum delivery.

Fetal oxygenation

With delivery of the head the volume of uterine contents is reduced and the uterus contracts down which diminishes or stops the blood flow and oxygenation to the intervillus space. Even though the infant's mouth and nose are delivered the fetal chest is compressed so that respiratory effort and oxygenation are impeded.

Complications

Fetal

- *Asphyxia* is progressive for the reasons outlined above. Provided the fetus is not hypoxic before shoulder dystocia occurs there should be 4–5 minutes before the possibility of permanent hypoxic damage.[2] Thus, there is time for the logical and systematic application of manoeuvres to safely deliver the infant before this occurs. On the other hand, if the fetus is already hypoxic when shoulder dystocia occurs the time to permanent hypoxic damage may be much shorter. In shoulder dystocia the combination of hypoxia, obstructed cerebral venous return and trauma during delivery renders the fetal brain vulnerable to damage.
- *Brachial plexus injury* is the most common of the serious fetal complications, occurring in 5–15% of neonates born after shoulder dystocia. The most common type is the Erb–Duchenne type involving C5 and 6 nerve roots. Rarely the whole brachial plexus will be injured, leading to a flail arm. Most cases of brachial plexus injury involve neuropraxia only, and in most series less than 10% have long-term disability. However, the range of disability is 5–50%.[3] Permanent brachial plexus palsy is one

of the commonest causes of obstetric litigation.

- *Fractures* are the most common complication, occurring in about 15% of infants with shoulder dystocia. The vast majority of these are clavicular, with fractures of the humerus accounting for less than 1%. Fracture or dislocation of the cervical spine is extremely rare but can be associated with desperate and ill-advised twisting manoeuvres of the fetal head. Fractures of the clavicle and humerus may be embarrassing to the accoucheur at the time, but they heal well with simple treatment and no long-term sequelae. It is the complications of fetal asphyxia and brachial plexus injury that potentially have the most serious sequelae, and management is therefore aimed at limiting these risks.

Maternal

- *Genital tract lacerations* are more common due to the tight feto-pelvic relationship and the additional room needed for the manoeuvres to overcome shoulder dystocia. Thus, extension of episiotomy and third and fourth degree tears are more common with shoulder dystocia. With more sphincter lacerations the potential exists for a higher incidence of long-term flatal and faecal incontinence.
- *Postpartum haemorrhage* is more common due to a combination of uterine atony and bleeding from lacerations.

Predisposing factors

Antepartum

There are a number of factors which increase the risk of shoulder dystocia and in most of these the common denominator is fetal macrosomia:

- Post-term pregnancy is associated with macrosomia. In addition, in the last weeks of pregnancy the fetal chest and shoulders continue to grow steadily while the biparietal diameter growth slows. This creates an unfavourable shoulder–head circumference ratio and increases the risk of shoulder dystocia.
- Both maternal obesity and excessive weight gain in pregnancy have been linked with large fetuses.
- Macrosomic infants of diabetic mothers have a singular risk of shoulder dystocia. The shoulder girth is composed of tissues that are insulin-sensitive and respond to hyperglycaemia and hyperinsulinism, while the head circumference and brain growth are less affected. As a result, infants of diabetic mothers tend to have a higher shoulder–head circumference ratio.

The association between excessive food intake and diabetes, obesity and weight gain in pregnancy has caused some to refer to shoulder dystocia as a 'disease of affluence'.

Intrapartum

Most cases of shoulder dystocia follow a normal progressive labour with spontaneous delivery or assisted low pelvic delivery and as such give no warning of impending trouble. However, the following patterns of labour increase the likelihood of shoulder dystocia:

- protraction/arrest in the late first stage of labour
- protraction/arrest of descent in the second stage of labour
- assisted mid-pelvis delivery.

The majority of cases of shoulder dystocia, however, occur in apparently normal labours with infants weighing less than 4000 grams. It seems likely that in many cases the cause may be a maladaptation between the descending shoulders and the pelvis, without an obvious anatomical abnormality in either.

Recurrent shoulder dystocia

The rate of repeat shoulder dystocia in a subsequent vaginal delivery has been reviewed in six series and the risk of recurrence ranges

Table 10.1 Recurrence of shoulder dystocia

Author	Years	Previous shoulder dystocia	Subsequent vaginal delivery	Recurrent shoulder dystocia Number	%
Smith et al[3]	1980–85	203	42	5	(9.8)
Baskett & Allen[4]	1980–89	254	93	1	(1.1)
Lewis et al[5]	1983–92	747	123	17	(13.8)
Flannelly & Simm[6]	1983–93	114	36	5	(13.9)
Olugbile & Mascarenhas[7]	1991–95	134	18	2	(11.1)
Ginsberg & Moisidis[8]	1993–99	602	66	11	(16.7)
Total		2054	378	41	(10.1)

from 1.1% to 16.7%.[4–9] The average recurrence rate was relatively low at 10.1% (Table 10.1). However, in a case with previous shoulder dystocia and brachial plexus injury or other complication, caesarean section could be justified in the next pregnancy.

Prediction and prevention

Unfortunately, attempts to find factors that will accurately predict shoulder dystocia and allow a practical prevention strategy have been unsuccessful. Most of the antepartum risk factors have fetal macrosomia as the underlying theme. Many of these risk factors are common, while the condition they predict, shoulder dystocia, is not. Furthermore, the risk of serious fetal injury associated with shoulder dystocia is rare. The hope that ultrasound prediction of fetal weight and more detailed ultrasound measurements such as shoulder width would provide an accurate level of risk have been unfulfilled. Indeed, for the macrosomic fetus clinical estimation of fetal weight is as accurate as that predicted by ultrasound. Even if one could predict fetal macrosomia accurately, this would be of limited value. About 95% of infants weighing over 4000 grams will not have shoulder dystocia. It has been suggested that elective caesarean section for fetuses weighing more than 4500 grams would reduce shoulder dystocia and fetal injury. A decision analysis model has shown that this strategy would be both clinically and cost ineffective; it was estimated that to prevent one permanent brachial plexus injury 3695 caesarean sections would be required.[10] Furthermore, the majority of cases of shoulder dystocia occur at fetal weight less than 4500 grams.

Thus, both the antepartum and intrapartum risk factors lack sensitivity and specificity. Having said that, there are individual cases with cumulative risk factors such as maternal diabetes and an estimated fetal weight > 4250 grams which may be best delivered by caesarean section. A combination of factors such as clinical fetal macrosomia with a protracted late first stage of labour and slow descent in the second stage requiring assisted mid-pelvic delivery may dictate that caesarean delivery would be more prudent.

Management

The important principle to remember is that the problem with the shoulders is at the level of the pelvic brim. Thus, traction or twisting movements involving the head are illogical, ineffective and potentially traumatic. It is extremely important not to put strong downward pressure on the fetal head as this is the most common iatrogenic cause of brachial plexus injury. Once the diagnosis of shoulder dystocia is made, summon assistance to help with positioning the woman for the necessary manoeuvres, and to provide neonatal resuscitation if required. Shoulder dystocia is one of the most panic-inducing situations in obstetrics and demands decisive equanimity from the obstetrician.

Analgesia

If the woman already has an epidural or pudendal block established, this should be sufficient analgesia for the required manoeuvres. If not, there is no time to establish these regional blocks, but rapid infiltration of the perineum with 1% xylocaine and inhalation analgesia can be provided.

McRobert's manoeuvre

With the woman in the recumbent position the maternal hips are slightly abducted and acutely flexed by bringing the knees towards the chest. This can be done by nursing personnel, family members, or even the patient herself by pulling behind both knees with her hands (Fig 10.1a). This manoeuvre does not increase the diameters of the pelvis but it does rotate the symphysis superiorly and straighten the lumbosacral angle. In so doing it facilitates descent of the posterior shoulder below the sacral promontory and, by flexing the fetal spine towards the anterior shoulder, helps dislodge the impacted shoulder. In addition, the angle of inclination of the pelvis is reduced so that the plane of the pelvic inlet is brought perpendicular to the expulsive forces (Fig 10.1b). The combination of these changes in the feto-pelvic relationship reduces the propulsion-extraction forces necessary to deliver the shoulders. This manoeuvre is simple and carries the least risk of trauma to mother and fetus. It is effective in the majority of mild to moderate cases of shoulder dystocia and is recommended as the first line of treatment.

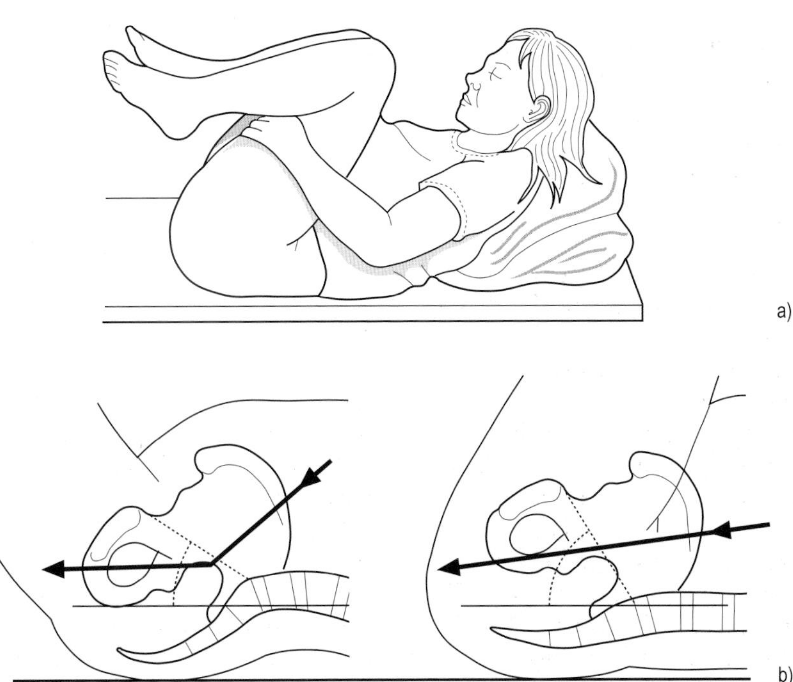

Figure 10.1 (a) McRoberts' manoeuvre. (b) Effect is to reduce both the lumbo-sacral angle and the angle of pelvic inclination.

Rotate fetal shoulders to the oblique diameter

The anteroposterior diameter of the pelvic brim is the narrowest so it is logical to try and rotate the fetal shoulders to the wider oblique and transverse diameters either as a prelude to, or in combination with other manoeuvres. Under no circumstances should one twist the head in an attempt to rotate the shoulders. It will not work and it risks trauma to the brachial plexus and cervical spine. Generally one cannot get one or two fingers up under the pubic symphysis to the anterior shoulder but the posterior shoulder has usually descended below the pelvic brim and is more accessible. Thus, with two fingers posteriorly in the vagina and with pressure on the posterior fetal axilla and scapula try and push the shoulder off the midline to the wider oblique and transverse diameters (Fig 10.2).

Suprapubic pressure

At the same time directed suprapubic pressure behind the fetal scapula can be provided by an assistant to push the shoulder off the midline, lateral and downwards. Pushing behind the scapula tends to adduct the shoulders which is a narrower diameter than the abducted shoulders. An assistant may use this technique in association with McRobert's manoeuvre (Fig 10.3)

If concomitant vaginal and suprapubic pressure is being applied the vaginal fingers push on the anterior fetal axilla, while the abdominal pressure is applied behind the scapula. If vaginal pressure alone is being used the pressure is best applied in the posterior fetal axilla to aid adduction and a reduction in the bisacromial diameter.

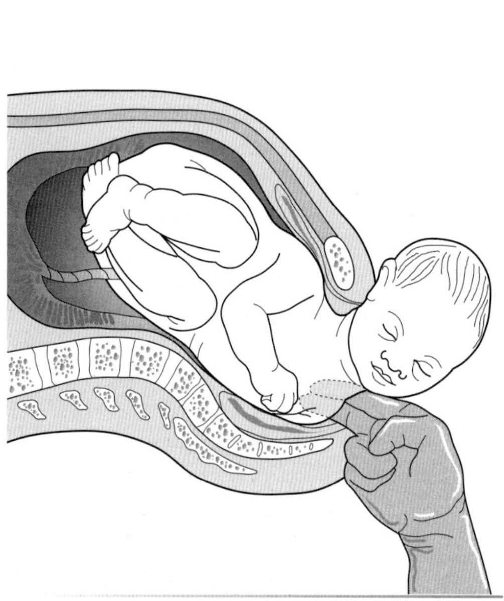

Figure 10.2 Rotation of fetal shoulders off the midline to the larger oblique diameter.

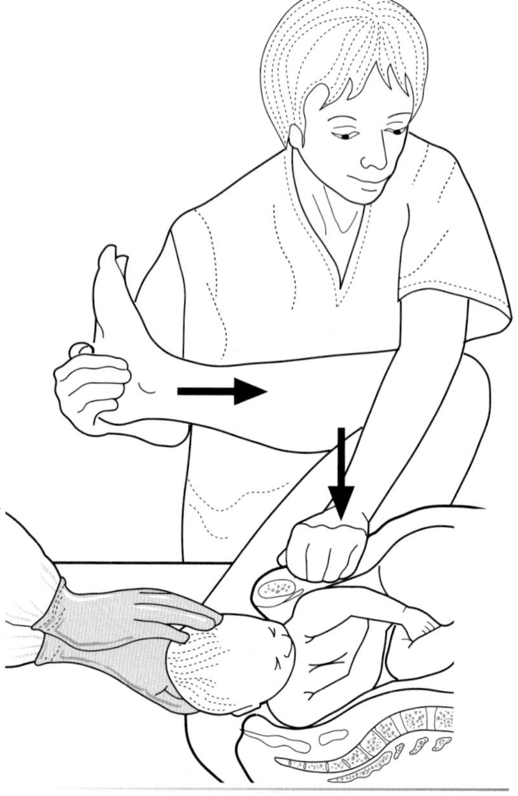

Figure 10.3 Assistant applies directed suprapubic pressure and facilitates McRoberts' manoeuvre.

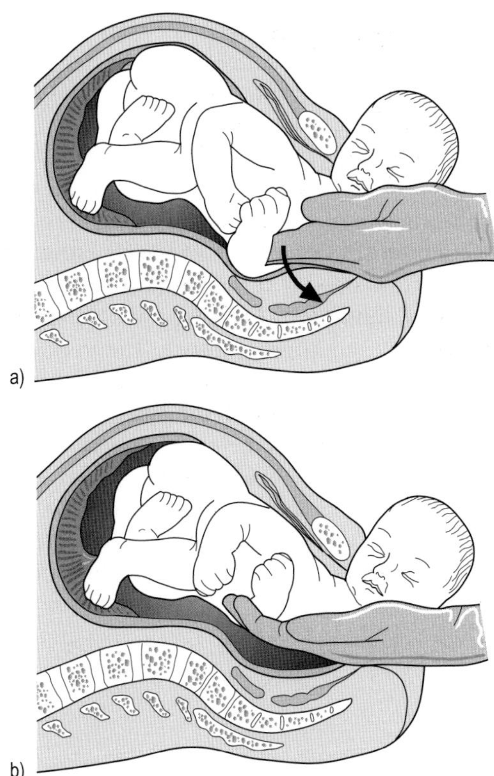

Figure 10.4 Delivery of the posterior arm.

Delivery of the posterior arm

Other than the very rare case of bilateral shoulder dystocia, the posterior shoulder will have descended beneath the sacral promontory into the sacral bay and be accessible. Pass the hand into the vagina, along with fetal humerus to the elbow. In Pinard's manoeuvre, pressure in the antecubital fossa should help flex the fetal forearm and bring it within reach. In practice, however, the fetus is so tightly lodged in the pelvis that this may not be successful. If so, one just has to reach further along the fetal forearm until one can grasp it and pull the arm across the fetal chest to delivery. Once the posterior arm has been delivered the transverse diameter of the shoulders is reduced and the trunk and anterior shoulder may deliver easily (Fig 10.4). If not, support the posterior shoulder and trunk of the fetus and rotate them 180° – which will bring the anterior shoulder round to become the posterior shoulder, below the level of the pelvic brim, and allow its delivery. Delivery of the posterior shoulder is one of the manoeuvres most likely to cause fracture of the clavicle and/or humerus. However, it is almost always successful in delivering the fetus and these fractures heal well without long-term sequelae; whereas the alternatives of fetal hypoxia, brachial plexus injury, and cervical spine injury may not.

Woods' screw manoeuvre

Some 60 years ago Woods studied the relationship between the fetal shoulders and the pelvic bony landmarks which they must traverse: symphysis, sacral promontory and coccyx.[11] Using wooden models he showed that the relationship between the fetal shoulders and these bony landmarks was

Woods' Screw Manoeuvre

'After the head has been born the shoulders of the baby resemble a longitudinal section of a screw engaged in three threads, the "pubic thread" the "promontory" thread and the "coccyx" thread. Any pulling on the baby's neck or axilla is mechanically incorrect because it violates a simple, well-known law of physics applicable to the screw ... A downward thrust is made with the left hand on the buttocks of the baby. At the same time, two fingers of the right hand, on the anterior aspect of the posterior shoulder, make gentle clockwise pressure upward around the circumference of the arc, and past 12 o'clock. The posterior shoulder is now delivered. With pressure applied downward from above with the left hand, the two fingers of the right hand make gentle counter-clock wise pressure upward around the circumference around the arc and past 12 o'clock, and the remaining shoulder is delivered.'

Charles E Woods
A principle of physics applicable to shoulder delivery. Am J Obstet Gynecol 1943; 45:796

similar to the threads of a screw. It is not possible to push or pull the shoulders through but they can be 'corkscrewed' through the pelvis by rotating the shoulders 180°. In this technique two fingers are placed in the vagina on the anterior aspect of the posterior fetal axilla and pushed off the midline to rotate the fetus 180° (Fig 10.5). Because the posterior shoulder is below the pelvic brim, as it rotates it remains at that level and once in the anterior position is accessible for delivery. During this 180° rotation the former anterior shoulder which started above the pelvic brim rotates to become the posterior shoulder and in so doing rotates below the level of the pelvic brim. Woods' screw manoeuvre correctly defines the relationship between the fetal shoulders and the pelvic brim and provides a logical solution, in the same manner that Løvset's manoeuvre does for delivery of extended arms in breech presentation.

All-fours manoeuvre

In this manoeuvre the woman is guided to the all-fours position on her hands and knees. In this position gravity should aid descent of the posterior shoulder downwards and forwards beneath the sacral promontory. Theoretically, the flexibility of the sacro-iliac joints may allow a 1–2 cm increase in the anteroposterior diameter of the pelvic brim. With gentle traction the posterior shoulder is delivered first. Assisting the woman into this position at this stressful and dramatic point of delivery, particularly with epidural analgesia, can require

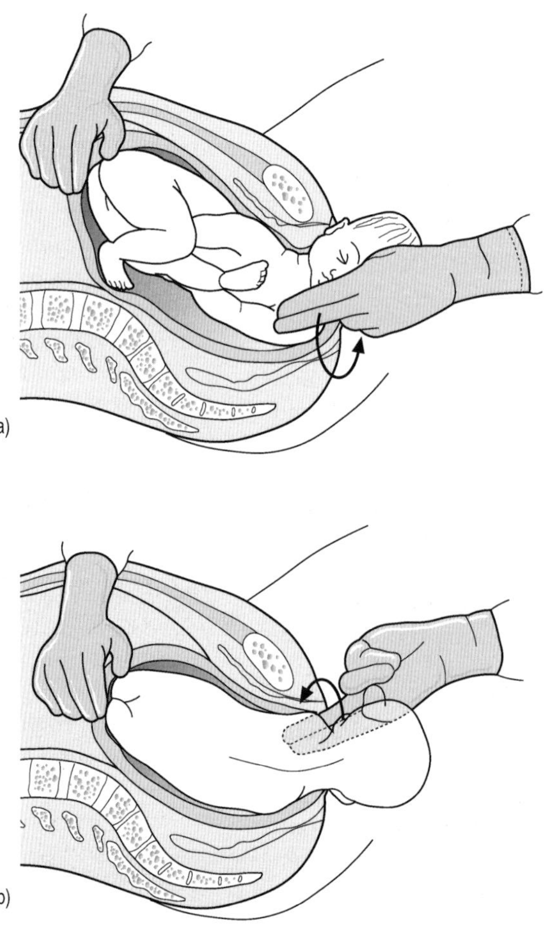

Figure 10.5 Woods' screw manoeuvre.

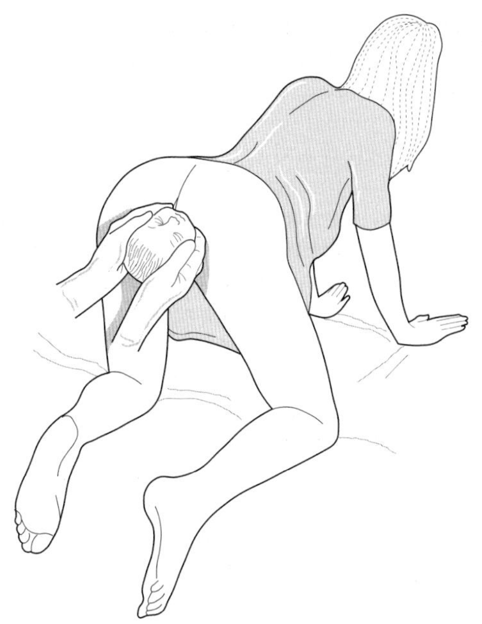

Figure 10.6 All-fours manoeuvre.

a number of personnel. It has been suggested that midwives may ask the woman to practise getting into this position during the first stage of labour in case it becomes necessary at delivery. This manoeuvre was originally observed by an American midwife working with indigenous midwives in Guatamala.[12] Experience with this technique is limited but promising, and it is worth a try if the standard manoeuvres have failed (Fig 10.6).

Cephalic replacement (Zavanelli manoeuvre)

This technique may have application in very rare circumstances in which bilateral shoulder dystocia exists or the more traditional methods of dealing with shoulder dystocia have failed. The normal mechanism of delivery of the fetal head is reversed by grasping the head, rotating it to the occipito-anterior position and flexing the head, which allows replacement in the vagina (Fig 10.7). In some cases, presumably those with bilateral shoulder dystocia, the head will return to the vagina with remarkable ease. In others it will be necessary to give uterine tocolysis to assist this manoeuvre. This would usually be done with intravenous nitroglycerine or terbutaline (see Chapter 26). Once the fetal head has been returned to the vagina the fetal heart is monitored and usually returns to normal. Preparations are then made for caesarean section.

While this technique is often successful there can be associated maternal morbidity with uterine rupture in up to 5% of cases and blood transfusion required in some 10%.[13,14] Perinatal death and morbidity from asphyxia and trauma are also encountered. These may have been due to the other methods tried and failed before cephalic replacement. This is a technique that should be remembered for the very rare occasion, perhaps once in a lifetime, that it will be required. If shoulder dystocia occurs and the sacral bay is explored and the posterior shoulder has not descended, this is probably the ideal case for cephalic replacement. If the other more traditional techniques fail it is important not to resort to trauma but to consider cephalic replacement.

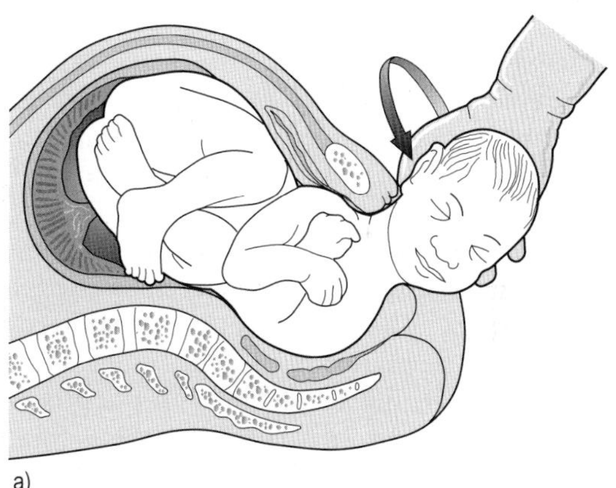

a)

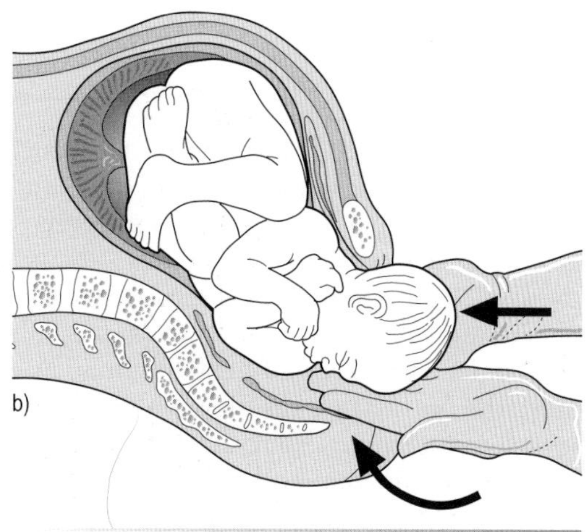

b)

Figure 10.7 Cephalic replacement.

Abdominal rescue

An even more rare alternative approach has been proposed for cases in which both the traditional manoeuvres and cephalic replacement have failed. Provided the infant is still alive a lower segment caesarean incision is performed. This allows elevation of the anterior shoulder and with manipulation the shoulder is rotated to the oblique position, facilitating descent of the posterior shoulder beneath the promontory where it can then be delivered directly. This is followed by rotation of the fetal body and rotation of the former anterior shoulder beneath the pelvic brim to allow its delivery also. This is an exceptionally rare endeavour and would really only be appropriate under remarkable circumstances, with the fetus still alive and bilateral shoulder dystocia unresponsive to cephalic replacement.

Symphysiotomy

Symphysiotomy continues to have a role in developing countries as an alternative to caesarean section in cases of cephalo-pelvic disproportion. Its use in cases of shoulder dystocia unresponsive to other methods of treatment has been suggested. However, there are no published series of its successful use for this purpose. The performance of symphysiotomy can be carried out rapidly under local anaesthesia by those familiar with the procedure (see Chapter 26). There may, therefore, be rare circumstances – both geographical and clinical – in which it may have application.

Cleidotomy

Deliberate fracture of the clavicle to reduce the bisacromial diameter and make the shoulders more flexible is an option. However, it is not always easy to deliberately fracture the clavicle of a term fetus. Furthermore, the underlying subclavian vessels are vulnerable to trauma. The increased flexibility may also make the brachial plexus more vulnerable to stretching and injury. Thus, cleidotomy is usually reserved for the dead fetus or an anomaly incompatible with life (e.g. anencephaly). It is usually performed using strong, straight scissors (see Chapter 26).

Fundal pressure

It is often stated, and cited in medicolegal cases, that fundal pressure should not be used as it is illogical and can only compound the problem by forcing the anterior shoulder against the unyielding symphysis. Used in isolation, fundal pressure is not indicated in cases of shoulder dystocia. However, in many instances, particularly with regional anaesthesia, maternal propulsive effort may be lacking. In such cases fundal pressure may be acceptable if it is used in conjunction with the other manoeuvres aimed at rotating and overcoming the shoulder dystocia.

Shoulder dystocia is one of those testing times in the life of an obstetrician. Most cases occur without identifiable risk factors in spontaneous or low pelvic assisted deliveries. Thus, all personnel who deliver babies must have an understanding of the rationale and techniques of the manoeuvres used to deal with this complication. There is much to be said for regular mannikin drills to achieve this level of preparedness.[5,15] There is no sequence of the accepted manoeuvres to deal with shoulder dystocia that has been shown to be superior. There is some logic, however, in starting with the indirect methods – McRoberts' manoeuvre and directed suprapubic pressure – before moving to methods that involve direct manipulation of the fetus. In most obstetric units all personnel working on labour wards are given recurrent CPR training, and yet the need to deal with shoulder dystocia is much more common than the need to apply CPR.

After a delivery involving shoulder dystocia it is essential that the personnel provide an immediate and detailed written report on the chart outlining the sequence of events and the manoeuvres used. This is necessary for both clinical audit and medicolegal reasons. The obstetrician should also review events with the woman and if there is a brachial plexus injury the appropriate follow-up should be arranged. This must include regular information and progress reports for the parents.[16]

The manoeuvres to deal with shoulder dystocia are outlined in Figure 10.8.

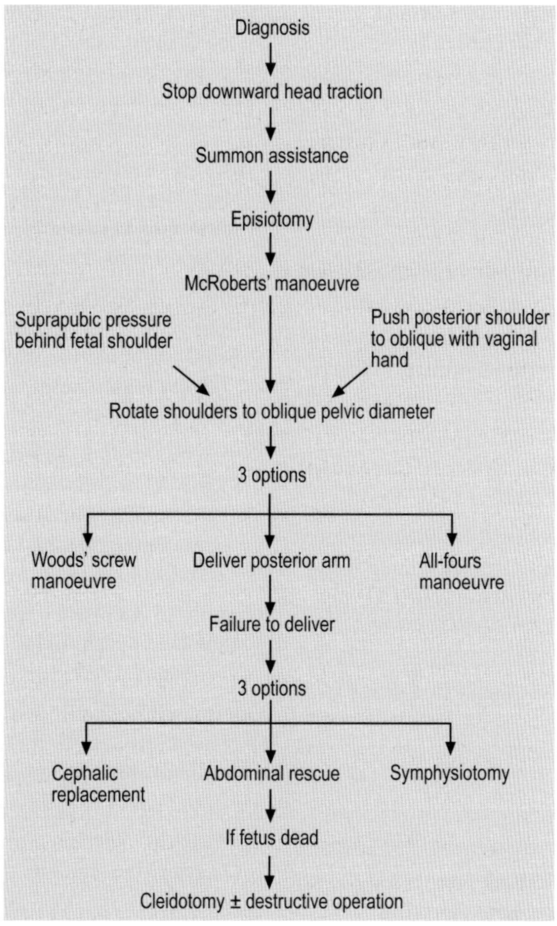

Figure 10.8 Management of shoulder dystocia.

References

1. Spong CY, Beall M, Rodrigues D, Ross MG. An objective definition of shoulder dystocia: prolonged head-to-body delivery intervals and/or the use of ancillary obstetric manoeuvres. Obstet Gynecol 1995; 86:433–441.
2. Wood C, Ng K, Hounslow D, Benning H. Time: an important variable in normal delivery. J Obstet Gynaecol Br Cwlth 1973; 80:295–298.
3. Pondaag W, Malessy MJA, Van Dijk JG, Thomeer RTW. Natural history of obstetric brachial plexus palsy: a systematic review. Develop Med Child Neurol 2004; 46:138–144.
4. Smith RB, Lance C, Pearson JF. Shoulder dystocia: what happens at the next delivery? Br J Obstet Gynaecol 1994; 101:713–715.
5. Baskett TF. Shoulder dystocia. Best Pract Res Clin Obstet Gynaecol 2002; 16:57–68.
6. Lewis DF, Raymond RC, Perkins MB. Recurrence rate of shoulder dystocia. Am J Obstet Gynecol 1995; 172:1369–1371.
7. Flannelly G, Simm A. A study of delivery following shoulder dystocia. British Congress of Obstetrics and Gynaecology, Dublin 4–7 July 1995. Abstract 516. London: Royal College of Obstetricians and Gynaecologists.
8. Olugbile A, Mascarenhas L. Review of shoulder dystocia at the Birmingham Women's Hospital. J Obstet Gynaecol 2000; 20:267–270.
9. Ginsberg NA, Moisidis C. How to predict recurrent shoulder dystocia. Am J Obstet Gynecol 2001; 184:1427–1430.
10. Rouse DJ, Owen J, Goldenberg RL, Cliver SP. The effectiveness and costs of elective

caesarean section for fetal macrosomia diagnosed by ultrasound. JAMA 1996; 276:1490–1496.

11. Woods CE. A principle of physics as applicable to shoulder delivery. Am J Obstet Gynecol 1943; 45:796–805.
12. Bruner JP, Drummond SB, Meenan AL, Gaskin IM. All-fours maneuver for reducing shoulder dystocia during labor. J Reprod Med 1998; 43:439–443.
13. Sandberg EC. Zavanelli maneuver: twelve years of recorded experience. Obstet Gynecol 1999; 93:312–317.
14. Vaithilingam N, Davies D. Cephalic replacement for shoulder dystocia: three cases. Br J Obstet Gynaecol 2005; 112:674–675.
15. Crofts JF, Attilakos G, Read M, Sibanda T, Draycott TJ. Shoulder dystocia training using a new birth training mannequin. Br J Obstet Gynaecol 2005; 112: 997–999.
16. Bellew M, Kay SP. Early parental experiences of obstetric brachial plexus palsy. J Hand Surg 2003; 28: 339–346.

Bibliography

Allen R, Sorab J, Gonik B. Risk factors for shoulder dystocia: an engineering study of clinician-applied forces. Obstet Gynecol 1991; 77:352–355.

Allen RH, Rosenbaum TC, Ghidini A, Poggi SH, Spong CY. Correlating head-to-body delivery intervals with neonatal depression in vaginal births that result in permanent brachial plexus injury. Am J Obstet Gynecol 2002; 187:839–842.

American College of Obstetricians and Gynecologists. Practice Bulletin No. 40. Shoulder dystocia. Washington, DC: ACOG 2002. (Obstet Gynecol 2002; 100:1045–1050).

Bager B. Perinatally acquired brachial plexus palsy – a persisting challenge. Acta Pediatr 1997; 86:1214–1219.

Baskett TF, Allen AC. Perinatal implications of shoulder dystocia. Obstet Gynecol 1995; 86:14–17.

Baskett TF. Prediction and management of shoulder dystocia. In: Bonnar J, ed. Recent advances in obstetrics and gynaecology. Vol. 21. Edinburgh: Church Livingstone, 2001:45–54.

Beall MH, Spong CY, Ross MG. A randomised controlled trial of prophylactic maneuvers to reduce head-to-body delivery time in patients at risk for shoulder dystocia. Obstet Gynecol 2003; 102:31–35.

CESDI (Confidential Enquiry into Stillbirths and Deaths in Infancy). 5th Annual Report. London: Maternal and Child Health Research Consortium, 1998:73–79.

Crofts JE, Bartlett C, Ellis D, Hunt LP, Fox R, Draycott TJ. Training for shoulder dystocia: a trial of simulation using low-fidelity and high-fidelity mannequins. Obstet Gynecol 2006; 108:1477–1485.

Deering S, Poggi S, Macedonia C, Gherman R, Satin AJ. Improving resident competency in the management of shoulder dystocia with simulation training. Obstet Gynecol 2004; 103:1224–1228.

Dimitry ES. Cephalic replacement a desperate solution for shoulder dystocia. J Obstet Gynaecol 1989; 10:49–50.

Gherman RB. Shoulder dystocia: an evidence-based evaluation of the obstetric nightmare. Clin Obstet Gynecol 2002; 45:345–362.

Gherman RB. A guest editorial: new insights to shoulder dystocia and brachial plexus palsy. Obstet Gynecol Surv 2002; 58:1–2.

Goodwin TM, Banks E, Miller LK, Phalen JP. Catastrophic shoulder dystocia and emergency symphysiotomy. Am J Obstet Gynecol 1997; 177:463–464.

Gonik B, Stringer CA, Held B. An alternative maneuver for management of shoulder dystocia. Am J Obstet Gynecol 1983; 145:882–884.

Gonik B, Allen R, Sorab J. Objective evaluation of the shoulder dystocia phenomenon: effect of maternal pelvic orientation on force reduction. Obstet Gynecol 1989; 74:44–48.

Gurewitsch ED, Kim EJ, Yang JH, Outland KE, McDonald MK, Allen RH. Comparing McRoberts' and Rubin's manoeuvres for initial management of shoulder dystocia: an objective evaluation. Am J Obstet Gynecol 2005; 192:153–160.

Hartfield VJ. Symphysiotomy for shoulder dystocia. Am J Obstet Gynecol 1986; 155:228.

Heazell AE, Judge JK, Bhatti NR. A retrospective study to determine if umbilical cord pH correlates with duration of delay between delivery of the head and body in shoulder dystocia. J Obstet Gynaecol 2004; 24:776–777.

Kwek K, Yeo GS. Shoulder dystocia and injuries: prevention and management. Curr Opin Obstet Gynecol 2006; 18:123–128.

Leigh TH, James CE. Medico-legal commentary: shoulder dystocia. Br J Obstet Gynaecol 1998; 105:815–817.

Mehta SH, Blackwell SC, Bujold E, Sokol RJ. What factors are associated with neonatal injury following shoulder dystocia? J Perinatol 2006; 26:85–88.

Menticoglou SM. A modified technique to deliver the posterior arm in severe shoulder dystocia. Obstet Gynecol 2006; 108:755–757.

Poggi SH, Spong CY, Allen RH. Prioritizing posterior arm delivery during severe shoulder dystocia. Obstet Gynecol 2003; 101:1068–1072.

Royal College of Obstetricians and Gynaecologists. Guidelines No. 42. Shoulder dystocia. London: RCOG Press, 2006.

Rubin A. Management of shoulder dystocia. JAMA 1964; 189;835–837.

11

Caesarean section

Caesarean section represents the most significant operative intervention in all of obstetrics. Its development and application has saved the lives of countless mothers and infants. On the other hand, its inappropriate use can be a direct and avoidable cause of maternal mortality and morbidity. For these reasons, caesarean section probably represents the largest source of controversy and debate in modern obstetrics. The frequency with which it is carried out continues to rise and has, in many maternity services, reached rates which Munro Kerr and his contemporaries would have found wholly perplexing. Twenty-five years ago Myerscough wrote in the last edition of this textbook that the incidence of caesarean section in UK National Health Service Hospitals was almost 6% and that figures of 15% or even more were not unknown. It would now be difficult to find many such hospitals with a rate less than 15% and figures of 30% or more are not unknown. Some national caesarean delivery rates even exceed 30%.

Historical Background

Caesarean section is almost certainly one of the oldest operations in surgery with its origins lost in the mists of antiquity and mythology – as historians are wont to say when they don't know. It has probably been performed by traumatic accident or postmortem for several millennia. Ancient myth and legend has it that Aesculapius and Bacchus, the Gods of Medicine and Wine respectively, were born by caesarean section.[1] *Thus, at least in legend, those born by caesarean section are in good company.*

Historical Background

The origin of the word 'caesarean' is unclear. The weak myth that Julius Caesar was born by this route is contradicted by the fact that his mother survived his birth by many years. It is likely that the term comes from the lex regia *or royal law legislated by one of the early kings of Rome, Numa Pompilius in 715 BC.*[2] *This law proclaimed that women who died before delivering their infant had to have the infant removed through the abdomen before burial. This law continued under the ruling Caesars when it was called* lex caesarea.

Traumatic caesarean sections have probably occurred throughout the course of history during war, acts of violence and accidents. Among the more well documented are those in which the horns of cattle have torn open the woman's abdomen and uterus.[3] *One of the best known cases was reported from Zaandam, Holland in 1647, in which a bull attacked a farmer and his wife tearing open her abdomen and uterus with its horn.*[4] *The woman and her husband later died but the infant survived. Self-performed caesarean section has probably been carried out for many centuries as some women, alone and in desperation, sought to relieve the unrelenting pain of non-progressive labour. Authentic cases are reported from the 18th century.*[1,5,6] *Caesarean section performed by lay persons also has a long history. One of the earliest reported cases in 1500 was by Jacob Nufer, a swine gelder, who delivered his wife after several days of apparent labour.*[1] *There was some doubt whether this was an abdominal pregnancy or a caesarean section. Apparently both the mother and infant survived.*[7] *In Northern Ireland in 1738 Mary Donnally, an illiterate but experienced lay midwife, carried out the first caesarean with survival of the mother in the British Isles.*[8]

The first witnessed and documented caesarean section by a physician was performed by Jeremias Trautmann in Wittenberg, Germany in 1610.[1] *However, a number of obstetric texts in the 16th and 17th centuries described the rare performance of caesarean section in cases of contracted pelvis. From the 16th to the 18th centuries the prevailing medical wisdom was strongly against caesarean section, with its almost inevitable fatal outcome for the mother. This viewpoint is summed up in the quote by the prominent Dublin obstetrician Fielding Ould (1710–1789) in 1742: 'Repugnant, not only to all rules of theory or practice, but even of humanity'.*[9]

The reasons for the high mortality in the pre-anaesthetic era was that caesarean sections were usually performed after prolonged labour on women who were dehydrated, exhausted and infected. In addition, after removal of the fetus the uterus was not sutured, adding haemorrhage to the morbidity equation. Lebas first advocated suturing the uterus in 1769 but his advice was not followed for a century.[2] *In addition to haemorrhage, sepsis was the commonest cause of death. Eduardo Porro (1842–1902) of Pavia, Italy, carefully studied this problem and, after experiments with animals, he performed a caesarean section followed by subtotal hysterectomy in 1876.*[10] *He sutured the cervical stump to the lower end of the abdominal wound to control the haemorrhage and to exteriorize any septic drainage. By controlling the haemorrhage and sepsis Porro dramatically reduced the maternal mortality by about half from its usual rate of 80–90%.*[11]

Historical Background

Throughout the 19th century obstetricians devised techniques to try and reduce the risk of sepsis and to preserve the uterus; including a lateral extraperitoneal approach by Ferdinand Ritgen (1787–1867) of Giessen in 1821.[12] Fritz Frank (1856–1923) modified the transperitoneal operation by suturing the edges of the incised lower uterine segment visceral peritoneum to the margins of the abdominal wall incision to contain any sepsis and promote its drainage.[12]

Ferdinand Kehrer (1837–1914) of Hiedelberg is one of the under-appreciated contributors to the development of the modern caesarean section.[4,12] In 1881 he performed a transverse lower segment caesarean section, virtually as it is done today.[13] He emphasized the need for careful suturing of the uterine muscle and a separate suture of the peritoneum over the lower uterine segment – the Doppelnaht *or 'double layer' technique. About a year later Max Sänger (1853–1903), working in Leipzig, emphasized the need for careful suturing of the uterine incision which he performed longitudinally in the uterus and called the classical caesarean incision.[11,14] It was Sänger's classical caesarean section that held sway while Kehrer's transverse lower segment technique was forgotten. The classical caesarean section was adopted in Britain, most notably by Murdoch Cameron in Glasgow. Cameron was confronted by a great demand for the procedure because his city had seen an enormous growth of population, especially of poor migrant workers. Many of his patients lived in conditions guaranteed to produce skeletal rickets. Poor housing, poor diet, atmospheric pollution and consequent lack of exposure to sunlight meant that Vitamin D deficiency was rife. In 1888 he began a series of elective classical caesarean sections on rachitic dwarfs which was immediately and dramatically successful. In the first 2 years, all but one of the 23 mothers and all the infants survived[15] (Fig 11.1).*

In addition to careful suturing of the classical uterine incision, Cameron owed his success to two factors. The first was his recognition that the procedure should be carried out before the mother's condition was compromised by exhaustion and the associated infection of a long obstructed labour. This required that the diagnosis of a hopelessly contracted pelvis should be made before, or at least early in labour. This required the refinement of the clinical science of pelvimetry in the era before x-rays, and depended on the digital assessment of the shape and capacity of the pelvis. The first case was the subject of fierce argument among Cameron and his colleagues, the pelvis being considered 'borderline' with an obstetric conjugate of 4 cm! Cameron's second advantage derived from his use of a vulcanized rubber ring which he effectively applied as a tourniquet around the lower part of the uterus after delivery of the infant, constricting the blood flow to the uterus while the wound was repaired. The success of this series of cases resounded across and beyond Europe and was a milestone in the operation's journey from a desperate and usually futile gesture to an acceptable clinical option.

Munro Kerr was a 20-year-old medical student when Murdoch Cameron began his celebrated series and would have undoubtedly attended the Glasgow Royal Maternity Hospital at around that time. He cannot possibly have been unaware of this dramatic development and seems likely to have been attracted

Historical Background

to obstetrics by the work of Cameron, whom he would succeed 39 years later as Regius Professor of Midwifery in that city. Indeed, it was Munro Kerr who would be largely responsible for the change from the classical incision to the low transverse incision. When Kehrer performed his low transverse procedure it was to reduce and contain the risk of sepsis. Kerr's main argument was that the healed incision was stronger and less liable to rupture in a subsequent pregnancy. As he wrote:

'I make no claims to originality as regards the incision and I recommend it only because I believe the cicatrix that results will be less liable to rupture. The advantages of the incision are that one cuts through a less vascular area … In the second place it is thin and consequently the surfaces can be readily brought together … The third advantage, and it is a very important one, is that the wound in this area is at rest during the early days of the puerperium. Lastly, there is great advantage that owing to the fact that the lower uterine segment does not become fully stretched until labour is well advanced, the scar is in a safer region than the ordinary longitudinal one.'[16]

Munro Kerr performed his first transverse lower segment caesarean operation in 1911 and reported his results in the 1920s and 30s. Acceptance came slowly and for many years he was a lone voice in his advocacy for the lower segment procedure, although he later had an ally in McIntosh Marshall (1901–1954) of Liverpool.[12] *Indeed, after its widespread adoption, the lower segment operation was known in Europe for many years as 'Kerr's operation'. Belated acknowledgement of Kerr's achievement in popularizing the lower segment procedure came at the time of the 12th British Congress of Obstetrics and Gynaecology, held in London in 1949, several years after he had retired from clinical practice. He was invited to the lecture platform and lauded for his achievement. In a dramatic response he raised his arms and declared: 'Alleluia! The strife is o'er, the battle done!'*

The role of caesarean section has been transformed in little more than a century from a procedure of desperation, performed only in the rarest and most terrible circumstances, to a commonplace frequently applied, especially in affluent society for what some would regard as trivial indications. During that time the operation has changed from one carrying terrifying risks in which the prospect of maternal survival was slim to one in which maternal death is an extreme rarity. During the last quarter of the 20th century in particular, caesarean section rates increased worldwide. A variety of reasons have improved the safety of caesarean section and increased the indications for its performance:

- The introduction of anaesthesia a century and a half ago – itself driven by the search for pain relief in labour, as well as to facilitate surgery.
- Continued improvement in anaesthetic techniques along with the emergence of specialists in obstetric anaesthesia has greatly increased the effectiveness and safety of this component of caesarean delivery.
- Improvements in blood transfusion, antibiotics and thromboprophylaxis have increased the perioperative safety.
- Improved surgical techniques have reduced not only the immediate

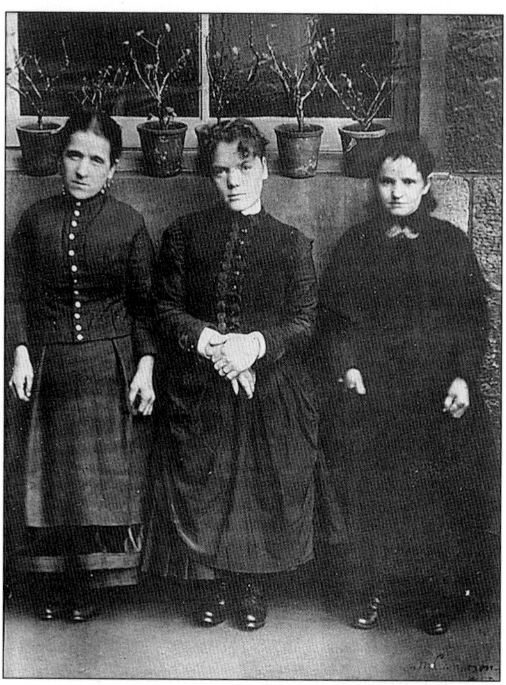

Figure 11.1 The first three cases in Murdoch Cameron's historic series of elective classical caesarean section performed on rachitic women with gross pelvic deformities. The photograph was taken outside Glasgow Royal Maternity Hospital and the windowsill on which the flowerpots stand is approximately one metre from the ground.

perioperative complications of caesarean section, but also lessened the risks in subsequent pregnancy.

- There is less experience with certain types of operative vaginal delivery and an unwillingness to accept even small increased risks associated with these techniques. Vaginal breech delivery is the most obvious but by no means only example of this.
- There are now social and medicolegal expectations of a perfect perinatal outcome, which has undoubtedly influenced obstetric care. It is almost unheard of for anyone to be sued for performing a caesarean section, but liability for not performing a caesarean section is not uncommon.
- Advanced maternal age, infertility and assisted reproductive technologies have led to a rise in the number of so-called 'premium' pregnancies. These women also tend to have more complications in pregnancy and labour.
- Although not common there is an increasing demand on the part of some women for elective delivery by caesarean section for what many regard as trivial clinical or social reasons. These may include a fear of labour and vaginal delivery, and the perceived benefits of reducing or eliminating rare fetal risks in labour and long-term sequelae of pelvic floor damage.
- Dramatic advances in neonatal care and outcome have lowered the gestational age at which intervention for fetal indications is appropriate.

As the risks to the woman have progressively diminished, the operation has been found to be justifiable for ever widening clinical and social indications. As more and more women enter second and subsequent pregnancies with a uterine scar it is important to emphasise the long-term potential for serious consequences of caesarean section, which are not often perceived by a short-sighted focus on the immediate decision concerning mode of delivery. It is worth reiterating the view of Myerscough in the 10th edition of this text (1982, p 296), written at a time when the tide of caesareans was at an early point in its inexorable rise:

> *'I do not doubt that this extension of caesarean section is in the main justified. The remarkable reduction in both maternal and fetal mortality rates bears this out. Nevertheless, I fear that today, more than ever before, there is a danger of abdominal delivery being regarded as the legitimate method of dealing with each and every obstetric abnormality. Although low, the maternal death rate is not negligible ... Nor should it be forgotten that a woman's obstetric future is prejudiced by the uterine scar ... The problem today is to select the cases best suited for delivery by caesarean section, having regard not only to the*

immediate needs of the mother and her unborn child, but also to her more remote obstetric future'.

Indications

The justification for caesarean section arises from clinical judgment that the interests of the mother, fetus or both are better served by resorting to caesarean delivery in order to avoid the continuation of pregnancy or the onset or the continuation of labour. The conditions that inform this judgment vary widely depending on the population served and the clinical skills and facilities available. As with a number of aspects which make obstetrics such a challenging discipline, the interests of the mother and those of the fetus can at times pull in opposite directions, so that careful assessment is demanded to reach the optimum solution. Recent trends have resulted in a radical change from the need to justify every caesarean against the stern criticism of the obstetric hierarchy to the orthodoxy of today which seems to preach 'if in doubt do a caesarean'. This attitude still needs to be challenged, however, if we are to avoid 'the easy way out', in more than one sense, becoming the norm. Obstetricians in training should be encouraged to develop clinical judgment which they can defend in the courts of the 'obstetric gods' as well as those of the legal system. Defensive obstetrics can be pernicious and must be resisted if we are to do the best for our patients rather than for ourselves. A degree of courage is required if we are not to find that trends in obstetric practice are to be led by external influences rather than clinical ideals.

The indications and proportions of caesarean delivery will vary from country to country and from hospital to hospital. Nonetheless, there are four main indications that account for 60–90% of all caesarean sections. These include: repeat caesarean section (35–40%), dystocia (20–35%), breech (10–15%) and fetal distress (10–15%).[17]

In many cases it is not one discreet indication but a combination of relative indications that necessitate caesarean delivery. For example, prolonged non-progressive labour in association with a non-reassuring fetal heart rate pattern may not represent absolute dystocia or definite fetal hypoxia, but relative degrees of each.

Most of the indications for caesarean section are discussed in the individual chapters of this book. However, it may be useful to consider them under three main categories:

Indisputable indications

- Placenta praevia, except possibly in the most minor degrees of this condition.
- Demonstrable fetal hypoxia or imminent fetal demise. Except in the second stage of labour when vaginal delivery may be a safer and quicker option, clear evidence of fetal hypoxia or its inevitability mandates immediate caesarean delivery. This includes antepartum or intrapartum asphyxia confirmed by fetal blood gas measurement or unequivocal cardiotographic evidence; umbilical cord prolapse; vasa praevia; uterine rupture; and severe abruptio placentae where the fetus is still viable.
- Unequivocal cephalopelvic disproportion, soft tissue obstruction or fetal malpresentation, not caused by gross fetal malformations incompatible with life.

Generally accepted indications

This includes many conditions which, depending on their severity, may present ranging from an absolute to a relative need for caesarean section.

- Previous caesarean section is one of the commonest indications. As outlined in the next chapter a variety of additional circumstances will dictate whether or not this is an absolute indication for repeat caesarean section or a trial for vaginal delivery. Within this category most would regard the woman with a previous classical caesarean scar as representing an absolute indication for repeat caesarean section.
- Breech presentation at term is now accepted as an indication for delivery by

caesarean section when safe facilities for this exist. This is discussed in Chapter 14.

- Dystocia, manifest by non-progressive labour, makes up an increasing proportion of all caesarean deliveries. Aspects of this diagnosis are discussed in Chapters 3 and 8.
- Fetal distress has been the indication for many caesarean sections for perceived fetal compromise, which was in fact quite misleading. This is discussed in detail in Chapter 4.
- Maternal indications are not common but there are a number of maternal disorders in which, depending upon the severity, it might be advisable to avoid labour. These include severe pre-eclampsia/eclampsia, cardiovascular disease and diabetes. In a number of these cases conditions may be favourable for vaginal delivery but in others caesarean delivery is warranted.

Marginal indications

This is a small category but has the potential to increase. Included here are those women who have a morbid fear of labour, possibly based on a previous bad experience. Another example is the woman who wants elective caesarean delivery to obviate the perceived risks of fetal injury or asphyxia during labour, or to minimize the risks of damage to her pelvic floor. Others may have worries about their body image or sexuality after vaginal delivery. Each of these women deserves a rational discussion and the provision of full information about the pros and cons of both routes of delivery. Often their concerns can be alleviated by the provision of balanced information, but if not, their wishes should be accommodated within the context of fully informed consent.

Classification of Urgency

In recent years a number of organizations have tried to establish guidelines for time limits within which caesarean section should be performed for urgent indications.[18] This debate has taken place within the context of clinical care, hospital accreditation and the spectre of litigation. A recent guideline[19] based on reasonable rationale and some validation has been proposed:[20,21]

- *Category 1* Immediate threat to the life of the woman or fetus. This will include caesarean sections for severe prolonged fetal bradycardia, fetal scalp blood pH < 7.2, cord prolapse, and uterine rupture. These caesareans should occur as quickly as possible and certainly within 30 minutes.
- *Category 2* Maternal or fetal compromise which is not immediately life-threatening. These include conditions such as antepartum haemorrhage and non-progressive labour with maternal or fetal compromise, but not to the degree of category 1. These cases should also be delivered within 30 minutes if possible but one has to take into account the potential risks in meeting this deadline. For example, the use of general anaesthesia with its increased risks to the mother compared to the slightly more time consuming institution of regional anaesthesia.
- *Category 3* No maternal or fetal compromise but early delivery required. This will include non-progressive labour without maternal or fetal compromise, and women booked for elective caesarean section who are admitted with ruptured membranes or in early labour. It is recommended that these women be delivered within 75 minutes. There are other cases with slowly worsening conditions such as pre-eclampsia and IUGR in which delivery is indicated. If they are preterm and induction of labour is deemed likely to fail an early caesarean delivery may be necessary.
- *Category 4* Elective planned caesarean section timed to suit the woman and staff.

Anaesthesia

Regional anaesthesia (epidural or spinal) should be chosen when possible as it has the least associated maternal and neonatal morbidity. General anaesthesia may be given if there is a need for extreme speed, such as in acute fetal distress; patient preference; and for women in whom regional anaesthesia fails (usually less than 5%).

Preoperative considerations

- Consent – it has to be admitted that informed consent for caesarean section can vary from the very brief statement of need in acute fetal distress to a much more considered and prolonged discussion in women requesting elective caesarean section for personal reasons. In general the indications for recommending caesarean delivery should be outlined along with the alternatives. The procedure and its complications should be reviewed in the context of the alternatives, which usually include allowing labour to continue or assisted vaginal delivery. The effect of caesarean delivery on future pregnancies should also be reviewed in relevant cases.
- Unless indicated by other medical complications, a complete blood count, blood group and antibody screen is adequate preoperative blood testing.
- A urinary (Foley) catheter is placed in the bladder once regional anaesthesia has been established.
- Antacid prophylaxis should be administered in the form of a histamine H_2 receptor blocker (ranitidine or cimetidine).
- The woman should be placed in a 15° left lateral tilt to avoid aorto-caval compression.
- Preoperative shaving of the incision site is not required. If the pubic hair over the proposed incision site is thick it can be clipped short, rather than shaved.

Perioperative care

- Antibiotic prophylaxis should be given in the form of a single dose of a first-generation cephalosporin or ampicillin. This is given for both elective and emergency caesarean sections and should be administered intravenously after the baby is delivered and the umbilical cord is clamped. In women with more prolonged labour and evidence of chorioamnionitis repeat doses of the same antibiotic can be given for the first 48 hours postoperatively.
- Thromboprophylaxis in the form of adequate hydration and early mobilization should apply to all postpartum women. Most women delivered by caesarean section should also receive subcutaneous heparin prophylaxis unless there is a contraindication. This can be administered after discussion with the anaesthetist and usually after removal of the epidural catheter or institution of spinal anaesthesia.
- The Foley catheter can be removed once regional anaesthesia has worn off and the woman is ambulant – usually about 12 hours post-caesarean.
- Postoperative analgesia is best achieved by intrathecal administration of diamorphine or morphine. Non-steroidal anti-inflammatory drugs can also be given, by suppository if necessary.
- Oral fluid and food intake should be administered when the woman feels thirsty or hungry, after confirming bowel peristalsis. In complicated cases, when the possibility of return to the operating theatre exists, oral intake should be withheld until her condition is stable.

Types of caesarean section

Low transverse caesarean section

In about 98% of cases a low transverse segment caesarean section can be performed. The uterine incision is confined to the lower uterine segment so that healing in this relatively non-contractile portion of the uterus in the puerperium is optimal. In addition, the risk of rupture in a subsequent pregnancy is lower than with the other types of caesarean section.

Low vertical caesarean section

This technique is rarely used. Its potential role is in those cases in advanced labour with a well-developed lower uterine segment but at an earlier gestational age, when the overall width of the uterine segment is reduced. In such cases an attempt at a transverse lower segment incision may extend into the major uterine vessels laterally and still not provide a large enough incision for atraumatic delivery of the infant. By making a vertical incision in the lower uterine segment it can be enlarged directly into the upper uterine segment should the size of the incision be inadequate for delivery of the infant. Those who advocate this technique feel that in these circumstances the advantages of the lower segment incision will be gained in most cases. However, most obstetricians feel that in many of these cases the upper uterine segment is entered, providing the same drawbacks to the classical incision in subsequent pregnancies.

Classical caesarean section

Classical caesarean section is undertaken when access to the lower segment is prohibited by extensive adhesions, uterine fibroids or, rarely, huge vascularity associated with placenta praevia with or without accreta. On rare occasions when extreme speed is deemed necessary to deliver the fetus a classical rather than a low transverse caesarean may be undertaken. With an experienced operator, the time saved in performing a classical over a low transverse caesarean is very little, so this indication is extremely rare. It would, however, have application in the very rare case of postmortem caesarean section (see later).

In most units classical caesarean section makes up < 2% of all caesarean deliveries. However, this figure is increasing modestly because of the falling gestational age at which caesarean section is performed.[22] This is particularly so in cases performed below 34 weeks gestation without labour. In such cases the lower segment may not be adequately formed to allow a transverse incision of sufficient size to accommodate atraumatic delivery of the fragile premature infant. It is best to take this decision after the abdomen has been opened and the lower uterine segment carefully inspected. In many cases it is possible to perform a low transverse caesarean section with adequate room to deliver the fetus. The advantages of this to the woman's future obstetric career are obvious. If after making the transverse incision one finds that it is of inadequate size then one has to add a vertical incision in the middle into the upper uterine segment. This will produce an inverted 'T' incision which in subsequent pregnancies will have to be treated as a classical caesarean scar. The advantage of this approach, however, is that in the majority of cases a low transverse incision will be achieved and in those cases in which the inverted 'T' has to be performed the morbidity to the mother and infant is no greater than for a classical caesarean section.[23]

Surgical techniques

For the majority of types of caesarean section the transverse Pfannenstiel incision or Joel–Cohen incision is appropriate. The main reason for using a lower midline incision instead is when speed of entry is paramount. This may be necessary with acute fetal compromise, massive haemorrhage, uterine rupture (in which speed is required both for fetal reasons as well as the extra room that may be needed for additional surgical manoeuvres) and the very rare case of perimortem caesarean delivery.[24]

During labour the bladder becomes an abdominal organ and therefore the peritoneal cavity should be opened as high as possible

> *'The abdominal incision should possess two qualities – it should be high and it should be sufficiently long … My rule is to make the incision 8 to 10 inches [20 to 25 cm] in length … two-thirds of this incision is made above and one-third below the level of the umbilicus'.*
>
> **Munro Kerr**
> *Operative Midwifery, 1908, p409*

and then extended down under transillumination. After opening the peritoneal cavity the uterus is checked for dextro- or laevo-rotation – the former is more common due to the sigmoid colon. This appraisal of the orientation of the uterus is very important in placing the uterine incision, otherwise it may be eccentric and extend into the uterine vessels on one side.[17] The loose utero-vesical peritoneum is identified. The attachment of this peritoneum, where it adheres to the surface of the uterus, is the upper margin of the lower uterine segment. This peritoneum should be divided about 2–3 cm below the level of this attachment in the midline and then extended laterally toward each side. The loose areolar tissue between the lower uterine segment and the bladder is gently separated with the forefinger and a Doyen or similar retractor placed to move the bladder down and keep it from the line of uterine incision.

In prolonged labour with disproportion the lower uterine segment is stretched and drawn up, forming a considerable portion of the lower uterus. It is important to identify the upper margin of the lower uterine segment where the utero-vesical peritoneum reflects from the uterus. The uterine incision is usually made about 2–3 cm below this point. If one does not use this landmark it is possible to place the uterine incision so low as to be in the vagina rather than the uterus. In making the uterine incision one should be constantly aware of the risk of laceration to the fetal presenting part. The risk is greatest in obstructed labour with a thin lower uterine segment stretched over the fetal head and face. Identify the midline and gently palpate with the fingers at the site of the proposed incision, which will give some idea of the thickness involved. Using a scalpel and with very gentle strokes make a 2 cm horizontal incision. After the first stroke and with each succeeding stroke sweep the index finger of the opposite hand across the incision so that the layers can be clearly seen. When the incision is partially through the muscle, press and release the centre of the incision with the forefinger – if the remaining layer is very thin this will usually raise a 'bleb' of membranes which can then be incised, almost like a blister, without risk to the underlying fetus. Alternatively, one can use the forefinger or the scalpel handle to 'burrow' through the final thin layer. Either way, obsessional attention to this point should almost eliminate the risk of fetal laceration.

Once the uterus is entered, the forefinger is placed between the fetus and the uterine muscle towards one side and the incision is continued with either curved Mayo or bandage scissors for about 2 cm on each side from the initial entry point with a slight curve upwards. Both fingers are then hooked into this incision and pulled laterally for the final extension of the incision. Once again, care should be taken to balance the pull on each side to avoid extension into the uterine vessels. In earlier gestation, when the width of the lower uterine segment may be marginal, the angles of the uterine incision can be directed upwards which will produce an enlarged 'trap-door' effect.

If the fetus is in cephalic presentation manual delivery of the head is, in most cases, straightforward. Insert the flat of the lower hand downwards between the head and the lower uterine segment. Using the lightly flexed fingers it should be possible to elevate the fetal head into the uterine incision. At the same time an assistant applies firm fundal pressure on the breech of the infant which facilitates delivery of the head (Fig 11.2). In elevating the head the occiput should be identified and the head flexed so that the narrowest diameter passes through the uterine incision. If there is difficulty in delivering the head manually, Simpson's or similar forceps can be used to guide the fetal head through the uterine incision. Make sure that the orientation of the head is appropriately identified so that the forceps can be placed correctly.

Once the head is delivered the oropharynx and nasal passages are cleared, if necessary with gentle suction. At this point the anaesthetist should give 5 units of oxytocin intravenously followed by an oxytocin infusion. Once the infant is completely delivered it should be rapidly dried and the cord double-clamped and a specimen kept for cord blood

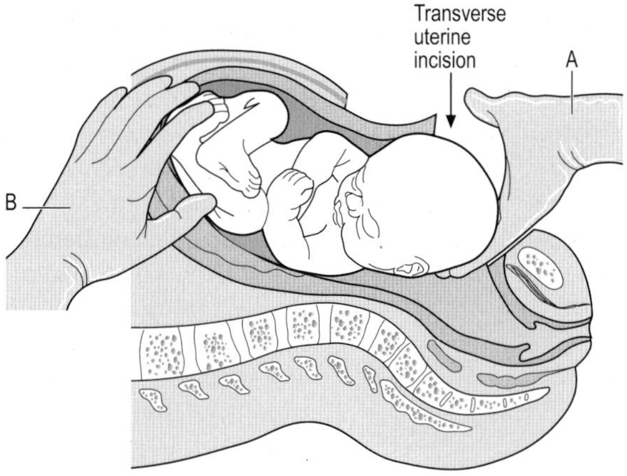

Figure 11.2 Manual delivery of the fetal head. Identify the occiput and flex the head (A) through the uterine incision with concomitant fundal pressure by an assistant (B).

pH analysis. The placenta should be removed by controlled cord traction once signs of separation have occurred. Routine manual removal of the placenta is discouraged as it increases blood loss and postoperative sepsis[24,25] and even occasionally acute uterine inversion.[26] Once the placenta has been delivered the uterine cavity should be checked to ensure there are no retained portions of placenta or membranes.

Exteriorization of the uterus should not routinely be carried out. In some women under regional anaesthesia this will cause nausea, vomiting and pain. With appropriate assistance and reasonable surgical skill it is quite possible to suture the uterine incision without this manoeuvre. On the other hand, if there is an extension of the uterine incision, or exposure is limited by heavy bleeding, then one should not hesitate to bring the uterus out of the abdominal incision to facilitate haemostasis and repair.

If there is more than slight bleeding from the cut edges of the uterine incision Green–Armytage or ring forceps can be used to compress the bleeding edges. Even if these are not required for bleeding it is useful to place at least one such forcep on the lower edge of the uterine incision for identification. The lower edge of the uterine incision often recedes inferiorly and may be obscured by blood. The posterior wall of the lower uterine segment may protrude forward and even mimic, to the unwary, the lower edge of the uterine incision.

Traditionally, closure of the uterine incision has been in two layers – although in the past decade an increasing number of obstetricians have moved to single-layer closure. This is usually with a continuous suture, either running or locked. In general this saves about 5 minutes operating time. There is as yet conflicting and inadequate data on the outcome of single- versus double-layer closure upon the integrity of the scar in subsequent labour.[18] One large cohort study showed a four-fold increase of uterine rupture in subsequent pregnancy for single- versus double-layer closure.[27] At least one large trial (CAESAR) is underway in an attempt to answer this question.[18] Until firm evidence is available the authors recommend two-layer closure. The first layer should include the cut edges of the muscle only and not the decidua. It should be a running suture, which avoids the bunching and elevation of tissues seen with a continuous locking suture, and facilitates the placement of the second layer which can be either running or locking (Fig 11.3). The second layer of sutures should raise a fold of muscle on the upper and lower side to cover the first layer of sutures. The most commonly used sutures are 0 or No. 1 polyglactin (Vicryl) or polyglycolic acid (Dexon).

Another change in surgical technique in recent years has been to omit closure of both the visceral peritoneum over the uterine segment and the parietal peritoneum. Reviews of the trials suggest that closure of neither of these layers is necessary and omission

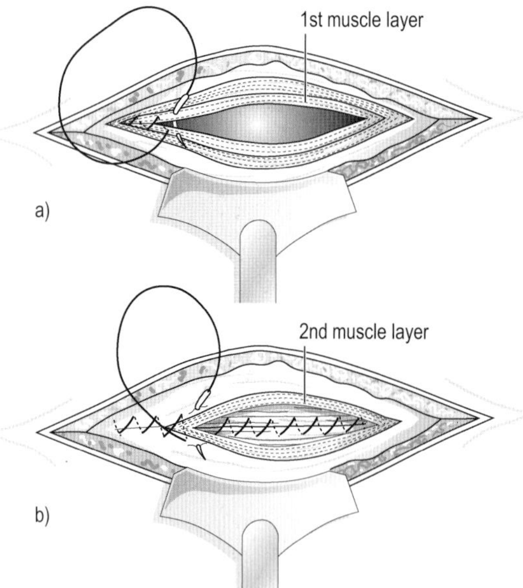

Figure 11.3 Two-layer lower segment uterine incision closure. The first running layer includes muscle but excludes the decidua. The second layer folds muscle over the first layer of sutures and can be a running or locking suture.

of this step is associated with a marginally shorter operating time and less postoperative pain.[18,24] However, a recent study has shown that closure of both these peritoneal layers significantly reduces adhesions found at subsequent caesarean section.[28] In addition, it is not uncommon to observe blood oozing from the peritoneal edge and underlying tissues of the uterovesical peritoneum, and in these cases closure with a simple running suture is recommended. The pros and cons of closing both the visceral and parietal peritoneum are unresolved and are being evaluated in the CAESAR trial.

For closure of the abdominal wall some will approximate the medial edges of the rectus muscles loosely with two or three interrupted and lightly tied sutures but many omit this step. The rectus sheath is closed with a running suture. It is unnecessary to place sutures in the subcutaneous fat as this does not improve healing and only serves to provide more foreign material for potential infection. The skin can be closed with staples, interrupted percutaneous sutures or a subcuticular suture. All caesarean sections are contaminated with vaginal flora and in women with prolonged labour it may be better not to use subcuticular closure. The problem with this technique is that it does not allow any serum to ooze from the wound and it is a bad surgical principle to seal a potentially infected space. In addition, should wound infection develop a subcuticular suture precludes drainage, in contrast to the simple removal of one or two staples or stitches. While the short-term cosmetic effect of subcuticular closure may be superior, the long-term cosmetic effect is no different with all three techniques. For the rare cases done through a low midline incision mass closure or a layered closure can be used.

A simplified variation of the above technique has been developed by Michael Stark at the Misgav Ladach Hospital in Jerusalem and named after that hospital. In the Misgav Ladach method the Joel–Cohen transverse skin incision is used, which is about 2–3 cm higher than the Pfannenstiel incision. The rectus sheath is incised, again higher than the traditional Pfannenstiel approach. At this level the rectus muscles move more freely beneath the fascia. The rectus muscles are pulled apart with the fingers. The parietal peritoneum is then stretched and entered bluntly as high as possible with the index finger. The lower uterine segment is identified and the uterovesical peritoneum divided as for the normal technique of transverse lower segment caesarean. A Doyen retractor is used to retract the bladder. The uterus is entered with a scalpel in the normal manner and the incision then enlarged with the fingers. After delivery of the fetus and placenta the uterus is closed in one layer. Neither the visceral or parietal peritoneum is closed, nor are the rectus muscles. The rectus sheath is closed with a running suture. This operative technique has been described in detail.[29] Experience with this method of caesarean section suggests that it results in a shorter operating time, less blood loss and less postoperative analgesic requirements.[30]

Complicated caesarean section

Classical caesarean section

The abdominal incision is the same as for a low transverse caesarean section. With appropriate retraction a classical caesarean section can be performed through a low transverse abdominal wall incision. Using a scalpel a 2–3 cm incision is made in the upper part of the lower uterine segment, with care taken to avoid the underlying fetus. Once the uterine cavity is entered two fingers are placed inside to protect the fetal parts and using either the scalpel or scissors the incision is extended 10–12 cm upwards in the longitudinal plane. Once the fetus and placenta have been delivered it is helpful to exteriorize the uterus as the classical incision is much more vascular and access to it is limited with the transverse abdominal wall incision. This allows the assistant's hands to encircle the incision with the fingers on one side and the thumbs on the other to compress the uterine incision and assist its closure (Fig 11.4). This manoeuvre of the assistant's hands is key in reducing blood loss and, by providing progressive compression, reduces the tension on the sutures as they are placed, facilitating closure of the thick gaping muscle. Depending on the thickness of the incised muscle, one or two running sutures may be required to bring together the deeper layers of the uterine muscle. This should aim to leave about 1 cm of the outer layer of uterine muscle gaping, which is closed by a final locking sero-muscular suture (Fig 11.5).

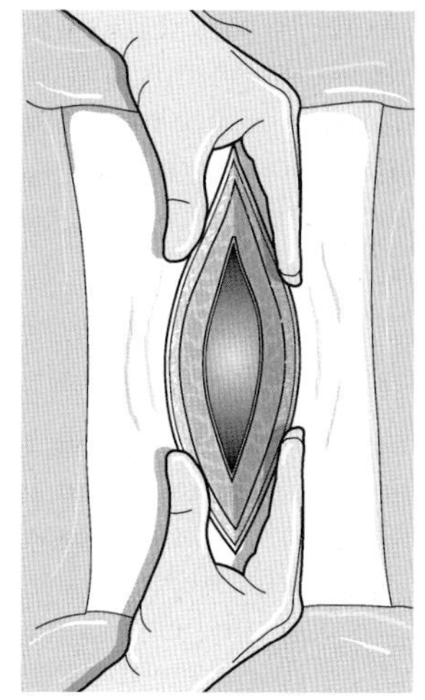

Figure 11.4 Classical caesarean section. The assistant's hands encircle the incision to reduce blood loss and facilitate its closure.

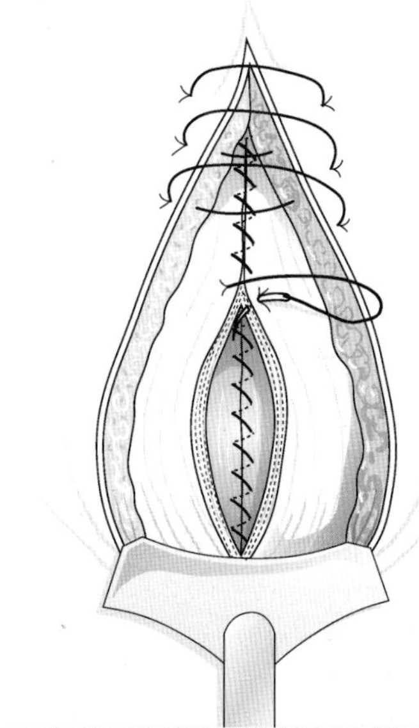

Figure 11.5 Suture closure of the classical caesarean incision. The deep layers are closed by 2–3 running sutures, with a final wide locking suture of the seromuscular layer.

Low vertical caesarean section

In low vertical caesarean section the uterine incision requires careful dissection of the bladder from the lower uterine segment. This dissection should not extend too far lateral or much bleeding will ensue from the vascular pillars of the bladder. An initial 2 cm vertical incision is made in the lower uterine segment in the midline with the same precautions for fetal protection as the low transverse incision. With the finger through the incision protecting the fetus, scissors are used to extend the incision downwards and upwards. One has to strike a balance between extending too far down and getting into the very vascular area of the vagina at the base of the bladder and too far upwards and extending into the upper uterine segment. In fact, in many cases extension to the upward uterine segment is necessary to provide a large enough incision for delivery of the fetus. The lower end of the incision should be captured with a stay suture in order to delineate the lower edge and, using traction on this stay suture, facilitate haemostatic closure of the lower part of the incision. Otherwise the incision is closed using the same principles as for the transverse lower segment incision.

Deeply engaged fetal head

Caesarean section at full cervical dilatation with the head deeply impacted in the pelvis can be associated with increased maternal and perinatal morbidity.[24,31] When the head is deeply engaged in the pelvis it may take considerable effort to elevate it up into the incision. This may be achieved by pushing the flat of the lower hand between the uterine incision and the fetal head deep into the vagina. Using the upper hand to grasp the wrist of the lower hand may aid in elevation of the lower hand and head without excessive levering movements of the lower hand, which risk extension of the uterine incision. If this is unsuccessful an assistant can place a hand vaginally and, cupping the fetal head in the hand, disengage it and elevate it upwards so that the hand of the abdominal operator can guide it through the uterine incision (Fig 11.6).[32]

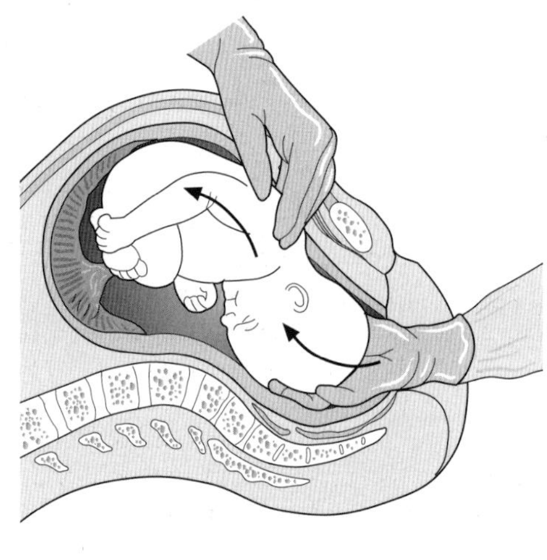

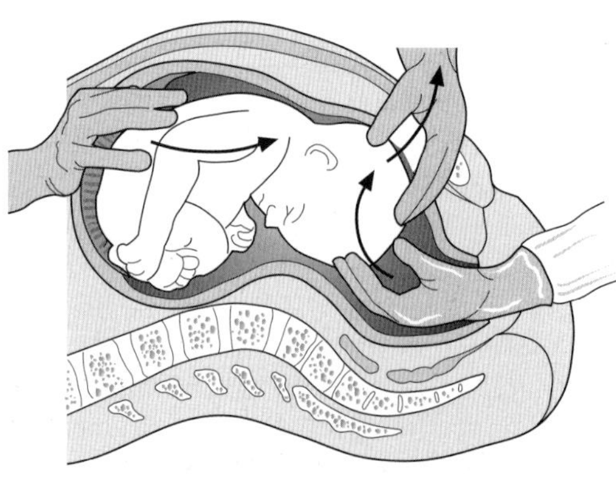

Figure 11.6 Vaginal elevation of the deeply engaged fetal head into the lower uterine segment.

Another option is to reach up and grasp the fetal feet and pull down, which elevates the fetal trunk and head. Continued traction, in essence, carries out an internal podalic version and the breech is delivered through the uterine incision first.[33,34] If the uterus is tightly contracted down around the fetus, as is often the case, tocolysis with intravenous nitroglycerine may aid the above manoeuvres (see Chapter 26).

Breech presentation

For breech presentation all of the manoeuvres are the same up until delivery of the fetus. In the preterm fetus, however, in which the body of the breech is significantly smaller than the head, there is the risk of entrapment of the fetal head by the uterine incision and contracted uterus after delivery of the body. This is particularly so with regional anaesthesia which does not cause any uterine relaxation. Thus, the anaesthetist should be forewarned and have intravenous nitroglycerine drawn up and ready to administer should this be necessary (see Chapter 14).

Transverse lie

With caesarean section for transverse lie the lower uterine segment may not be well developed due to the absence of a presenting part in the pelvic brim. Once the abdomen has been opened a careful assessment of the development and capacity of the lower uterine segment should be made. In some cases it is possible to turn the fetus to a longitudinal lie and find that the lower uterine segment is sufficiently developed to carry out a transverse lower segment incision. Alternatively, internal podalic version followed by breech extraction through a lower segment incision may be feasible. If the lower segment is inadequately developed, a vertical incision will have to be made, starting low and extending into the upper uterine segment.

Placenta praevia

There are a number of potential complications of caesarean section specific to placenta praevia and placenta praevia accreta. These are covered in Chapter 17.

Documentation

After every caesarean delivery a detailed note should be recorded in the chart. This should include a summary of events in labour, the indication, and surgical details of the operation. This is necessary for audit purposes and so that the information is available to those who may look after the woman in a subsequent pregnancy. The perioperative decisions and procedures should also be reviewed with the woman during her postpartum stay in hospital.

Postmortem and perimortem caesarean section

As outlined in the historical background of this chapter, postmortem caesarean section has a long history and associated rich mythology.[4] Almost invariably the infant did not survive.[4] Within 6 minutes of cessation of cerebral blood flow in the mother there is neurological injury.[35] Thus, if the mother dies the fetus ideally should be delivered within 5 minutes. If delivery cannot be achieved within 10–15 minutes then it should not be attempted, as the chance of a normally surviving infant is remote.

> POSTMORTEM CAESAREAN
>
> *'It is, indeed, possible to save a child by the caesarian operation, or cutting it out of the womb of its mother just expired; but what man in his senses would put his character upon this footing.'*
>
> **Edmund Chapman**
> *A Treatise on the Improvement of Midwifery. London: L. David and C. Reymers, 1759:xiv*

The term perimortem caesarean section has been used to describe the situation in which the mother has had cardiac arrest but is being actively resuscitated. Cardiopulmonary resuscitation is most effectively carried out with the woman in the supine position. Up to 26 weeks gestation the uterus does not reach above the bifurcation of the aorta so that aorto-caval compression does not occur. Thus, up to 26 weeks gestation resuscitation of the woman in the supine position can occur, and at this gestation caesarean section will not help the mother and is unlikely to result in a surviving infant. This is particularly so when the circumstances arise, as they most commonly do at this gestation, far from the immediate availability of a neonatal intensive care unit.[36] It bears emphasis that at this gestation no personnel or resources should be diverted from maternal resuscitation.

In the third trimester of pregnancy the uterus will cause aorta-caval compression so that CPR should be performed in the head down lateral tilt position, which is more difficult. If adequate CPR cannot be achieved in this position then classical caesarean section through a lower midline incision, preferably within 5 minutes of starting CPR, is advantageous – both to the mother and the infant.[35,37] A recent review of perimortem caesarean sections has shown this principle to be appropriate, with half of the cases showing a marked improvement in haemodynamic status immediately after the uterus was emptied by caesarean section.[35] Thus, this approach benefits both the mother and the infant.

References

1. Young JH. Caesarean section. The history and development of the operation from earliest times. London: H. K. Lewis, 1944.
2. Fasbender H. Geschichte der geburtshulfe, Jena: Gustav Fisher, 1906:979–1010.
3. Harris RP. Cattle-horn lacerations of the abdomen and uterus in pregnant women. Am J Obstet Dis Women Child 1887; 20:673–685.
4. Trolle D. The history of caesarean section. Copenhagen: C. A. Rietzel, 1982.
5. Cawley T. London Med J 1785; 6:372.

6. Mosley B. Tropical diseases. London, 1795.
7. Pickrell KL. An inquiry into the history of cesarean section. Bull Soc Med Hist Chicago 1935; 4:414–453.
8. Stewart D. Edin Med Essays and Observ 1771; 5:37.
9. Ould F. A treatise of midwifry. Dublin: O. Nelson, 1742:xxiii.
10. Porro E. Della amputazione utero-ovarica come complemeno di talio cesareo. Ann Univ Med Chir (Milan) 1876; 237:289–350.
11. Baskett TF. On the shoulders of giants: eponyms and names in obstetrics and gynaecology. London: RCOG Press, 1996:101–102, 109, 213–215.
12. Marshall CM. Caesarean section lower segment operation. Bristol: John Wright, 1939.
13. Kehrer FA. Ueber ein modificintes verfahren biem kaiserschnitte. Arch Gynakol 1882; 19:177–209.
14. Sänger M. Zur rehabilitirung des classischen kaiserschnitte. Arch Gynakol 1882; 19:370–399.
15. Dow DA. The Rottenrow, the history of the Glasgow Royal Maternity Hospital 1834–1984. Lancaster: Parthenon Press, 1984.
16. Kerr JM. The lower uterine segment incision in conservative caesarean section. J Obstet Gynaecol Br Emp 1932; 28:475–487.
17. Baskett TF, Arulkumaran S. Intrapartum care. London: RCOG Press, 2002:93–102.
18. National Institute for Clinical Excellence. Clinical guideline: caesarean section. London: RCOG Press, 2004.
19. The National Sentinel Caesarean Section Audit Report. London: RCOG Press, 2001.
20. National Confidential Enquiry in Perioperative Deaths. Report of the National Confidential Inquiry into Perioperative Deaths 1992–3, London: HMSO, 1995.
21. Lukas DN, Yentis SM, Kinsella SM, et al. Urgency of caesarean section: a new classification. J R Soc Med 2000; 93:346–350.
22. Bethune M, Pemezel M. The relationship between gestational age and the incidence of classical caesarean section. Aust NZ J Obstet Gynaecol 1997; 37:153–155.
23. Patterson LS, O'Connell CM, Baskett TF. Maternal and perinatal morbidity associated with classical and inverted 'T' cesarean sections. Obstet Gynecol 2002; 100:633–637.
24. Hema KR, Johanson R. Techniques for performing caesarean section. Best Pract Res Clin Obstet Gynaecol 2001; 15:17–47.
25. Baska A, Kalan A, Ozkan A, Baksu B, Tekelicoglu M, Goker N. The effect of placental removal method and site of uterine repair on postcesarean endometritis and operative blood loss. Acta Obstet Gynecol Scand 2005; 84:266–269.
26. Baskett TF. Acute uterine inversion: a review of 40 cases. J Obstet Gynaecol Can 2002; 24:953–956.
27. Bujold E, Bujold C, Hamilton EF, Harel F, Gauthier RJ. The impact of single-layer or double-layer closure on uterine rupture. Am J Obstet Gynecol 2002; 186:1326–1330.
28. Lyell DJ, Caughey AB, Hu E, Daniels K. Perinatal closure at primary cesarean delivery and adhesions. Obstet Gynecol 2005; 106:275–280.
29. Holmgren G, Sjoholm L, Stark M. The Misgav Ladach method for cesarean section: method description. Acta Obstet Gynecol Scand 1999; 78:615–621.
30. Darj E, Nortstrom ML. Misgav Ladach method for cesarean section compared to the Pfannenstiel method. Acta Obstet Gynecol Scan 1999; 78:37–41.
31. Allen VM, O'Connell CM, Baskett TF. Maternal and perinatal morbidity of caesarean section at full cervical dilatation compared with caesarean delivery in the first stage of labour Br J Obstet Gynaecol 2005; 112:986–990.
32. Londesman R, Graber EA. Abdominovaginal delivery: modification of the cesarean operation to facilitate delivery of the impacted head. Am J Obstet Gynecol 1984; 148:707–710.
33. Levy R, Chernomoretz T, Appelman Z, Levin D, Or Y, Haggy ZJ. Head pushing versus reverse breech extraction in cases of impacted fetal head during caesarean section. Eur J Obstet Gynecol Reprod Biol 2005; 121:24–26.
34. Fasubaa OB, Ezechi OC, Orji EO. Delivery of the impacted head of the fetus at caesarean section after prolonged obstructed labour: a randomized comparative study of two methods. J Obstet Gynaecol 2002; 22:375–378.
35. Katz V, Balderstan K, DeFreest M. Perimortem cesarean delivery: were our assumptions correct? Am J Obstet Gynecol 2005; 192:1916–1921.
36. Baskett TF. Trauma in pregnancy. In: Essential management of obstetric emergencies. 4th ed. Bristol: Clinical Press Ltd, 2004:271–272.
37. Whitten M, Irvine LM. Post-mortem and perimortem caesarean section: what are the indications? J R Soc Med 2000; 93:6–9.

12

Vaginal birth after caesarean section

Once a caesarean always a caesarean

'One thing must always be borne in mind, viz., that no matter how carefully a uterine incision is sutured, we can never be certain that the cicatrized uterine wall will stand a subsequent pregnancy and labor without rupture. This means that the usual rule is, once a Caesarean always a Caesarean. Many exceptions occur ... The general rule holds, however, that we cannot depend upon a sutured uterine wall, whether it is done in a Caesarean section or a myomectomy, hence I believe the extension of Caesarean section to conditions other than dystocia from contracted pelvis or tumours should be exceptional and infrequent.'

Edwin Craigin
Conservatism in obstetrics. NY Med J 1916; 104:1–3

One of the most common dictums in obstetrics was put forward some 90 years ago by Edward Craigin: 'once a caesarean always a caesarean'. The main purpose of Craigin's presentation was to point out the maternal risks of caesarean section with a plea that it should be used only for the most stringent indications. In the early 20th century the most common indication for caesarean section was disproportion and contracted pelvis, and the type of caesarean section was classical with its associated significant risk of uterine rupture in a subsequent pregnancy. Thus, when Craigin proposed his dictum it was appropriate, as it would be now under the same circumstances. Craigin's main point was that caesarean section was a dangerous operation and that once it was performed the woman would be subject to the dangers of repeat caesarean section in a subsequent pregnancy. He did, however, point out that vaginal delivery after previous caesarean section was feasible and reported one of his own patients who had three vaginal deliveries after one caesarean section.

As the low transverse caesarean section became more common in the 1930s and 40s, and the indications for caesarean section widened to include non-recurrent reasons, the approach to women previously delivered by caesarean section changed in many countries. The risk of subsequent rupture of low transverse caesarean section was small and increasing numbers of women were encouraged to undergo labour and vaginal delivery. By the late 1970s and 1980s there were many reports of large series showing that spontaneous labour and vaginal delivery following a single low transverse caesarean section was a safe and reasonable option with appropriate safeguards. Consensus statements embraced and encouraged labour and vaginal delivery with a previous caesarean section under these circumstances.

However, as is so often the case in obstetrics, the pendulum of opinion swings too far and labour and vaginal delivery was pursued for widening indications – including more than one previous caesarean section, induction of labour, and augmentation of non-progressive labour. Not surprisingly, an increasing number of cases of uterine rupture were reported, some of which resulted in fetal death or severe neonatal neurological damage, as well as maternal morbidity, sometimes including hysterectomy. These rare but tragic outcomes and the associated medicolegal sequelae caused the pendulum to swing rapidly back in the opposite direction. Revised national guidelines suggested more stringent facility and personnel requirements in order to conduct labour and vaginal delivery following previous caesarean section.[1,2] Some hospitals, fearing institutional liability, forbade labour and vaginal delivery following previous caesarean section. The most sensible, practical and safest clinical course lies in the middle ground.

The term 'trial of labour' has been applied incorrectly to these cases. Trial of labour is a well-established obstetric principle when labour is undertaken in the face of suspected disproportion, which is contraindicated in a woman with a uterine scar. The term 'trial of scar' should also be avoided. The correct term is 'trial for vaginal delivery'.

This chapter will outline the factors that need to be considered in helping women reach a decision whether or not to undertake labour with a view to vaginal delivery after previous caesarean section.

Selection criteria for vaginal birth after caesarean section (VBAC)

The previous obstetrical record should be reviewed so that details of the labour, indications for caesarean section, operative details and postoperative recovery can be appraised. There are several factors that need to be evaluated in assessing the level of medical risk and, indeed, medicolegal risk so that the appropriate informed consent can be obtained.

Type of uterine scar

- *Classical caesarean section scars* are about 10 times more likely to rupture during labour than lower segment caesarean incisions and may rupture before the onset of labour. The rupture rate for a previous classical scar is approximately 3–5%. In addition this type of scar rupture is potentially much more lethal to both fetus and mother as they tend to give way suddenly and this may be before labour or early in labour. As a result the woman is often not in hospital when the rupture occurs. This is in contrast to the lower segment caesarean scar which is most likely to rupture after some hours of labour when the woman is in hospital and appropriate medical intervention can be undertaken without delay.

- *Low vertical caesarean sections* are rarely performed. The indication is usually in earlier gestation when the lower uterine segment has formed to a degree but its transverse dimensions are felt to be inadequate for the normal transverse incision. In these cases the low vertical incision has been advocated as an alternative to classical caesarean section. However, in many instances the lower segment is not sufficiently developed, even vertically, to allow a big enough incision without encroaching on the upper uterine segment. Thus, these scars, while having a slightly smaller risk of rupture than a classical caesarean scar, are probably best treated in the same manner.
- *Extensions of a transverse lower segment caesarean incision* should be appraised by careful scrutiny of the operative report. If there was any marked extension of one or both angles, or a 'T' extension into the upper uterine segment, these scars are best not subjected to labour.
- *Hysterotomy* scars are not commonly seen in modern obstetrics with medical methods for second trimester termination. However, if present they should be treated in the same manner as a classical caesarean scar and repeat elective caesarean section chosen.
- *Myomectomy* incisions require individual consideration. If the incisions are extensive, and particularly if the uterine cavity was entered, they are probably best not subjected to labour. Similarly, hysteroscopic myomectomy incisions, if associated with perforation of the uterus would be best managed by elective caesarean section. Otherwise, hysteroscopic myomectomies not associated with perforation or deep myometrial excision can be allowed to labour.
- *Previous rupture* of any type of uterine scar in a previous pregnancy is obviously a contraindication to subsequent labour.

In some cases it is impossible to obtain the previous operative record. From the history it is often possible to work out the type of the previous uterine incision. For example, if the previous caesarean section was done at term, and particularly if it was for dystocia, one can reasonably assume that it was a transverse lower segment caesarean section. On the other hand, if the caesarean section was done at less than 32 weeks gestation and not in labour the chances are more likely that a classical caesarean section was done.

Labour with the previous caesarean section

If the previous caesarean section was carried out electively without labour, or in the early latent phase of labour, the pattern of uterine activity in the subsequent labour is likely to be of the nulliparous type, requiring stronger and longer uterine work to efface and dilate the 'nulliparous' cervix.[3] In contrast, those who had previous caesarean section in active labour are more likely to show a multiparous pattern in a subsequent labour with less uterine work and less strain on the uterine scar.

Previous vaginal delivery

If the woman had a previous vaginal delivery, either before or after the caesarean section, her chances of a successful and safe VBAC are enhanced. This is one of the most positive factors in favour of trial for vaginal delivery.[4]

Uterine incision closure

One large retrospective review showed a significant increase of subsequent scar rupture in those women in whom the initial caesarean had a single-layer versus a double-layer closure.[5] However, this finding has not been noted in other hospitals and there are many who have not shown an increase in scar rupture rates since changing to single-layer closure.[6]

Postoperative infection

Postpartum endomyometritis may interfere with adequate healing of the uterine scar and increase the risk of subsequent rupture in labour.[7] The practical clinical point here is that many cases of postpartum fever are not due to endomyometritis. Thus, it is inappropriate to exclude all women who have had a postpartum fever following the previous caesarean delivery. However, if there is good clinical evidence in the record that the sepsis was intrauterine it may be prudent to avoid labour in a subsequent pregnancy.

Recurrent indications for caesarean section

One of the most common reasons for primary caesarean section is dystocia or cephalo-pelvic disproportion, although a true diagnosis of the latter is rare. These diagnoses are not necessarily a recurrent indication and many will labour and deliver successfully after a previous caesarean for these indications. Overall, however, they have a slightly lower success rate than for other 'non-recurrent' indications.

Inter-pregnancy interval

Pregnancy and delivery within 12 months of a previous caesarean section may be associated with an increased risk of scar rupture in that pregnancy.[8]

Twins

There are a number of small series that show successful VBAC in twin pregnancy.[9] However, to some extent twin pregnancies have potentially double the price to pay for subsequent scar rupture. In addition, over-distention of the uterus associated with multiple pregnancy and the possible need for intrauterine manipulation for delivery of the second twin increase the risk of scar rupture. These are cases in which other selection criteria and individual considerations have to be weighed very carefully and cautious prudence remains the guiding principle.

More than one previous caesarean delivery

There are a number of series that have shown success in achieving vaginal delivery in women with two previous caesarean sections. However, the risk of uterine rupture is approximately doubled and the woman should be so informed.[10,11]

Measurement of lower uterine segment thickness

Small studies using ultrasound to measure the thickness of the lower uterine segment in the third trimester of pregnancy have suggested that those women with a very thin lower uterine segment have an increased risk of scar rupture.[12] This work is preliminary but promising and it is possible that there may be a critical measurement below which trial for vaginal delivery carries too great a risk.

Hospital facilities and personnel

Trial for vaginal delivery can only be undertaken in a hospital which has immediately available midwifery, nursing, anaesthesia and obstetric staff along with the appropriate operating theatre, laboratory and blood transfusion services. These criteria have been reviewed in national guidelines.[1,2]

There are a number of so-called 'soft factors' which, in addition to the above, may influence the decision. These include maternal age, secondary infertility, the desire for more pregnancies and previous maternal morbidity.

It is essential that the woman and her partner understand and accept the principles involved in a trial for vaginal delivery. From a review of the above selection criteria certain increased risks may be identified and these must be discussed with the woman, along with the advantages of a successful trial for vaginal delivery. It is quite inappropriate to apply any coercion, however subtle, towards labour.

Management of trial for vaginal delivery

Antenatal care

This should be routine other than the detailed review of the previous delivery record and of the selection factors noted above.

Induction of labour

This is one of the more contentious areas in the debate on VBAC. Obviously, spontaneous labour is the most desirable and induction of labour should only be considered when the indication is compelling. If the cervix is favourable, amniotomy is the method of choice and adds no additional risk to spontaneous labour. If amniotomy fails to induce labour, oxytocin may be cautiously used, which only very slightly increases the risk of uterine rupture. If the cervix is unfavourable and prostaglandins are chosen the level of risk rises.[13] This is greatest with misoprostol but also significantly higher with the prostaglandin E2 gels.[14] The use of these gels to ripen the unfavourable cervix should only be considered in hospital with on-site anaesthesia, obstetrics and immediate operating theatre facilities. Even then it is doubtful that this level of increased risk is acceptable and perhaps only in very unusual circumstances (such as fetal death). The woman should be advised that this method of induction does carry a small but significantly increased risk of uterine rupture.[15,16] The risk associated with misoprostol, even in a small series, has shown an unacceptably high rate of uterine rupture and this agent should not be used.[17]

Labour

The woman who selects trial of vaginal delivery should be advised to come into hospital early after labour starts. On admission, blood should be taken for group and screen. It is reasonable to allow the woman to ambulate in early labour. Once labour is established, however, an intravenous drip should be established and external fetal heart rate monitoring instituted. The latter is wise because fetal heart rate abnormalities are the earliest warning sign of uterine rupture.[18] If requested, epidural analgesia is not contraindicated and fears that it would mask the signs and symptoms of uterine rupture have not been substantiated.

The progress of labour should be carefully monitored and, provided this is satisfactory, an optimistic outcome can be expected. Early signs and symptoms of uterine rupture should be sought. These are discussed in Chapter 13. There is increasing experience with oxytocin augmentation of non-progressive labour but this does carry an increased risk of uterine rupture.[13] This should only be undertaken in hospitals with on-site anaesthesia and obstetric staff and the woman should understand that this does increase the risk. If oxytocin augmentation is chosen one should expect a smooth and progressive response. If this does not occur discretion is the better part of valour and caesarean section should be performed.

The second stage of labour is the time of maximal strain to the lower uterine segment and this may be shortened with assisted vaginal delivery by forceps or vacuum if the second stage is prolonged and the head is low in the pelvis. The conduct of the third stage of labour is normal. There are those who advocate routine exploration of the caesarean scar following delivery. In fact this can be carried out fairly easily with a vaginal examination through the cervix and feeling across the lower uterine segment for the V-shaped gutter of the scar to assess its integrity. However, most large series have shown that if uterine rupture occurs at the time of delivery the mother will have symptoms that draw attention to this diagnosis. If there are no such signs and symptoms scar rupture that would require treatment has not occurred and the manual exploration itself may cause perforation of the scar.

Rising caesarean section rates worldwide mean that in some countries 10–12% of the obstetric population have previously been delivered by caesarean section. This, then, is one of the most common complications of pregnancy. In some hospitals about 70% of women who undertake a trial for vaginal delivery will achieve their desired result. However, even in hospitals with a well-established policy of VBAC only about 30–40% of all women previously delivered by caesarean section choose and achieve vaginal delivery.

No large randomized trial has compared trial of vaginal delivery with elective repeat caesarean section. A meta-analysis from the 1990s shows a slightly increased risk of uterine rupture and neonatal mortality and morbidity with trial for vaginal delivery and increased rates of maternal morbidity with elective caesarean section.[19] The essence of the selection for and management of VBAC is to avoid the extremes. The majority of women with one previous transverse low segment caesarean section and spontaneous progressive labour will achieve vaginal delivery with safety for themselves and their infant. Once exceptions are made to this and additional risks undertaken – such as labour after more than one previous caesarean section, induction of labour and augmentation of non-progressive labour – the risk to both mother and infant increases. There comes a time in this equation when discretion is the better part of valour and it is not appropriate to take additional risks when the chances of increasing the rate of safe vaginal delivery are relatively low and the chances of uterine rupture and its sequelae increase.[20]

From a maternal point of view the safest outcome is spontaneous labour and spontaneous vaginal delivery, while the outcome associated with the greatest morbidity (other than uterine rupture) is a failed trial for vaginal delivery resulting in caesarean section.[21,22] Compared with caesarean section after a failed trial, elective caesarean section carries much less morbidity for both mother and infant. Careful clinical appraisal should delineate the probability of either of these two extremes occurring and, along with the woman's wishes, provide a sensible guide to either trial of vaginal delivery or repeat elective caesarean section. Blind adherence to either one of these clinical options is not appropriate. For the woman who wants to have more than 2–3 children, the cumulative morbidity of repeated elective caesarean sections will make trial for vaginal delivery a more attractive prospect. However, excessive zeal in the pursuit of vaginal delivery after previous caesarean section, most often manifest in those with limited experience, can put the woman and her infant at unreasonable risk.

References

1. American College of Obstetricians and Gynecologists. Vaginal birth after previous cesarean delivery. Practice Bulletin No. 55. Washington, DC: ACOG, 2004.
2. Society of Obstetricians and Gynaecologists of Canada. Guidelines for vaginal birth after previous caesarean birth. Clinical Practice Guideline No. 155. Ottawa: SOGC, 2005.
3. Arulkumaran S, Gibb DMF, Ingemarson I, Kitchener S, Ratnam SS. Uterine activity during spontaneous labour after previous lower segment caesarean section. Br J Obstet Gynaecol 1989; 96:933–938.
4. Zelop CM, Shipp TD, Repke JT, Cohen A, Lieberman E. Effect of previous vaginal delivery on the risk of uterine rupture during a subsequent trial of labour. Obstet Gynecol 2001; 183:1184–1186.
5. Bujold C, Hamilton EF, Harel R, Gauthier RJ. The impact of single-layer or double-layer closure on uterine rupture. Am J Obstet Gynecol 2002; 186:1326–1330.
6. Durnwald C, Mercer B. Uterine rupture, perioperative and perinatal morbidity after single layer closure at cesarean delivery. Am J Obstet Gynecol 2003; 189:925–929.
7. Shipp TD, Zelop C, Cohen A, Repke JT, Lieberman E. Post-cesarean delivery fever and uterine rupture in a subsequent trial of labour. Obstet Gynecol 2003; 101:136–139.
8. Esposito MA, Menihan CA, Mallee MP. Association of interpregnancy interval with uterine scar failure in labor: a case-control study. Am J Obstet Gynecol 2000; 183:1180–1183.
9. Delaney T, Young DC. Trial of labour compared to elective caesarean in twin gestation with a previous caesarean delivery. J Obstet Gynaecol Can 2003; 25:289–292.
10. Caughey AB, Shipp TD, Repke JT, Zelop CM, Cohen A, Lieberman E. Rate of uterine rupture during a trial of labor in women with one or two prior cesarean deliveries. Am J Obstet Gynecol 1999; 181:872–876.
11. Bretalle F, Cravello L, Shojair R, Roger V, D'Ercole C, Blanc B. Childbirth after two previous caesarean sections. Eur J Obstet Gynecol Reprod Biol 2001; 94:23–26.

12. Rozenberg P, Goffinet F, Phillipe HJ. Thickness of the lower segment: its influence in the management of patients with previous cesarean sections: Eur J Obstet Gynecol Reprod Biol 1999; 87:39–45.

13. Lydon-Rochelle M, Hoet VL, Easterling TR, Martin BP. Risk of uterine rupture during labor among women with a prior cesarean delivery. N Engl J Med 2001; 345:3–8.

14. Ravasi DJ, Wood SL, Pollard JK. Uterine rupture during induced trial of labor among women with previous cesarean delivery. Am J Obstet Gynecol 2000; 183:176–179.

15. McDonagh MS, Osterweil P, Guise JM. The benefits and risk of inducing labour in patients with prior caesarean delivery: a systematic review. Br J Obstet Gynaecol 2005; 112:1007–1015.

16. Kayani SI, Alfirevic Z. Uterine rupture after induction of labour in women with previous caesarean section. Br J Obstet Gynaecol 2005; 112:451–455.

17. Wing DA, Lovett K, Paul RH. Disruption of prior uterine incision following misoprostol for labor induction in women with previous cesarean delivery. Obstet Gynecol 1998; 91:828–830.

18. Ridgeway JJ, Weyrich DL, Benedetti TJ. Fetal heart rate changes associated with uterine rupture. Obstet Gynecol 2004; 103:506–512.

19. Mozurkewich EL, Hutton EK. Elective repeat cesarean delivery versus trial of labor: a meta analysis of the literature from 1989 to 1999. Am J Obstet Gynecol 2000;83: 1187–1197.

20. Guise JM, Berlin M, McDonagh M, Osterweil P, Chan B, Helfand M. Safety of vaginal birth after cesarean: a systematic review. Obstet Gynecol 2004; 103:420–429.

21. Allen VM, O'Connell CM, Liston RM, Baskett TF. Maternal morbidity associated with cesarean delivery without labor compared with spontaneous onset of labor at term. Obstet Gynecol 2003; 102:477–482.

22. Allen VM, O'Connell CM, Baskett TF. Maternal morbidity associated with cesarean delivery without labor compared with induction of labor at term. Obstet Gynecol 2006; 108:286–294.

Bibliography

Allen VM, O'Connell CM, Baskett TF. Cumulative economic implications of initial method of delivery. Obstet Gynecol 2006;108: 549–555.

American College of Obstetricians and Gynecologists Committee Opinion No 342. Induction of labor for vaginal birth after cesarean delivery. Obstet Gynecol 2006;108: 465–467.

Appelton B, Targett C, Rasmusen M, Readman E, Sale F, Rermezal M. Vaginal birth after caesarean section: an Australian multi-centre study. Aust NZ J Obstet Gynaecol 2000; 40:87–91.

Beckett PA, Regan L. Vaginal birth after caesarean: the European experience. Clin Obstet Gynecol 2001; 44:594–603.

Buhimschi CS, Buhimschi IA, Patel S, Malinow AM, Weiner CP. Rupture of the uterine scar during term labour: contractility or biochemistry? Br J Obstet Gynaecol 2005; 112:38–42.

Coassolo KM, Stamilio D, Pare E, et al. The safety and efficacy of vaginal birth after caesarean attempts at or beyond 40 weeks of gestation. Obstet Gynecol 2005; 106:700–706.

Guise JM, McDonagh MS, Osterweil P, Nygren P, Chan BKS, Helfand M. Systematic review of the incidence and consequences of uterine rupture in women with previous caesarean section. BMJ 2004; 329:19–23.

Landon MB, Spong CY, Thom E, Hauth JC, Bloom SL, Varner MW, et al. Risk of uterine rupture with a trial of labor in women with multiple and single prior cesarean delivery. Obstet Gynecol 2006; 108:12–20.

Patterson LS, O'Connell CM, Baskett TF. Maternal and perinatal morbidity associated with classical and inverted 'T' cesarean sections. Obstet Gynecol 2002; 100:633–637.

Socol ML. VBAC – is it worth the risk? Semin Perinatol 2003; 27:105–111.

Smith GCS, Pell JP, Cameron AD, Dobbie R. Risk of perinatal death associated with labor after previous cesarean delivery in uncomplicated term pregnancies. JAMA 2002; 287:2684–2690.

Turner MJA, Agnew G, Langan H. Uterine rupture and labour after a previous low transverse caesarean section. Br J Obstet Gynaecol 2006; 113:729–732.

Zinberg S. Vaginal delivery after previous cesarean delivery: a continuing controversy. Clin Obstet Gynecol 2001; 44:561–570.

13

Uterine rupture

Uterine rupture is a life threatening condition for both mother and fetus. The profile of causes and mortality varies between developed and developing countries. However, the limitation of health services in the latter and a rising caesarean section rate in the former means that uterine rupture is increasing in most areas of the world. The hospital-based incidence of uterine rupture varies from 1 in 100–500 deliveries in developing countries to 1 in 3000–5000 in hospitals with well-developed health services.[1–3] Maternal death from uterine rupture is rare in developed countries but severe maternal morbidity associated with haemorrhage and emergency obstetric hysterectomy is common.[4–7] In developing countries maternal mortality from uterine rupture may be 5–15% and fetal loss can exceed 80%.[8]

Types

- *Complete uterine rupture* involves the full thickness of the uterine wall.
- *Incomplete rupture* occurs when there is disruption of the muscle but the overlying visceral peritoneum remains intact. The most benign type of incomplete uterine rupture is dehiscence of a previous lower uterine segment caesarean scar. This is often found incidentally at the time of repeat caesarean section and in those circumstances carries little or no threat to mother or fetus. However, in some cases incomplete ruptures may extend laterally and bleed extensively into the broad ligament, even though the overlying peritoneum remains intact.

The site of rupture in the previously scarred uterus is usually the scar itself. In the intact uterus rupture is more likely to occur in the lower uterine

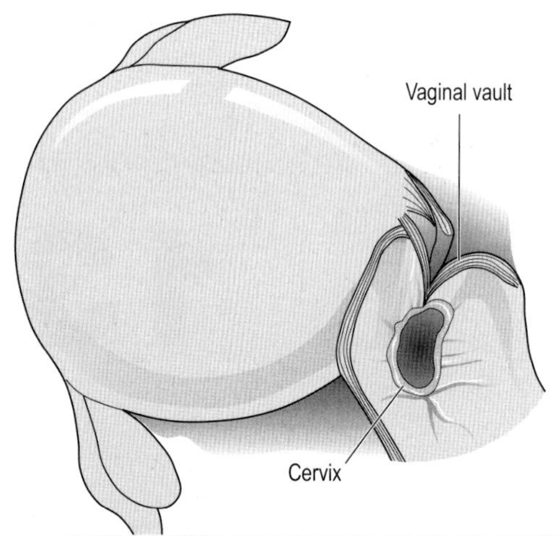

Figure 13.1 Laceration of lower uterus, cervix and vaginal vault (colporrhexis).

segment and more often in the anterior portion. With rupture of the lower uterine segment, particularly if scarred, the bladder may also be torn. When the cause of uterine rupture is traumatic vaginal delivery both the lower part of the uterus including the cervix and the vaginal vault may be involved (colporrhexis) (Fig 13.1). Damage to branches of the uterine and vaginal arteries may cause considerable haemorrhage into the broad ligament and paravaginal tissues.

Causes

Spontaneous rupture before labour

Spontaneous rupture of the normal uterus before the onset of labour is extremely rare, and almost unknown in the primigravid woman.[5,9] However, cases are described with spontaneous rupture of the uterus in the second or third trimester occurring without apparent previous instrumentation of the uterus or congenital anomaly.

Uterine scar

This is by far the commonest cause in the developed world and the rising caesarean section rate is the main reason that uterine rupture is also increasing.[10]

Caesarean section

The classical caesarean section scar in the upper uterine segment is much more prone to rupture than the lower segment caesarean section scar. In the puerperium the upper uterine segment actively contracts and may disrupt the sutured incision, interfering with healing. During a subsequent pregnancy the upper uterine segment is more contractile and Braxton Hicks contractions may further disrupt the scar. If the placenta is implanted over the scar, a much more likely event in the upper uterine segment, the invading trophoblast and poor decidual response may further weaken the scar.

Hysterotomy

There is not much experience with pregnancy and labour after hysterotomy. However, the hysterotomy scar seems to have a similar propensity to rupture as the classical caesarean scar.[11]

Myomectomy

The uterine scar of abdominal myomectomy is not encountered frequently in modern obstetrics. If the scar or scars are not extensive, and particularly if the uterine cavity was not entered, subsequent uterine rupture in labour is uncommon. Similarly, hysteroscopic myomectomy, particularly if the fibroid was polypoid and mainly submucous, may not impair the integrity of the uterine wall. However, many of these patients have had associated infertility, are older and may be regarded as 'premium' pregnancies. For a combination of these and other reasons they are often delivered by elective caesarean section.

Metroplasty

The abdominal excision of a uterine septum and reconstruction of the uterus has largely been replaced by hysteroscopic resection. In women who have had an abdominal metroplasty, especially to unify a bicornate uterus, the scar should be treated like that of a classical caesarean section.

Salpingectomy with cornual resection

A simple salpingectomy carried out flush with the uterine wall does not increase the risk of subsequent rupture. If, however, cornual resection was undertaken – possibly in association with a previous cornual ectopic – this, the thinnest part of the myometrium, would be vulnerable to rupture in a subsequent pregnancy and labour.

Previous uterine perforation

This may occur with a number of intrauterine manipulations including: dilatation and curettage (pregnant or non-pregnant); insertion of intrauterine contraceptive device; diagnostic and operative hysteroscopy; and manual removal of the placenta – particularly if there were accretic areas 'clawed off' the uterine wall with the hand.

Cervical scar

Cervical amputation or conisation, deep cervical lacerations and cervical cerclage are rare causes of rupture of the lower uterine segment and vaginal vault.

Oxytocic drugs

The inappropriate use of oxytocic drugs is an important and ideally preventable cause of uterine rupture. The prostaglandin agents have a longer action than oxytocin and their use for induction of labour is associated with an increased risk of uterine tachysystole and hypertonous with the potential for uterine rupture – particularly in the presence of a previous uterine scar (see Chapter 12).

The use of oxytocin augmentation for non-progressive labour in the multiparous woman requires caution and judgement.[5] Augmenting uterine contractions in the presence of cephalo-pelvic disproportion in a multiparous woman risks uterine rupture.

Obstructed labour

Neglected obstructed labour is a significant contributor to uterine rupture in developing countries. A distinction should be made between the primiparous and multiparous woman. The primigravid uterus responds to obstruction with exhaustion and diminution of contractions, whereas the multiparous uterus will often 'redouble its efforts' in the face of obstruction, culminating in rupture. Indeed, multiparity is a predisposing cause to all types of uterine rupture. Repeated pregnancy leads to an increase of fibrous tissue in the uterus and a thinning of the uterine muscle.

Bandl's ring

'The upper parts of the uterus were uniformly hard, the lower somewhat softer. A shallow, transverse furrow, an inch below the umbilicus indicated the boundary between the uterine corpus and the cervix (lower uterine segment) ... The head and shoulders were partly palpable through the abdominal wall, covered only by a very thin layer. The whole cervix (lower uterine segment) was uniformly paper-thin and enormously stretched out, so that it must surely have contained half the infant while the body of the uterus and fundus sat on the infant like a cap ... The conditions in this case were obviously most favorable for rupture of the uterus. It would have taken only one or two additional contractions of the uterus or the increased pressure of the physician's hand or an instrument to bring it about ...'

Ludwig Bandl
Über Ruptur der Gebärmutter und ihre Mechanik. Vienna: Czermak, 1875

Obstetric manipulation

Internal version and breech extraction of a neglected shoulder presentation carries the highest risk of uterine rupture. In these cases the lower uterine segment is stretched to its maximum and the additional manipulation is often the final straw, culminating in a longitudinal rupture up the lateral side of the uterus. The lower uterine segment, cervix and vaginal vault are often collectively ruptured in this manoeuvre. Thus, the only acceptable role for internal version and breech extraction in modern obstetrics is in delivery of the second twin.

Forceps delivery can cause uterine rupture, but only with the type of forceps delivery – carried out at a higher level in the pelvis (at spines or above) – that is unacceptable in modern obstetrics. Of these, forceps rotation is more likely to cause uterine rupture, particularly with the classical application of the anterior blade of Kielland's forceps.

Manual removal of the placenta is an uncommon cause of uterine rupture. However, if it is done following a prolonged labour, the lower uterine segment may be very thin and the junction with the contracted and retracted upper uterine segment is vulnerable to perforation by the exploring hand. Rupture of the uterus can also occur during over-energetic 'clawing' at the uterine wall, particularly if there are accretic portions of placenta.

Fetal destructive operations may breach the uterine wall, particularly if the lower segment is over-distended by, for example, fetal hydrocephalus or shoulder presentation (see Chapter 26).

Uterine manipulation used with excessive force, such as fundal pressure and suprapubic pressure with shoulder dystocia or manipulations associated with external version, may rarely cause rupture.

Trauma

Direct trauma to the maternal abdomen and uterus leading to uterine rupture can occur with motor vehicle accidents, assault and accidental falls.

Miscellaneous

A number of other rare causes of uterine rupture include cornual pregnancy, gestational trophoblastic disease, placenta percreta and uterine anomalies.

Clinical features

There is a broad spectrum of clinical presentation with uterine rupture, from mild non-specific signs and symptoms to an obvious haemorrhagic intra-abdominal catastrophe. The classical symptoms and signs of complete uterine rupture are a sudden feeling of something giving way, cessation of uterine contractions, alteration in the shape of the abdominal swelling, severe abdominal pain, haemorrhage and collapse. At the other end of the clinical spectrum rupture of the relatively avascular lower segment caesarean scar may occur with no symptoms and labour continuing normally, only for the rupture to manifest itself postpartum, if at all. The following symptoms and signs of impending or early uterine rupture are relevant:

Tenderness over the site of the uterine scar is often cited as a sign of imminent rupture; seldom, however, is it encountered in practice. Tenderness over the lower uterine segment in between contractions is not uncommon in normal labour with an intact unscarred uterus. That said, persistent and increasing point tenderness should not be ignored.

Lower abdominal pain occurs to a varying degree. This may be limited or non-existent in the case of incomplete rupture of a lower segment caesarean scar. In obstructed labour, as the expulsive forces try in vain to expel the fetus, the patient becomes restless and complains of constant pain over the lower part of the uterus, while the uterine contractions become more and more tetanic. This is associated with increasing vertical stretching and thinning of the lower uterine segment, such that there is a thick band of muscle at the junction between the upper and lower uterine segments. This is known as a 'retraction ring' (Bandl's ring). Such a late sign should not be seen in modern obstetrics but can occur in cases of neglected obstructed labour and may be visible and palpable on abdominal examination in thin women.

Cessation of uterine contractions will occur if the uterus ruptures sufficiently for the fetus to be extruded into the abdominal cavity. It may be difficult for the patient to distinguish between the pain of uterine contractions and the pain from scar rupture and intraperitoneal bleeding.

Alteration in the shape of the abdominal swelling will occur only if the child passes in whole or in part outside the uterus – this does not happen as often as is supposed.

When it does, two abdominal swellings can be differentiated, the one representing fetal parts which have escaped and the other the retracted uterus. If, however, the retracted uterus is displaced behind or in front of the fetus it may not be possible to distinguish the two swellings. Generally speaking if this sign is elicited there are other obvious signs of intra-abdominal bleeding and shock.

Vaginal bleeding can vary from none, to little, to heavy. Often a previous caesarean scar, classical or lower segment, is quite avascular and ruptures with minimal bleeding either externally or internally. On other occasions there may be heavy bleeding but this is confined to the peritoneal cavity or into the broad ligament and retroperitoneal space, without a lot of vaginal bleeding. If there is lateral rupture of the lower uterine segment and the vaginal vault the bleeding *per vaginam* may be profuse.

Bladder symptoms and signs are important. In early rupture of the lower uterine segment there may be bladder tenesmus and haematuria. This is particularly so in the case of rupture of a previous lower segment scar which is often adherent to the posterior bladder wall.

Maternal tachycardia, hypotension and syncope will accompany intraperitoneal bleeding.

Fetal heart rate abnormalities such as tachycardia, variable, late and prolonged decelerations are common, and among the most reliable early warning signs of uterine rupture.

Management

Treat hypovolaemic shock if required (see Chapter 22).

Laparotomy

If the diagnosis is one of potential early scar rupture with a stable fetal heart and maternal condition (e.g. with a previous lower segment caesarean section) one may enter through a Pfannenstiel incision. In most cases, however, the degree of urgency either for fetal or maternal condition, or both, will warrant the most rapid method of entry by lower midline incision. Once the abdomen is entered the fetus should be immediately delivered if partially or completely extruded from the uterus. If the fetus remains in the uterus it should be delivered with dispatch. In some cases both the fetus and the placenta are extruded into the peritoneal cavity and both should be removed. (Before closing the abdomen, always remember to account for the placenta, which can be forgotten during the sometimes hectic surgical endeavours.)

The uterus should be brought out of the incision. The assistant can aid by placing the hands behind the uterus, pulling it up and with the fingers and thumbs occluding the uterine vessels. Green–Armytage or ring forceps should be applied swiftly to the bleeding edges of the lacerated uterine muscle.

If the bleeding is torrential, which is quite rare, manual compression of the aorta may be useful as a stop gap measure to allow suction and mopping away of the blood to delineate the extent of the damage.

If it is clear that the uterus is ruptured beyond repair and that hysterectomy will be required two large straight clamps should be applied across the adnexal structures (round ligament, utero-ovarian ligament and fallopian tube) and close to the uterine body. This will stop the source of bleeding from the ovarian arteries. If the rupture is in the upper uterine segment a catheter, penrose drain, or portion of intravenous tubing can be passed around the lower uterine segment, just above the cervix and tightened to occlude the uterine arteries (see Chapter 26).

Surgical options

After securing haemostasis the choice of definitive surgery will depend on the type of rupture and a number of other factors including the patient's condition, facilities available, experience of the surgeon, and the woman's desire to retain the uterus and possible future fertility.[12]

Repair of laceration

Provided the laceration is simple, and this is most likely with rupture of a previous caesarean scar (either lower segment or classical), repair is appropriate and straightforward.[13–15]

In the case of ruptured caesarean scars there is often little bleeding due to the avascular nature of the scar, unless there has been extension into the adjacent unscarred myometrium or broad ligament. In repairing avascular caesarean scars it is a good idea to trim the scarred edges and re-suture the more viable adjacent tissues. Any subsequent pregnancy is at increased risk of scar rupture and should be delivered by elective caesarean section at 37 weeks gestation.

Repair of laceration plus tubal ligation

If the rupture is simple and uninfected then this is the simplest and safest treatment. Only if the woman has a strong desire to retain her fertility would one omit tubal ligation after simple repair of a laceration. This assumes one has been able to discuss this preoperatively with the woman to obtain appropriate consent.

Subtotal hysterectomy

If there is no overt sepsis, and no involvement of the cervix or paracolpos, subtotal hysterectomy is the procedure of choice. This can be done more rapidly and, compared with total hysterectomy, carries less risk of damage to the ureters or bladder (see Chapter 26).

Total hysterectomy

This procedure is necessary if the cervix and paracolpos are involved or if there is sepsis associated with the rupture (see Chapter 26).

In all cases involving the lower uterine segment it is essential to clarify the position and integrity of the bladder. The bladder must be identified and retracted well clear of the surgical field. With lower segment ruptures, particularly those of previous lower caesarean scars, the bladder wall is often lacerated because of its adherence to the lower uterine segment. The integrity must be carefully checked as outlined in Chapter 26.

All of the above procedures should be covered with perioperative antibiotics and thromboprophylaxis.

References

1. Aboyeji AP, Ijaiya MDA, Yahaya VR. Ruptured uterus: a study of 100 consecutive cases in Ilorin, Nigeria. J Obstet Gynaecol Res 2001; 27:341–348.
2. Al-Sakka M, Harusho A, Khan L. Rupture of the pregnant uterus: a 21 year review. Int J Gynecol Obstet 1998; 63:105–108.
3. Kafkas S, Toner CE. Ruptured uterus. Int J Gynaecol Obstet 1991; 34:41–44.
4. Eden RD, Parker RT, Gall SA. Rupture of the pregnancy uterus: a 53 year review. Obstet Gynecol 1986; 68:671–673.
5. Gardeil F, Daly S, Turner MJ. Uterine rupture in pregnancy reviewed. Eur J Obstet Gynecol Reprod Biol 1994; 56:107–110.
6. Turner MJ. Uterine rupture. Best Prac Res Clin Obstet Gynaecol 2002; 16:69–79.
7. Yap OWS, Kim ES, Laros RK. Maternal and neonatal outcomes after uterine rupture in labor. Am J Obstet Gynecol 2001; 184:1576–1581.
8. Hofmeyer GJ, Say L, Gülmezoglu AM. WHO systematic review of maternal mortality and morbidity: the prevalence of uterine rupture. Br J Obstet Gynaecol 2005; 112:1221–1228.
9. Miller DA, Goodwin TM, Gherman RB, Paul RH. Intrapartum rupture of the unscarred uterus. Obstet Gynecol 1997; 89:671–673.
10. Kieser KE, Baskett TF. A 10-year population-based study of uterine rupture. Obstet Gynecol 2002; 100:749–753.
11. Clow N, Crompton AC. The wounded uterus: pregnancy after hysterotomy. BMJ 1973; 1:21–23.
12. Mokgokong ET, Marivate M. Treatment of the ruptured uterus. S Afr Med J 1976; 50:1621–1624.
13. O'Connor RA, Gaughan B. Pregnancy following simple repair of the ruptured gravid uterus. Br J Obstet Gynaecol 1989; 96:942--944.
14. Solton MH, Khashoggi T, Adelusi B. Pregnancy following rupture of the pregnant uterus. Int J Gynecol Obstet 1996; 52:37–42.
15. Lim AC, Kwee A, Bruinse HW. Pregnancy after uterine rupture: a report of 5 cases and a review of the literature. Obstet Gynecol Surv 2005; 60:613–617.

14

Breech delivery

'If the feet of the child come foremost, you must take care to baptize them immediately …'

Paul Portal
The Compleat Practice of Men and Women Midwives. London: J. Johnson, 1763, p23

The fetus in breech presentation has a higher perinatal mortality and morbidity due mainly to prematurity, congenital anomalies, birth asphyxia and trauma. At 28 weeks gestation the incidence of breech presentation is approximately one in five. At term, 3–4% of all fetuses are in breech presentation, making this the commonest malpresentation.

Over the past 25 years there has been a worldwide trend to deliver a greater proportion of breech presentations by caesarean section. In 2000 an international multicentre randomized controlled trial of planned vaginal delivery versus planned elective caesarean section for uncomplicated term breech presentation confirmed that perinatal mortality and serious neonatal morbidity were significantly lower in the planned caesarean group.[1] Secondary analysis of the Term Breech Trial showed that prelabour caesarean and caesarean during early labour were associated with the lowest adverse perinatal outcome due to labour or delivery and that vaginal delivery had the highest risk of adverse outcome.[2] As a result, although the conclusions of this trial have been disputed,[3–6] where appropriate facilities exist caesarean section for the term breech has become a standard of care in many hospitals.[7] For the preterm breech there is no conclusive evidence that caesarean delivery is safer than a carefully conducted vaginal delivery, however, the majority of obstetricians choose caesarean section for the viable preterm breech.

The above notwithstanding, there are still occasions when vaginal breech delivery will have to be undertaken, for the following reasons:

1. Labour may proceed so rapidly that there is inadequate time to perform caesarean section. Even in the Term Breech Trial almost one in 10 of those assigned to delivery by caesarean section were delivered vaginally.[1]
2. Labour and delivery may occur in a setting where caesarean section is unavailable or carries greater risks than are justified by the perceived perinatal benefit.
3. From erroneous observation or lack of opportunity the diagnosis of breech presentation may not be made until late in the second stage of labour, when it is too late to perform caesarean section.
4. The woman, although informed of the increased perinatal risks, may still choose to proceed with labour and vaginal delivery.

In addition, while caesarean section may reduce the risks of fetal trauma, it is still necessary to know and perform the appropriate manoeuvres required to safely deliver the fetus through the uterine incision. This applies particularly to the after-coming head of the fetus. These manoeuvres are similar to those required for atraumatic vaginal breech delivery. Thus, it remains essential for the accoucheur to acquire and retain the skills necessary to protect the fetus during vaginal delivery. In units where very few breeches are delivered vaginally these skills may still be acquired by careful teaching and mannikin drills, and with the routine and systematic application of appropriate manoeuvres during caesarean delivery of the fetus in breech presentation through the uterine incision.[8,9]

Intrapartum fetal risks

The main reasons for the poor outcome of the breech presentation, compared with the fetus in cephalic presentation, are prematurity and congenital anomalies. It is also possible that there are subtle neurological abnormalities that cause the fetus to lie in breech presentation and which may contribute to a poorer outcome irrespective of the method of delivery. During labour and delivery the fetus in breech presentation is subjected to the following risks:

- A higher incidence of cord entanglement or cord prolapse, especially in the footling breech, may lead to asphyxia. In addition, when the after-coming head of the breech enters the pelvic brim the associated cord compression can cause asphyxia if there is undue delay in descent and delivery of the head.
- The fetal buttocks and trunk have a smaller diameter than the head. This is particularly exaggerated in the preterm fetus. Thus, there is a danger that the buttocks and trunk will slip through an incompletely dilated cervix causing entrapment of the arms and/or the head, leading to trauma and asphyxia.
- Fracture or dislocation of limbs may occur and this is most likely with extended or nuchal displacement of the arms.
- Damage to intra-abdominal organs may be sustained, especially the liver and spleen, if the hands of the accoucheur are placed above the pelvis and encircle the abdomen during manipulations.
- Cervical spine dislocation or fracture due to excessive traction during delivery of the head, particularly if there is hyperextension of the neck because of undue elevation of the body of the fetus while the head is still in the pelvis.
- Brachial plexus injury due to inappropriate and excessive traction on the shoulders in an attempt to deliver the head.
- Traction on the fetal trunk while the head remains in the pelvis may tend to pull the base of the fetal skull away from the vault.
- As the fetal head descends across the pelvic floor and perineum there is compression and, if delivery of the fetal head is not carefully controlled, sudden decompression as the head delivers. This may cause a tentorial tear and intracranial haemorrhage, risks which are increased when there is concomitant hypoxia.

In essence, the job of the obstetrician is to protect the fetal brain during labour and delivery, and nowhere is this duty more critical than in breech delivery. The key is to apply a well-rehearsed sequence of manoeuvres and achieve the balance between excessive haste leading to traumatic delivery and undue delay with its risk of asphyxia. In most cases a minimal amount of interference is required but there should always be active control and protection of the fetal head at delivery.

Anaesthesia

For some women a combination of narcotic, inhalation and pudendal block will provide adequate analgesia and allow the most natural progression of the first and second stages of labour. Epidural block provides the best pain relief and also has the advantage of blunting the maternal bearing-down effort in the late first stage of labour. In the nulliparous woman epidural block may be required for adequate pain relief, but can prevent the desired maternal bearing-down effort in the second stage of labour. This may lead to uncertainty as to whether such failure of descent is due to impaired maternal propulsive effort or due to feto-pelvic disproportion. In carefully selected cases oxytocin augmentation may be used, but with extreme caution. On the other hand, the multiparous woman often receives adequate pain relief with narcotic, inhalation and pudendal block, but epidural analgesia has the benefit of blunting her bearing-down reflex which may occur prematurely in the late first stage of labour. The ideal, therefore, is a selective epidural block that allows retention of motor activity, while providing a humane degree of sensory block. Ideally an anaesthetist should be present at all breech deliveries, either to supervise the regional block or to provide rapid general anaesthesia and/or uterine relaxation if necessary.

First stage of labour

In general the frank and complete types of breech presentation fill the lower uterine segment and are well applied to the cervix. In contrast, the footling breech (Fig 14.1) may not and there is a much higher incidence of cord prolapse. For this reason, and the propensity of the footling breech to slip through

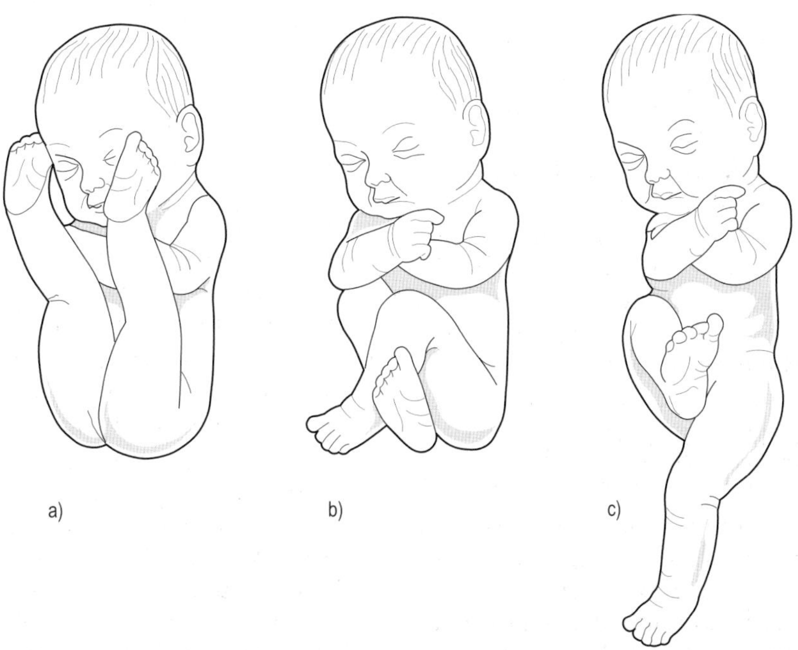

Figure 14.1 Types of breech presentation. (a) Frank, (b) complete and (c) footling.

the incompletely dilated cervix, labour is best avoided with a footling breech presentation unless there is no alternative. The frank or complete breech at term, of reasonable size (2000–3800 g), is most likely to result in a safe vaginal delivery if the first stage of labour is smooth and progressive.

Oxytocin augmentation is permissible, particularly in the nulliparous breech, for similar indications to cephalic presentation. However, this would only be undertaken in cases where caesarean delivery is not a realistic alternative. Amniotomy in labour is acceptable if the breech is well applied to the cervix. In general, however, one tries to leave the membranes intact as long as possible. X-ray pelvimetry is of no proven value for management of the breech in labour.

When the membranes rupture spontaneously during labour an immediate pelvic examination should be done to exclude cord prolapse.

It is essential to be sure that the cervix is fully dilated and not palpable before encouraging maternal bearing-down effort. Because the breech is usually smaller than the aftercoming head it is possible, even at term, for the breech to appear at the introitus before the cervix is fully dilated. The early appearance of male external genitalia can also be misleading. It is therefore a cardinal rule that one must check for full cervical dilatation before proceeding with delivery.

Conduct of breech delivery

Delivery of the breech and legs

With uterine contractions and maternal effort the breech should be allowed to descend to the perineum. The woman can then be placed in the lithotomy position and, if epidural analgesia has not already been established, a pudendal block is performed along with local anaesthetic infiltration of the perineum. The guiding principle at this time is 'keep your hands off the breech', be patient, and await the appearance of critical anatomical landmarks (Fig 14.2). The most helpful manoeuvres involve flexion and rotation but not traction. The following sequence should be observed:

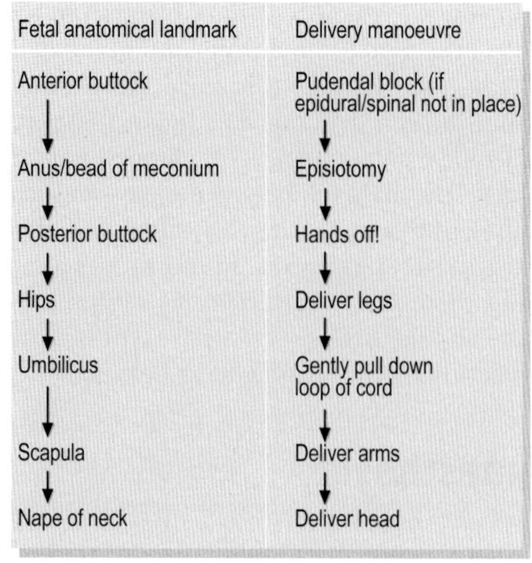

Fetal anatomical landmark	Delivery manoeuvre
Anterior buttock ↓	Pudendal block (if epidural/spinal not in place) ↓
Anus/bead of meconium ↓	Episiotomy ↓
Posterior buttock ↓	Hands off! ↓
Hips ↓	Deliver legs ↓
Umbilicus ↓	Gently pull down loop of cord ↓
Scapula ↓	Deliver arms ↓
Nape of neck	Deliver head

Figure 14.2 Breech delivery: fetal anatomical landmarks and sequence of manoeuvres.

- As the breech descends it meets the obstruction of the perineum. With further maternal effort the anterior buttock of the fetus 'climbs up' the perineum until the fetal anus is visible over the fourchette – usually manifest by a bead of meconium. The breech does not recede in between contractions. At this point the combination of descent and lateral flexion of the fetus has reached its maximum and further progress will only occur when the obstruction of the perineum is removed. This, therefore, is the point at which episiotomy is performed, with special care to avoid injury to the fetal genitalia. The comparable timing for a footling breech presentation is when the fetal buttocks reach the perineum.
- A combination of the above observations and testing the distention of the perineum with a finger will guide the precise timing of episiotomy, with particular care taken to avoid cutting fetal soft tissues. Wait until the beginning of a contraction and then perform the episiotomy, which ensures maternal effort throughout the entire uterine contraction to help deliver the buttocks and legs. With a complete breech, maternal effort alone will usually deliver the legs and lower trunk.
- With a frank breech presentation the extended legs often require assistance in

the form of slight abduction at the hip and flexion of the knee for delivery. One hip is usually anterolateral and two or three fingers should be placed along the fetal thigh above the knee to slightly abduct and flex the hip followed by flexion of the knee on the fetal body. The more 'splinting' fingers that can be placed along the thigh to conduct this manoeuvre the greater the distribution of force, which lessens the chance of fracture of the femur. This principle applies to all manoeuvres involving the limbs. Once the anterior leg has been flexed and delivered the breech should be gently rotated so that the other hip is anterolateral and the same procedure repeated on the other side (Fig 14.3).

- The remainder of the abdomen and lower thorax will usually deliver with maternal effort alone. At this point gently bring down a loop of umbilical cord so it is not under tension for the remainder of the delivery.

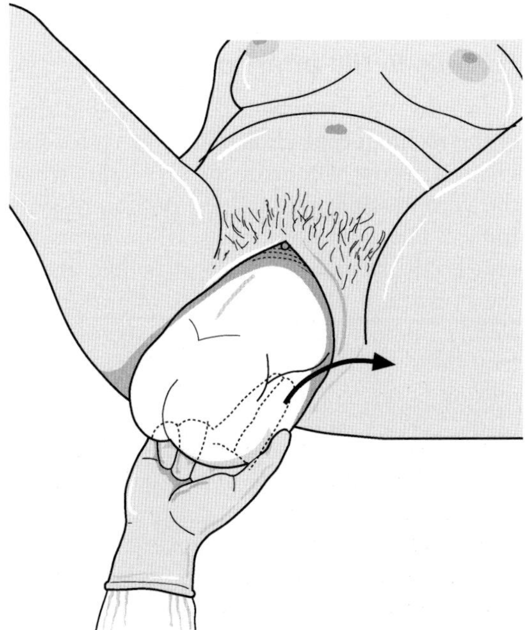

Figure 14.3 Assisted delivery of extended legs. The fingers splint the femur, slightly abduct the thigh and then flex the hip and knee.

- Throughout delivery of the legs, abdomen and lower thorax there should be minimal or no traction, which is likely to cause extension of the arms and fetal head – both undesirable. Other than assisting the delivery of extended legs with flexion and ensuring that the fetal back remains anterior, one should rely on maternal effort alone.

Delivery of the shoulders and arms

A critical stage of the delivery has now been reached. As the fetal trunk delivers and descends the fetal head will enter the pelvic brim, causing compression of the umbilical cord. Ideally the rest of the delivery should be accomplished within 2–3 minutes, to avoid asphyxia. On the other hand one must not panic and employ undue haste, potentially leading to trauma of the arms, brachial plexus, cervical spine and brain. Although it may not seem so, 2–3 minutes is ample time to systematically and carefully go through the manoeuvres to effect safe delivery:

- With maternal effort alone the lower border of the more anterior scapula will become visible under the pubic arch. Provided no undue traction has been applied the arms are usually flexed across the fetal chest. Using two fingers pass them over the fetal shoulder and down along the humerus, splinting and sweeping it across the chest to deliver the elbow and forearm. The fetus is then rotated 90° to bring the other scapula into view and the same procedure is repeated.
- When rotating the fetus for this and other purposes it is important to avoid gripping the fetal abdomen. The obstetrician's hands should grasp the thighs with the thumbs over the sacrum and the index fingers around the iliac crest. In this way the intra-abdominal contents will not be traumatized. The use of a small sterilized towel will assist the correct placement and help maintain the grip (Fig 14.4).

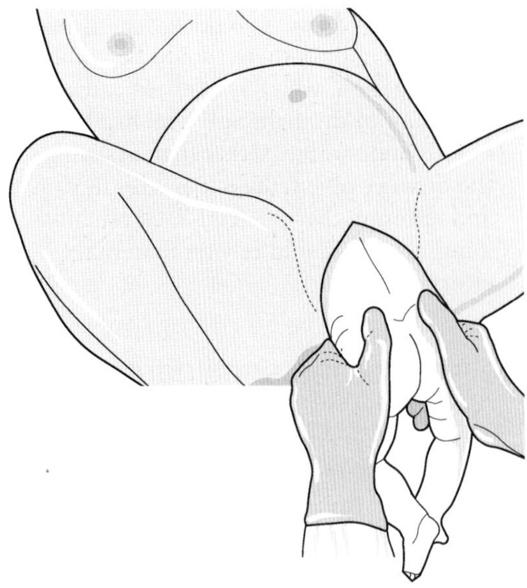

Figure 14.4 The manner of grasping the breech for rotation and traction.

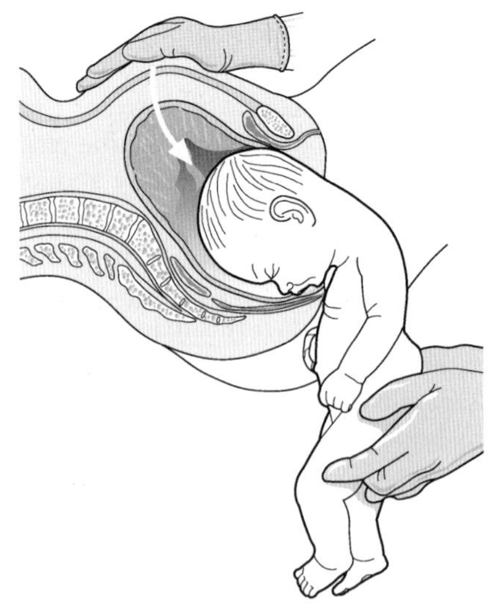

Figure 14.5 The fetus suspended vertically, partially supported by the operator's hands. An assistant provides suprapubic pressure. This combination promotes descent and flexion of the fetal head.

Delivery of the head

At this point the obstetrician becomes actively involved to protect the fetal head during delivery. The key factors are gentle descent and flexion of the fetal head, protection of the cervical spine from excessive traction or hyperextension, and protection of the fetal brain from the compression and sudden decompression forces during delivery over the perineum. It is this sudden decompression, or 'champagne cork' delivery, that can lead to tentorial tears and intracranial haemorrhage. The following sequence is recommended:

- After delivery of the arms, descent and flexion of the fetal head are encouraged by allowing the infant's body, partially supported by the operator's hands, to hang vertically. An assistant applies mild suprapubic pressure to help promote descent and flexion (Fig 14.5). It is important that the infant should not hang by its own weight unsupported as this may promote extension of the head or, in a small infant, allow completely uncontrolled delivery of the head.
- When the hair line on the back of the infant's head (the nape of the neck) is visible under the pubic arch the head has descended adequately and the time has come for its assisted delivery.

In all cases delivery of the head should be carefully controlled. There have been many techniques described for this purpose but the two main ones will be described here.

Forceps to the after-coming head

If facilities and assistance are available this is the technique of choice as it provides the greatest degree of control and protection from the compression and sudden decompression forces. The operator kneels while an assistant holds the infant's body at or just above the horizontal plane. It is very important to clearly instruct the assistant not to hold the fetal body higher than this plane as hyperextension of the fetal neck can cause dislocation of the cervical spine, bleeding in the venous plexus around the cervical spinal cord, and even quadriplegia.

Piper's forceps were designed particularly for the after-coming head of the breech, but any of the long handled forceps can be used. The reason the operator kneels is to see under the trunk of the infant and also because the plane of application of the forceps is in a slightly upward manner following the curve of the sacrum. Hold one forcep by the handle

First use of forceps to the after-coming head of the breech

'In the year 1755, I was called to a case ... but after the body was delivered, the head of the child stuck at the brim of the pelvis, on which I made several trials to bring it down into the vagina ... I was afraid of overstraining the neck if I repeated these trials and increased the force. The patient being in a supine position, I introduced a blade of the long forceps, curved to one side, up along each side of the pelvis, while an assistant held up the body of the child to give more room for the application; and having fixed them on the head, and joined the blades of the instrument together, I introduced two fingers of my left hand, and fixed them on each side of the child's nose, while my right hand pulled the head with the instrument and delivered it safely.'

William Smellie
The Collection of Preternatural Cases and Observations in Midwifery. Vol 3. London: D. Wilson and T. Durham, 1764, p193

with the tips of the fingers of the second hand placed at the end of the blade. The blade is then inserted between four and five o'clock and the tips of the fingers guide the insertion alongside the fetal head. A similar procedure is done with the other forcep blade inserted between 7 and 8 o'clock. Particular care should be exercised in applying the forceps blades. Because the episiotomy has already been performed there is a danger that the tip of the blade can track into the paravaginal tissues under the apex of the episiotomy.

Another advantage of the forceps is that gentle traction promotes flexion of the fetal head, reducing the diameter and aiding descent. During initial descent of the fetal head the body of the fetus must remain in the horizontal plane (Fig 14.6a). Once the chin and mouth are visible over the perineum then the forceps, body and legs of the fetus are raised in unison

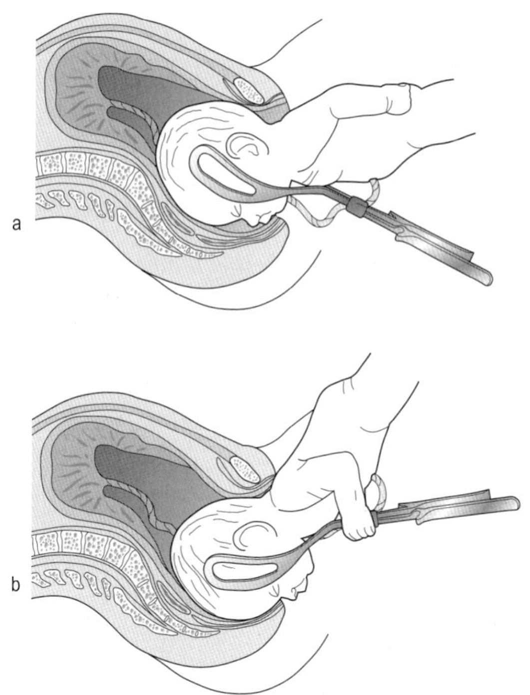

Figure 14.6 Forceps to the after-coming head. (a) During initial descent and flexion of the head the fetal trunk is kept horizontal. (b) As the fetal chin is delivered the forceps and body are raised in unison.

to complete delivery (Fig 14.6b). The combination of flexion and safe traction on the fetal head, plus the cradling effect of the forceps which provides protection from compression and decompression, make this an ideal method for safe delivery of the head.

Mauriceau–Smellie–Veit manoeuvre

This technique is invaluable when delivery happens rapidly, there is no assistance, or no time to apply the forceps. The operator's forearm is placed under the fetal body with a fetal leg on either side. The forefinger and middle finger of this hand are placed on the maxilla beside the nose to promote flexion of the fetal head. It is permissible initially to gently flex the lower jaw to bring the maxilla into reach. However, no undue traction should be placed on the lower jaw of the fetus as it risks dislocation and is not as effective in flexing the fetal head as the safer position of the fingers on the maxilla. The other hand is placed on the fetal back with the middle finger pushing up the occiput, to promote flexion, and the other fingers resting on the fetal shoulders. With this grip, the cervical

First description of what was to become the Mauriceau-Smellie-Veit manoeuvre

'I therefore passed my fingers up the child's mouth supporting the breast with my wrist and arm, putting one finger into the mouth, and two others upon the cheeks, I pulled towards me, and at the same time drawing with my other hand above the shoulders, brought out the head.'

William Giffard
Cases in Midwifery. London: Motte, 1734

Mauriceau-Smellie-Veit manoeuvre

'Then I brought the body lower, but finding that the head stopped at the upper part of the pelvis, I insinuated my hand up along the breast, and introduced a finger into the mouth, and by pulling gently brought the forehead into the concave part of the sacrum: being afraid of overstraining the underjaw, I quitted that hold and placed a finger on each side of the nose; then I laid the body of the child on that arm, and by slipping the fingers of my other hand over the shoulders and on each side on the neck, I got the head safely extracted'.

William Smellie
The Collection of Preternatural Cases and Observations in Midwifery. Vol 3. London: D. Wilson and T. Durham, 1764, p72

spine is splinted and protected while flexion of the fetal head is promoted (Fig 14.7). Gentle traction in a downward and backward plane should help guide the head over the perineum and control delivery to avoid sudden decompression. Only gentle traction should be used with this technique and its role is usually that of slowing down and controlling the delivery, rather than providing traction. If traction is necessary to cause descent of the fetal head, forceps to the after-coming head is the safer technique.

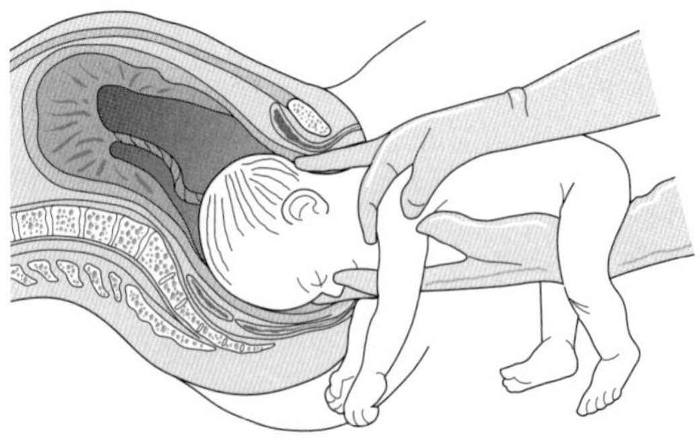

Figure 14.7 Mauriceau–Smellie–Veit manoeuvre.

Complications of breech delivery

Extended arms

Extension of the arms usually occurs when there has been inappropriate traction up to this point in the delivery. It also may occur if the trunk has passed through an incompletely dilated cervix. There are two techniques for dealing with extended arms.

Løvset's manoeuvre

'The theoretical basis for this procedure is that the posterior shoulder is always the lower one, owing to the pelvic inclination and the direction of the birth axis in the pelvic outlet ... If the body of the foetus is turned 180° with its back to the front, the shoulder will appear under the pubis if the body descends sufficiently during the last 90° to 130° of the manoeuvre. To make this possible the posterior shoulder must be below the promontory when the rotation begins, whether spontaneously or by traction.'

Jørgen Løvset
Shoulder delivery by breech presentation. J Obstet Gynaec Br Emp 1937; 44:696-701

Løvset's manoeuvre

The principle of this elegant manoeuvre is based on the fact that the inclination of the pelvis is such that the posterior shoulder enters the pelvic cavity in advance of the anterior shoulder. Using the pelvic grip on the fetus the trunk is gently drawn downwards with its back in the oblique anterior position. The body is then lifted to cause upward and lateral flexion, which promotes descent of the posterior shoulder below the sacral promontory. Using gentle traction and rotation the posterior shoulder is rotated through 180° to become the anterior shoulder. As it started below the pelvic brim it will remain at that level as it rotates to become the anterior shoulder, where it will be easily accessible below the symphysis pubis and the humerus can be swept down across the fetal chest and delivered. Keeping the back uppermost the body is then rotated back 180° bringing the other shoulder into the anterior and accessible position for delivery (Fig 14.8).

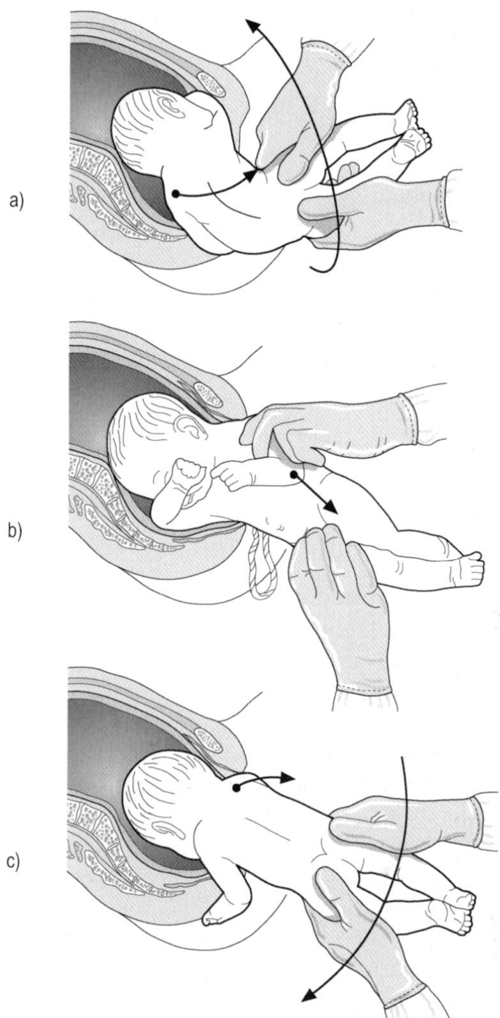

Figure 14.8 Løvset's manoeuvre. (a) The fetus is elevated slightly to facilitate descent of the posterior shoulder below the sacral promontory and then rotated 180°. (b) The posterior shoulder has been rotated to the anterior position and can be delivered. (c) Keeping the back uppermost the body is rotated 180° to allow delivery of the other arm.

Bringing down the posterior arm

This is an alternative to Løvset's manoeuvre, but requires full regional or general anaesthesia. If the fetal back is toward the mother's right side the operator's right hand grasps the fetal legs and pulls them gently up and over to the mother's left side, which serves to promote descent of the posterior shoulder. The operator's left hand is passed along the spine of the fetus, over its shoulder and laid along the humerus (Fig 14.9). Having reached the fetal shoulder, the index and middle fingers should be placed along the upper arm as far as the bend of the elbow and the arm pushed down across the fetal face. This should bring the humerus and elbow into range to be grasped, splinted and delivered by the whole hand. In the initial manoeuvre it is important not to try and hook the humerus down with one or two fingers or you risk fracture. By pushing it down across the fetal face flexion of the elbow should make the arm more accessible.

Nuchal arm

On rare occasions, usually because of inappropriate traction and rotational manoeuvres, the shoulder is extended and elbow flexed with the forearm trapped behind the occiput. Attempts to hook down the trapped arm will usually result in fracture of the humerus. Correct treatment is to rotate the fetus in the direction in which the hand is pointing. The occiput slips past the forearm and the friction of the rotation causes the shoulder and

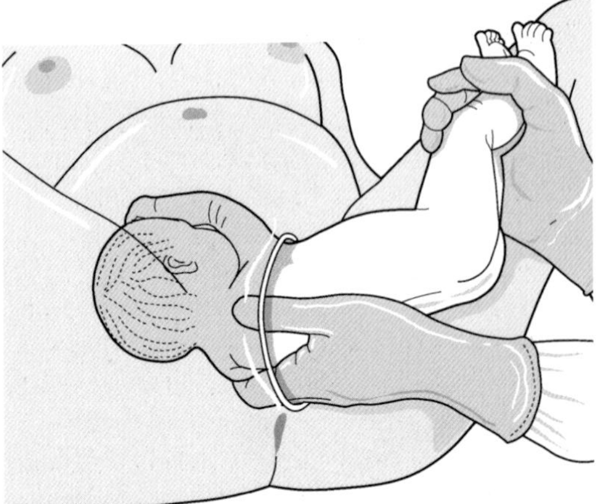

Figure 14.9 Bringing down the posterior extended arm.

elbow to flex and become accessible for delivery (Fig 14.10). In the very rare event of bilateral nuchal arms this type of rotation will assist in releasing one arm but worsen the situation of the other. Thus, gentle rotation is tried in either direction to find which arm can be more easily released first. Rotation in the opposite direction should then allow delivery of the other arm. Bilateral nuchal displacement of the arms is exceptionally rare and can be very difficult to rectify.

Posterior rotation of the trunk and head

This complication should not occur if a competent accoucheur has been in attendance throughout delivery and corrected any tendency of the back to rotate posteriorly. It can happen when the fetal trunk is born before assistance arrives, when of necessity one has to deal with an occipito-posterior position of the head. Even at this stage rotation may often be accomplished using the Mauriceau–Smellie–Veit manoeuvre to elevate and rotate the fetus to the occipito-anterior position. It is very important that the head and trunk are rotated together. If this is accomplished the delivery can be completed either by the Mauriceau–Smellie–Veit manoeuvre or with forceps to the after-coming head.

If rotation is impossible because the head is too firmly fixed low in the pelvis it may be delivered in the occipito-posterior position using the Mauriceau–Smellie–Veit manoeuvre or with forceps. The other alternative is to use the reverse Prague manoeuvre with one hand exerting gentle traction downwards and backwards on the shoulders, while the other lifts the feet to flex the infant and aid delivery of the occiput (Fig 14.11).

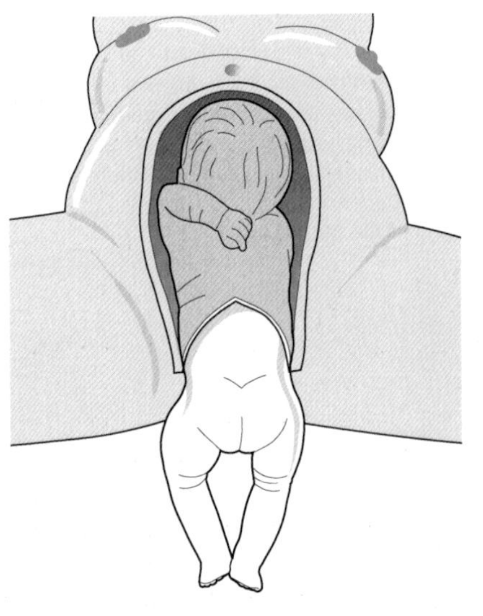

a)

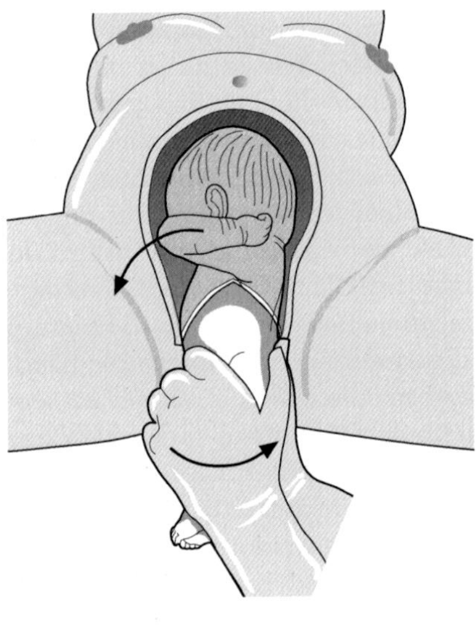

b)

Figure 14.10 (a) Nuchal arm. (b) The body is rotated 90° freeing the forearm from the occiput.

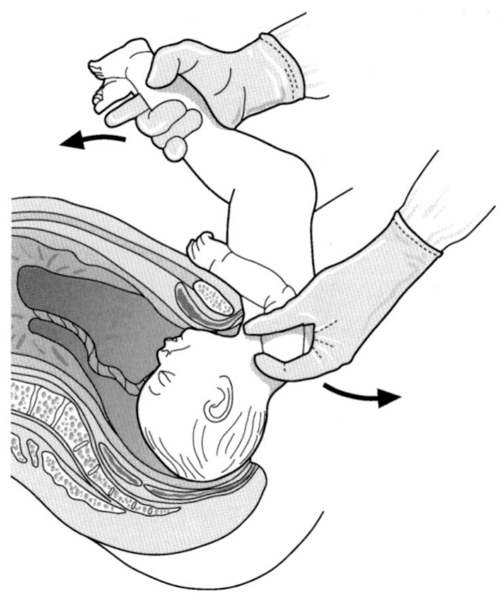

Figure 14.11 Reverse Prague manoeuvre to deliver the after-coming head when the occiput is posterior.

Head entrapment by incompletely dilated cervix

This is one of the most feared complications and, as previously mentioned, all steps should be taken to ensure that the cervix is fully dilated before breech delivery. It is more common in the preterm breech where the small body may easily slip through an incompletely dilated cervix. Should this occur before the head has descended enough to compress the umbilical cord, every effort should be made to prevent descent of the breech. In a number of these cases, cervical dilatation is occurring quite rapidly and only a few minutes stalling may be required.

If, however, the head has descended so that the cervix encloses the head and chin, the cord will be compressed and delivery must be effected rapidly. If the cervix is sufficiently distensible, forceps may be carefully slipped through the cervix and placed around the head to cradle and protect it while traction guides the head through the cervix to delivery. If the cervix is rigid and unyielding, it will have to be incised at the 4 and 7 o'clock position with long scissors so that the cervix is sufficiently open, but any extension of the incision does not extend upwards and tear the uterine vessels.

Breech extraction

Other than in selected cases of the second twin (Chapter 15) this procedure is rarely required in modern obstetrics. It is only justifiable if there is delay in the second stage together with a contraindication to caesarean section, or if the fetus is already dead. Exceptionally, in some geographical circumstances, breech extraction may be performed for cord prolapse at full dilatation in a multiparous patient.

The procedure should be carried out under anaesthesia with uterine relaxation. If the breech has arrested low in the pelvis, groin traction may be all that is required to make the legs accessible and accomplish the rest of the delivery in the manner of an assisted breech delivery. If only the anterior groin is accessible, traction may be provided with the forefinger passed over the thigh and the traction made against the trunk of the fetus. The amount of traction can be increased if the wrist is grasped by the other hand (Fig 14.12). If both the anterior and posterior fetal groins are accessible then a forefinger in each groin is more effective (Fig 14.13). Traction should be applied during a uterine contraction and a generous mediolateral episiotomy performed.

If the breech is higher in the pelvis, such that groin traction will not make the legs accessible, one has to bring down one or both legs. Under anaesthesia and profound uterine relaxation the hand should be passed up along the anterior thigh to beyond the bend of the knee. The lower tibia and foot are then grasped (Fig 14.14). Pinard's manoeuvre, which involves flexing the knee against the fetal abdomen and chest, may help make the foot more accessible (Fig 14.15). When reaching up for the ankle the operator should feel for the cord and try and manoeuvre it to the outer side of the hand, so that it lies between the hand and the uterine wall and is less likely to be entangled as the leg is brought down. If possible the posterior leg should also be brought down. If not, the anterior leg is adequate and if only one leg can be brought down it should always be the anterior one. If only the posterior leg is brought down the anterior buttock may be caught up on the symphysis pubis (Fig 14.16).

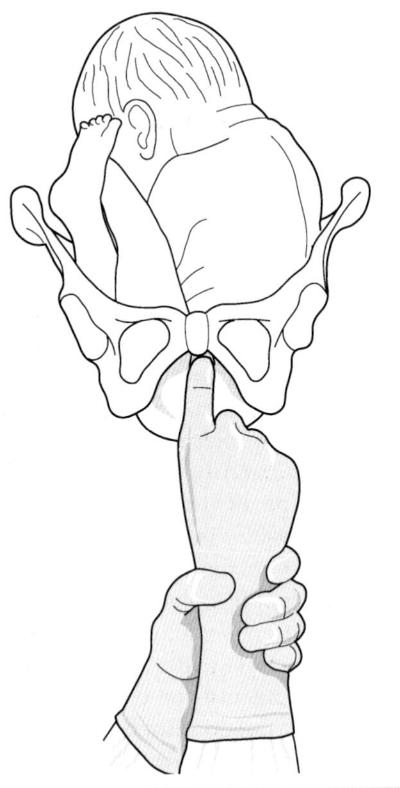

Figure 14.12 Breech extraction: traction with forefinger in the anterior groin. The other hand grasps the wrist to allow stronger traction.

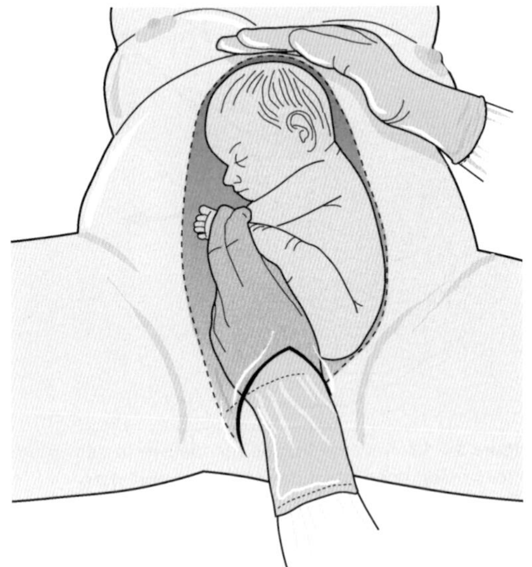

Figure 14.14 Breech extraction: bringing down the anterior leg.

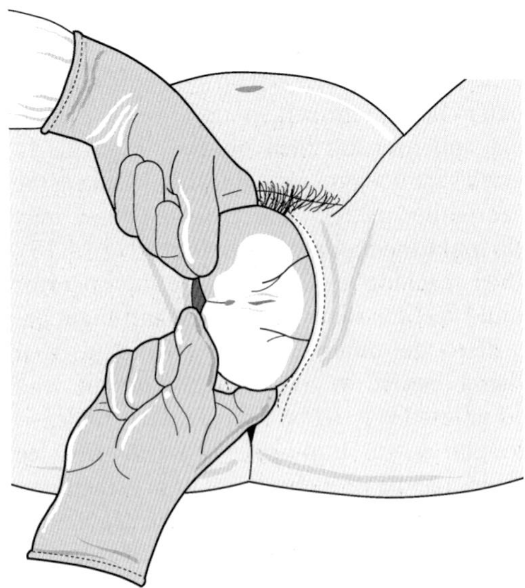

Figure 14.13 Traction with a forefinger in each groin.

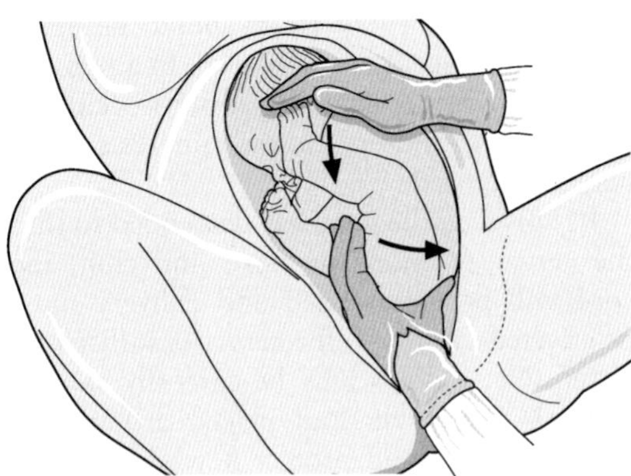

Figure 14.15 Breech extraction: Pinard's manoeuvre to make the foot more accessible.

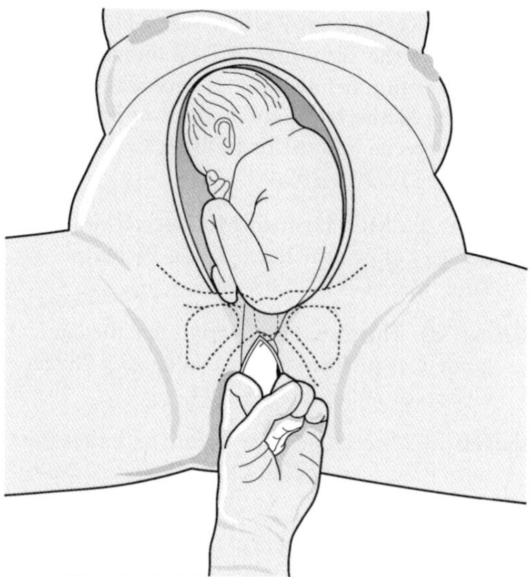

Figure 14.16 Breech extraction: if only the posterior leg is brought down, the anterior buttock may be caught up on the pubic symphysis.

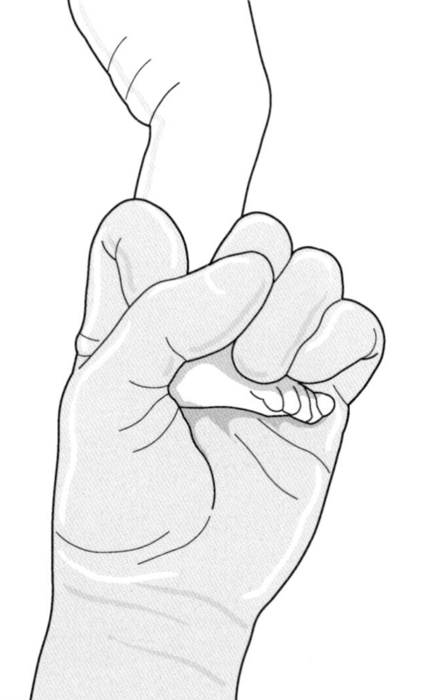

Figure 14.17 Breech extraction: method of grasping the foot.

Once the anterior or both feet have been brought down the foot or feet are grasped in the manner shown in Figure 14.17. Steady traction should be exerted downwards and backwards in line with the axis of the upper pelvis. If only the anterior leg has been delivered, traction is exerted until the fetal pelvis has been delivered. Rotate the infant so that the posterior hip becomes anterior and the leg is then delivered with the fingers splinting the femur and flexing the hip and knee upon the fetal abdomen. The remainder of the delivery is performed as for an assisted vaginal delivery. However, because of the traction employed extended arms are more likely to be encountered.

If the posterior leg has been brought down in error, the leg is rotated 180° in a wide arc during downward traction to become the anterior leg.

While this chapter has stressed that the modern standard of care for the term breech is delivery by caesarean section, careful selection and conduct of labour and vaginal breech delivery can bring good perinatal results with less risk to the mother. Depending on circumstances and facilities the obstetrician may be faced with no alternative but to conduct a breech vaginal delivery. Because most breech presentations are now delivered by caesarean section it is important that obstetricians organize a programme of external cephalic version in their practice or hospital in order to reduce the number of infants presenting by the breech. Details of external cephalic version are to be found in Chapter 26.

References

1. Hannah ME, Hannah WJ, Hewson SA, Hodnett ED, Saigal S, Willan AR. Planned caesarean section versus planned vaginal birth for breech presentation at term: a randomised multi-centre trial. Term Breech Trial Collaborative Group. Lancet 2000; 356:1375–1383.
2. Su M, Hannah WJ, Willan A, Ross S, Hannah ME. Planned caesarean section decreases the risk of adverse perinatal outcome due to both labour and delivery complications in the Term Breech Trial. Br J Obstet Gynaecol 2004; 111:1065–1074.
3. Van Roosmalan J, Rosendaal F. There is still room for disagreement about vaginal delivery of breech infants at term. Br J Obstet Gynaecol 2002; 109:967–969.
4. Hauth J, Cunningham FG. Vaginal breech delivery is still justified. Obstet Gynecol 2002; 99:1115–1116.

5. Alarab M, Regan C, O'Connell MP, Keane DP, O'Herlihy C, Foley ME. Singleton vaginal breech delivery at term: still a safe option. Obstet Gynecol 2004; 103:407–412.
6. Glegeman M. Five years to the term breech trial: the rise and fall of a randomized controlled trial. Am J Obstet Gynecol 2006; 194:20–25.
7. Royal College of Obstetricians and Gynaecologists. The management of breech presentation. Guideline No. 20. London: RCOG, 2001.
8. Baskett TF. Trends in operative obstetrical delivery: implications for specialist training. Ann R Coll Phys Surg Can 1988; 1:119–121.
9. Deering S, Brown J, Hodor J, Satin AJ. Simulation training and resident performance of singleton vaginal breech delivery. Obstet Gynecol 2006; 107:86–89.

Bibliography

American College of Obstetricians and Gynecologists. Mode of term singleton breech delivery. Committee Opinion No. 265. Obstet Gynecol 2001; 98:1189–1190.

Burke G. The end of vaginal breech delivery. Br J Obstet Gynaecol 2006; 113:969–972.

Canadian Consensus on Breech Management at Term. SOGC Policy Statement. J Obstet Gynaecol Can 1994; 16:1839–1848.

Cheng M, Hannah M. Breech delivery at term: a critical review of the literature. Obstet Gynecol 1993; 82:605–618.

Halmeskami E. Vaginal breech delivery: a time for reappraisal? Acta Obstet Gynecol Scand 2001; 80:187–190.

Kotaska A. Inappropriate use of randomized trials to evaluate complex phenomena. BMJ 2004; 329:1039–1042.

Menticoglou SM. Symphysiotomy for the trapped after coming parts of the breech: a review of the literature and a plea for its use. Aust NZ J Obstet Gynaecol 1990; 30:31–39.

Porter R. Breech delivery: the dilemma. Br J Obstet Gynaecol 2006; 113:973–974.

Queenan JT. Teaching infrequently used skills: vaginal breech delivery. Obstet Gynecol 2004; 103:405–406.

Rietberg CC, Stinkens PME, Visser GHA. The effect of the Term Breech Trial on medical intervention behaviour and neonatal outcome in The Netherlands: an analysis of 35,453 term breech infants. Br J Obstet Gynaecol 2005; 112:205–209.

Tunde-Byass MO, Hannah ME. Breech vaginal delivery at or near term. Semin Perinatol 2003; 27:34–45.

Turner MJ. The term breech trial: Are the clinical guidelines justified by the evidence? J Obstet Gynaecol 2006; 26:491–494.

Vidaeff AC. Breech delivery before and after the term breech trial. Clin Obstet Gynecol 2006; 49:198–210.

Young PF, Johanson RB. The management of breech presentation at term. Curr Opin Obstet Gynaecol 2001; 13:589–593.

15

Twin and triplet delivery

On Twins: 'It is a constant rule, to keep patients, who have born one child, ignorant of there being another, as long as it can possibly be done'.

Thomas Denman
An Introduction to the Practice of Midwifery. London: J. Johnston, 1795

The advent of assisted reproductive technology in developed countries over the past 25 years has resulted in a doubling of the incidence of twin pregnancy, along with a 10-fold increase in triplet deliveries.[1] In many countries twins now constitute about 2% of all deliveries. Compared with singleton pregnancies the perinatal mortality, morbidity and long-term neurodevelopmental disability is increased 5–10-fold in twins and even more for triplets and higher order multiple pregnancies. Prematurity, low birth weight, congenital anomalies, twin-to-twin transfusion and intrauterine growth restriction are the main contributors to the raised perinatal mortality and morbidity. Intrapartum asphyxia and trauma are additional risks, with malpresentation of one or both twins being present in 60% of deliveries. While there is no evidence that planned caesarean section for all twins will result in lower perinatal mortality and morbidity the caesarean delivery rate for twins has increased worldwide. A multicentre randomized controlled trial to compare methods of delivery is under way.

Obstetric factors

Malpresentations

In 60% of twin pregnancies one or both of the twins is in malpresentation at the time of delivery. The most common combinations are, in decreasing order of frequency (Twin A/Twin B):

- vertex/vertex
- vertex/breech
- breech/vertex
- breech/breech.

These combinations constitute 90% of twin deliveries, with the rest involving transverse lie of one or both fetuses. Overall the most common combinations are:

- vertex/vertex (40%)
- vertex/non-vertex (35–40%)
- non-vertex/other (20–25%).

The main factor in considering labour and vaginal delivery is the presentation of the first twin. In 75–80% of cases the first twin is in the favourable cephalic presentation. In this decision the presentation of the second twin is not relevant. If it is favourable at the start of labour it may not be when the first twin has delivered. Alternatively, if it is unfavourable at the onset of labour it may become favourable after the delivery of the first twin. In about 20% of cases an unfavourable lie in the second twin at the onset of labour converts spontaneously to a favourable lie after the first twin has been delivered.

Second twin

There are a number of reasons why the second twin is at increased risk during labour and delivery:

- After delivery of the first twin partial separation of the placenta, or interference with placental circulation consequent to partial emptying of the uterus, may reduce oxygen transfer and cause asphyxia. The longer the interval following delivery of the first twin the greater this risk. The ability to apply electronic fetal heart rate monitoring to the second twin should ensure early detection of such a trend.[2,3]
- The second twin is more likely to be a malpresentation and is therefore vulnerable to trauma associated with the required intrauterine manipulations for delivery. The careful application of external cephalic version and, in rare cases, the ability to perform caesarean section for the second twin will reduce this risk.

Individual considerations

In each case there are a number of factors which will influence the decision for or against labour and vaginal delivery:

- General maternal considerations such as age, parity, infertility, medical complications.
- Potential fetal compromise including, fetal growth restriction, twin-to-twin transfusion, abnormal tests of fetal wellbeing.
- Estimated fetal weight. Although there is no evidence to support planned caesarean section for low birth weight twins, many obstetricians will deliver by caesarean those infants less than 33 weeks gestation or with an estimated fetal weight < 1500 g.
- Weight discrepancy between twins. If there is a significant weight discrepancy (> 750 g), particularly if twin B is bigger than twin A.
- Monoamniotic twins are rare but the risk of cord and fetal entanglement is high enough to warrant delivery of all such cases by elective caesarean.
- Appropriate facilities and skilled personnel should be available. This involves an obstetrician, anaesthetist and neonatal personnel plus equipment capable of looking after two or more infants.

Maternal risks

Although most of the emphasis in multiple pregnancies is on fetal and neonatal risks there are also increased maternal complications. These include a higher incidence of anaemia, hypertension and pre-eclampsia, gestational diabetes, caesarean delivery, postpartum haemorrhage and thromboembolism. In addition, with the high incidence of preterm labour the mother is exposed to the potential risks of tocolytic therapy (see Chapter 7).

Anaesthetic factors

For the uncomplicated twin delivery narcotic, inhalation and pudendal block anaesthesia may be adequate. However, the ideal is an epidural anaesthetic. This obviates the need for narcotic analgesia which is less desirable in the pre-term fetus – more common with twins. In addition, should intrauterine manipulation or caesarean delivery become necessary during the second stage of labour the mother is saved the hazards of rapid induction of general anaesthesia. It is important that the anaesthetist understand the potential need for acute uterine relaxation during delivery of the second twin, should internal podalic version and breech extraction be required. Epidural analgesia provides no uterine relaxation and the anaesthetist should be prepared at a moment's notice to provide uterine relaxation with agents such as nitroglycerine or terbutaline (see Chapter 26).

First stage of labour

The first stage of labour should be managed as in a singleton pregnancy. If the presentation of twin A is other than cephalic, caesarean section will be chosen in most cases. If twin A is cephalic, induction of labour and augmentation with oxytocin can be carried out with the same principles as for a singleton. Ideally both twins should receive electronic fetal heart rate monitoring. An intravenous infusion should be started early in labour and, if available and appropriate, epidural analgesia is established.

Second stage of labour

The necessary anaesthetic, obstetric and neonatal equipment and personnel should be marshalled. There may be an advantage in conducting the second stage of labour in a delivery room with the capability of immediate recourse to caesarean section should this become necessary. The neonatal equipment should be made ready to receive two infants with potential needs for resuscitation and early support.

With over-distention of the uterus the maternal bearing-down effort may be reduced, but in general the first twin is delivered spontaneously or assisted by forceps or vacuum for the same indications as a singleton. Once delivered the cord of the first twin should be clamped and 'tagged' in case there are anastomotic vascular connections between the twins' placental circulations.

Once the first twin has delivered there is usually a period of uterine inertia for several minutes. Thus, in advance one should have prepared a solution of 5 units oxytocin in 500 ml crystalloid which can then be 'piggy-backed' to the main intravenous line.

Delivery of the second twin

Once the first twin has been delivered, handed off and the cord securely clamped, the lie of the second twin should be established. It is here that an obstetric assistant using ultrasound may help delineate the lie in cases of doubt. However, in general, abdominal palpation and vaginal examination will accurately confirm the lie and presentation. The following management is recommended:

> *'Being convinced there is a second child, the membranes must be immediately broke without waiting for pains; and introducing the hand into the womb, to find out the feet, the child must be brought forth by them'.*
>
> **Fielding Ould**
> *A Treatise of Midwifry. Dublin: O. Nelson, 1742, p52*

- If the presentation is cephalic or breech check vaginally to rule out cord presentation.
- Provided there is no cord, steady the presenting part over the pelvic brim and start the oxytocin infusion at 10 drops per minute, gradually working up until uterine contractions occur. Once regular contractions are established rupture the membranes and apply the fetal scalp electrode to the presenting part. Before this the fetal heart rate can be monitored externally.
- Provided the fetal heart rate is normal one can wait for spontaneous delivery of the second twin – either cephalic or an assisted breech delivery (see Chapter 14).
- If the second twin is an oblique or transverse lie external cephalic version should be attempted and some will use the ultrasound transducer to assist this manoeuvre, with pressure behind the fetal head and neck while allowing monitoring of the fetal heart simultaneously (Fig 15.1). If cephalic version is unsuccessful then try external podalic version. If either of these succeeds then continue with the management of the longitudinal lie as above.

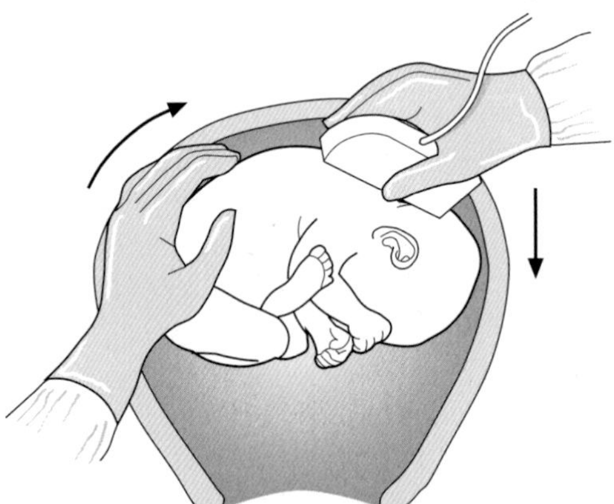

Figure 15.1 Use of ultrasound transducer to assist external cephalic version of twin B, while providing continuous observation of the fetal heart rate.

- If external version is unsuccessful, or if the second twin is a footling breech, then consideration should be given to immediate internal podalic version and/or breech extraction. Provided the obstetrician is skilled at this procedure and there is good anaesthesia and uterine relaxation this is a reasonable choice and attended by good results.[4–6] The technique of breech extraction is outlined in Chapter 14 and that of internal version in Chapter 26.
- If the skill is not available to safely perform internal podalic version and breech extraction, or if difficulty is encountered (and this will usually be because of inadequate uterine relaxation), then caesarean section for the second twin may have to be chosen. This may be seen by some as an 'obstetrical defeat'. However, it is, on rare occasions, better to accept this than risk trauma or asphyxia of the fetus.[7–9]
- If there is a non-reassuring fetal heart rate pattern, intrapartum bleeding or cord prolapse delivery of the second twin will have to be accelerated. If the fetus is in low vertex presentation, forceps or vacuum assisted delivery should be feasible. If the fetal head is at a higher station in the mid-pelvis or at the pelvic brim the vacuum is the better option. It is essential that the vacuum be placed over the flexion point so that the narrowest diameter is presented (see Chapter 8). If the fetus is a breech presentation then breech extraction should be considered. In either of these cases individual factors may push the obstetrician to consider caesarean section of the second twin, although usually assisted vaginal delivery will be safely feasible. A summary of the intrapartum management is outlined in Figure 15.2.

Third stage of labour

The over-distended uterus with twins is very prone to uterine atony in the minutes and hours after delivery. Thus, active management of the third stage of labour should be carried out and intravenous oxytocin kept running for 8 hours.

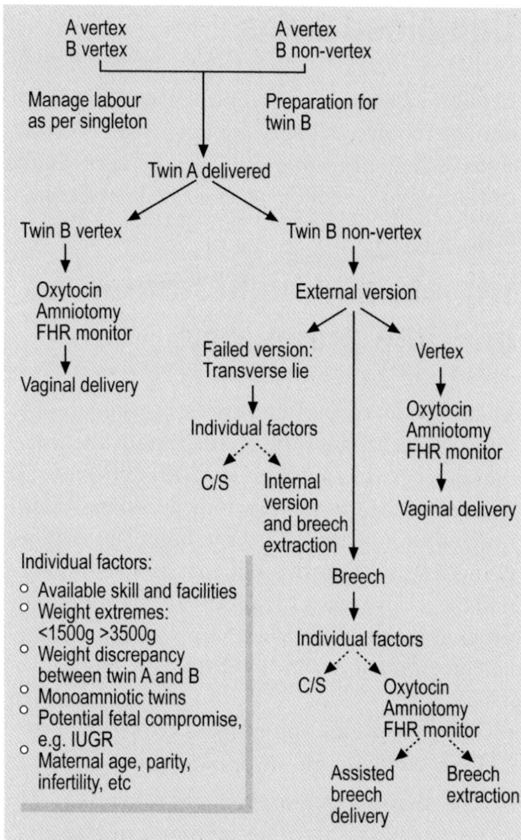

Figure 15.2 Intrapartum management of twin pregnancy (reproduced with permission from: Baskett TF. Essential management of obstetric emergencies. 4th ed. Bristol: Clinical Press, 2004).

'The method of extracting the second immediately after the first child, is never practised by the female adventurers in the art of midwifery; for they leave it all to nature; cutting the funis, tying it to the mother's thigh; they wait for a new labour; and the waters gathering which the poor patient is seldom able to undergo, being much weakened and fatigued by what she has already suffered; yet it sometimes happens, that she has a full week between the bringing forth of two children, and frequently two to three days'.

Fielding Ould
A Treatise of Midwifry. Dublin: O. Nelson, 1742, p55

Locked twins

This is an extremely rare condition occurring in about 1 in 1000 twin gestations. It is most likely to occur with small fetuses which descend together. The most common combinations are, in decreasing order of frequency (twin A/twin B): breech/vertex (Fig 15.3); vertex/vertex (Fig 15.4); and a variety of combinations with vertex, breech or transverse.

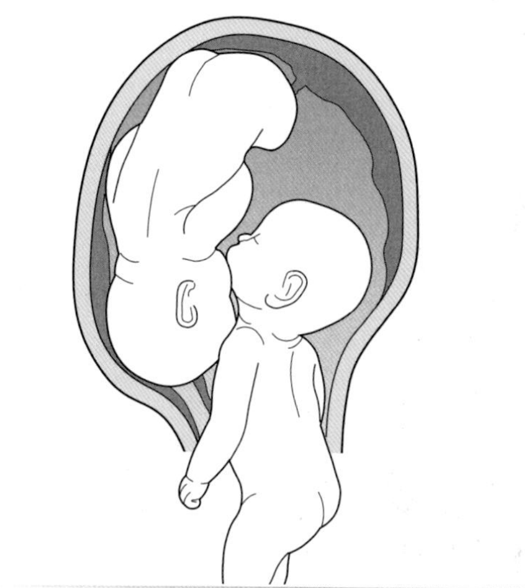

Figure 15.3 Locked twins: breech/vertex.

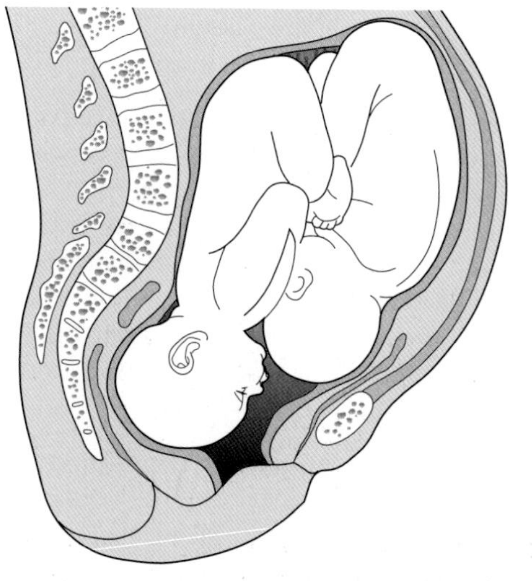

Figure 15.4 Locked twins: locked fore-coming heads.

The most common variety, breech/vertex, is unlikely to be encountered in modern obstetrics as most viable twins with the first fetus presenting as a breech will be delivered by caesarean section. However, should one be confronted with this situation there are three options:

1. Under anaesthesia and with profound uterine relaxation it may be possible to disimpact the interlocking heads by elevating the first twin and pushing away the head of the second twin. This would be followed by breech extraction of the first twin (see Chapter 14). Should the first twin be dead, and the operator have the skill to perform it, decapitation of the first twin using the Blond–Heidler saw would allow delivery of the first twin's body followed by assisted delivery of the cephalic second twin, probably using the vacuum or, if the head has descended, low forceps. The head of the first twin can then be retrieved (see Chapter 26). Obviously, this manoeuvre is associated with risk of rupture of the lower uterine segment and potential asphyxia and trauma to the second twin. Depending on the geographical location, the available facilities and the implications in subsequent pregnancies, caesarean section would be chosen. This will almost certainly need to be of the classical variety to allow room for atraumatic delivery of each twin.
2. In the case of locking of two fore-coming heads, this usually occurs in relatively small fetuses. It may be possible, therefore, under appropriate anaesthesia and uterine relaxation, to elevate the head of the second twin to allow descent and assisted delivery of the first. Unless this is technically easy, caesarean section should be chosen.
3. For most of the other varieties of locked twins, caesarean section, often requiring a classical incision in the uterus, is the safest method of delivery.[10]

Conjoined twins

Conjoined twins are exceptionally rare and, if viable, require delivery by caesarean section. Even if they are not viable, unless very small, caesarean may still be necessary for dystocia.[11]

Triplets and higher-order multiple pregnancy

In many developed countries assisted reproductive techniques have increased the incidence of triplets to 1 in 500–1000 of all deliveries. Maternal morbidity and perinatal morbidity and mortality are higher in triplets compared with both singleton and twin pregnancies.[12] In many hospitals all viable triplet pregnancies are delivered by elective caesarean section for a combination of reasons:

- The first presenting fetus of triplets is other than vertex in about one-third of cases.
- The chances of a malpresentation requiring intrauterine manipulation of the second and third of triplets is high.
- It can be technically difficult to monitor the fetal hearts of three fetuses simultaneously.
- As the majority of triplets come into labour and deliver preterm the need for three neonatal teams at delivery is easier to marshal for an elective rather than an emergency delivery.

It is difficult to compare the outcome of triplets delivered vaginally versus those born by caesarean section. Few centres have enough experience to provide adequate comparison groups. However, there is no proof that caesarean delivery brings better perinatal outcome. Individual hospitals will have to make their own decisions based on local facilities, personnel and experience.[13–15]

Vaginal delivery of triplets may be considered at 32 weeks gestation and beyond, with no signs of compromise of any of the fetuses, the ability to monitor all three fetal hearts in labour and with the first triplet presenting as a vertex. Otherwise the principles of management for the first stage of labour will be normal and delivery of the first triplet either spontaneous or by low assisted vaginal delivery. It is better not to delay the delivery of the second and third fetuses. If they present by the vertex the membranes of each sac can be ruptured and delivery be either spontaneous or by low assisted delivery. If the lie is breech or transverse then breech extraction or internal podalic version and breech extraction should be carried out. Here again it is emphasized that adequate uterine relaxation must be available for these intrauterine manipulations to be carried out with safety.

For viable quadruplets and higher order multiple pregnancies, elective caesarean section will be chosen.

References

1. Van Voorhis BJ. Outcomes from assisted reproductive technology. Obstet Gynecol 2006; 107:183–200.
2. Leung TY, Tam WH, Leung TN, Lok IH, Lau TK. Effect of twin-to-twin delivery interval on umbilical cord blood gas in the second twin. Br J Obstet Gynaecol 2002; 109:63–67.
3. Leung TY, Lok IH, Tam WH, Leung TN, Lau TK. Deterioration in cord blood status during the second stage of labour is more rapid in the second twin than in the first twin. Br J Obstet Gynaecol 2004; 111:546–549.
4. Adam C, Allen AC, Baskett TF. Twin delivery: influence of the presentation and method of delivery on the second twin. Am J Obstet Gynecol 1991; 165:23–27.
5. Barrett JFR, Ritchie JWK. Twin delivery. Best Prac Res Clin Obstet Gynaecol 2002; 16:43–56.
6. Boggess KA, Chisholm CA. Delivery of the nonvertex second twin: a review of the literature. Obstet Gynecol Surv 1997; 52:728–735.
7. Pschera H, Jonasson A. Is cesarean section justified for delivery of the second twin? Acta Obstet Gynecol Scand 1988; 67:381–382.
8. Persad VL, Baskett TF, O'Connell CM, Scott HM. Combined vaginal-cesarean delivery of twin pregnancies. Obstet Gynecol 2001; 98:1032–1037.
9. Wen SW, Fung KF, Oppenheimer L, Demissie K, Yang Q, Walker M. Occurrence and predictors of cesarean delivery for the second twin after vaginal delivery of the first twin. Obstet Gynecol 2004; 103:413–419.
10. Saad FA, Sharara HA. Locked twins: a successful outcome after applying the Zavanelli manoeuvre. J Obstet Gynaecol 1997; 17:366–367.
11. Bianchi A, Maresh M, Rimmer S. Conjoined twins. In: Hillard T, Purdie D, eds. The Yearbook of Obstetrics and Gynaecology. Vol 11. London: RCOG Press, 2004:37–47.
12. Cassell KA, O'Connell CM, Baskett TF. The origins and outcomes of triplet and quadruplet pregnancies: 1980 to 2001. Am J Perinatol 2004; 21:439–445.
13. Wildshut HIJ, Van Roosmalen J, Van Leeuwen E, Keirse MJNC. Planned abdominal compared with planned vaginal birth in triplet pregnancies. Br J Obstet Gynaecol 1995; 102:292–296.
14. Dommergues M, Mahieu-Caputo D, Mandelbrot L, Huon C, Moriette C, DumezY. Delivery of uncomplicated triplet pregnancies: is the vaginal route safer? A case-control study. Am J Obstet Gynecol 1995; 172:513–517.
15. Dommergues M, Mahieu-Caputo D, Dumez Y. Is the route of delivery a meaningful issue in triplets and higher order multiples? Clin Obstet Gyneol 1998; 41:25–29.

Bibliography

American College of Obstetricians and Gynecologists. Practice Bulletin No. 56. Multiple Gestation: Complicated twin, triplet, and high-order multi-fetal pregnancy. Washington, DC: ACOG 2004 (Obstet Gynecol 2004; 104:869–883).

Armson BA, O'Connell C, Persad V, Joseph KS, Young DC, Baskett TF. Determinants of perinatal mortality and serious neonatal morbidity in the second twin. Obstet Gynecol 2006; 108:556–566.

Carroll MA, Yeomans ER. Vaginal delivery of twins. Clin Obstet Gynecol 2006; 49:154–166.

Healy AJ, Gaddipati S. Intrapartum management of twins: truths and controversies. Clin Perinatol 2005; 32:455–473.

Hogle KL, Hutton EK, McBrien KA, Barrett JFR, Hannah ME. Cesarean delivery for twins: a systematic review and meta-analysis. Am J Obstet Gynecol 2003; 188:220–227.

Ledger WL, Anumba D, Marlow N, Thomas CM, Wilson ECF. The costs to the NHS of multiple births after IVF treatment in the UK. Br J Obstet Gynaecol 2006; 113:21–25.

Lee YM, Cleary-Goldman J, D'Alton ME. Multiple gestations and late preterm (near-term) deliveries. Semin Perinatol 2006; 30:103–112.

MacKay AP, Berg CJ, King JC, Duran C, Chang J. Pregnancy-related mortality among women with multifetal pregnancies. Obstet Gynecol 2006; 107:563–568.

Ramsey PS, Repke JT. Intrapartum management of multifetal pregnancies. Semin Perinatol 2003; 27:54–72.

Robinson C, Chauhan SP. Intrapartum management of twins. Clin Obstet Gynecol 2004; 47:248–262.

Smith GCS, Shah I, White IR, Pell JP, Dobbie R. Mode of delivery and the risk of delivery – related perinatal death among twins at term: a retrospective cohort study of 8073 births. Br J Obstet Gynaecol 2005; 112:1139–1144.

Stone J, Eddkeman K, Patel S. Controversies in the intrapartum management of twin gestations. Obstet Gynecol Clin North Am 1999; 26:327–343.

Yokoyama Y, Shimizu T, Hayakawa K. Prevalence of cerebral palsy in twins, triplets and quadruplets. Int J Epidemiol 1995; 24:943–948.

16

Cord prolapse

'Yet sometimes the navel string falls down and comes before it; for which cause the child is in much danger of death ... As soon as 'tis perceived, you must immediately endeavor to put it back, to prevent the cooling of it, behind the child's head, lest it be bruised ... But sometimes, not withstanding all these cautions, and the putting back of it, it will yet come forth every pain; then without further delay, the chirurgeon must bring the child forth by the feet, which he must search for, tho the infant comes with the head; for there is but this only means to save the child's life.'

Francois Mauriceau
The Diseases of Women with Child, and in Child-Bed. London: John Darby, 1663, p255

Prolapse of the umbilical cord represents one of the most urgent emergencies in obstetrics. It occurs when the membranes are ruptured and part of the cord lies below the presenting part of the fetus. Cord presentation is the same situation with intact membranes – a much rarer diagnosis. Over the past century the incidence of cord prolapse had decreased from about 1 in 150 to 1 in 500 deliveries. Similarly, in well-equipped hospitals, the perinatal mortality has fallen over the past 50 years from 50–60% to 2–15%.

The risk to the fetus is the loss of umbilical blood flow to and from the placenta with consequent hypoxia due to physical compression of the blood vessels in the cord, or spasm of the blood vessels due to the colder temperature if the cord prolapses outside the vagina.

Predisposing factors

The following conditions may interfere with the close application of the fetal presenting part to the lower uterine segment and cervix and therefore predispose to cord prolapse.

Fetal

- Malpresentations such as complete and footling breech, transverse and oblique lie.
- Prematurity: the premature fetus is more likely to lie in malpresentation and, in addition, the small size of the presenting part may facilitate prolapse of the cord.
- Fetal anomaly: the abnormal fetus is more likely to lie in an abnormal position and may have an irregular presenting part (e.g. anencephaly).
- Multiple pregnancy has a higher association with prematurity and malpresentations.

Maternal

- High parity, associated with lax uterine musculature and a high presenting part.
- Contracted pelvis.
- Pelvic tumours, such as a cervical fibroid.

Placental

- Minor degree of placenta praevia. The lower edge of the placenta elevates the fetal presenting part and the insertion of the umbilical cord is nearer the cervix and more prone to prolapse.

Amniotic fluid

- Polyhydramnios is more often associated with malpresentation or a high presenting part. In addition, the cascade of a large volume of amniotic fluid when the membranes rupture increases the likelihood of washing down the cord.
- Prelabour rupture of the membranes.
- Amniotomy to induce or augment labour is often given as a risk factor, but provided it is appropriately carried out is no more likely to lead to cord prolapse than spontaneous rupture of the membranes. Furthermore, should cord prolapse occur it is better that it is detected and managed as soon as possible.

Cord

- Long umbilical cord.

Obstetric manipulation

- Manual or forceps rotation of the fetal head.
- Version.
- Amnioinfusion.

Many of the above factors are interrelated with the main culprits being prematurity, malpresentations and multiple pregnancy.

Diagnosis

On rare occasions, cord prolapse may be obvious with the dramatic appearance of a loop of umbilical cord at the introitus, usually shortly after spontaneous rupture of the membranes. The most common method of diagnosis is by vaginal examination and this should be carried out in all women with predisposing factors to cord prolapse. Thus, all women with breech presentations should have a vaginal examination immediately after spontaneous rupture of the membranes. Similarly, when fetal heart rate abnormalities are noted, particularly the cord compression pattern of variable deceleration, a vaginal examination should be undertaken to exclude cord prolapse. A loop or loops of cord may be obvious on vaginal examination but, on occasions, the presentation can be quite subtle with a loop just beside and barely below the presenting part (Fig 16.1).

With the increased availability of ultrasound on labour wards, the diagnosis of cord presentation can be made in cases with predisposing factors before rupture of the membranes. Occasionally, loops of cord can be felt through the intact membranes below the presenting part.

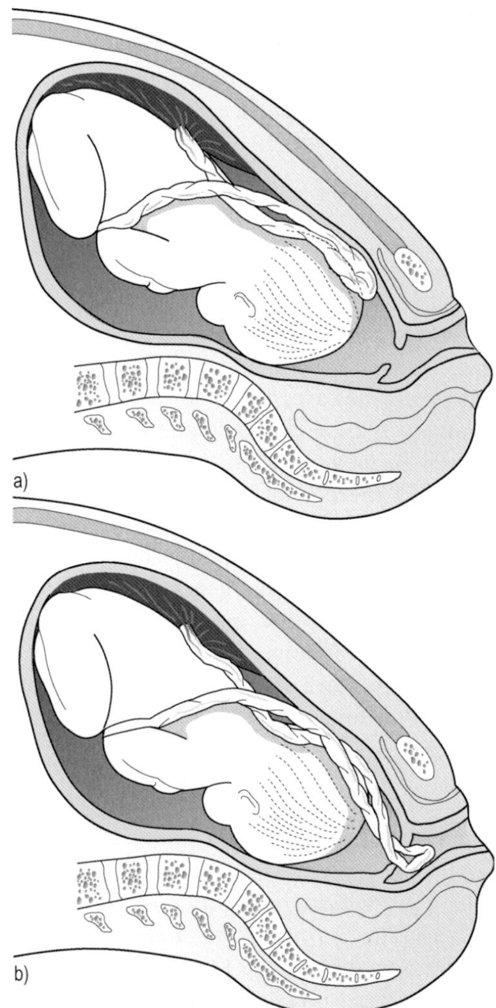

Figure 16.1 (a) Occult cord prolapse. (b) Prolapsed cord.

Management

In general, the perinatal outcome is related to the detection–delivery interval, although with the application of the techniques outlined below, longer delays can be associated with good results.

Immediate relief of cord compression

This is the first approach in all cases. If the cord has prolapsed outside the vagina it is gently cradled in the hand and replaced in the vagina. Even if the cord has only prolapsed into the vagina, similar gentle cradling should be performed to relieve pressure on the cord from the vaginal walls. The tips of the fingers are further advanced through the cervix to the presenting part to ensure that it is not compressing the cord against the cervix or bony pelvis. The cord must be handled as gently as possible as excessive manipulation may cause spasm of the vessels (Fig 16.2).

In addition to this manual replacement and protection of the cord the patient should be placed in the knee–chest position so that gravity also becomes an assistant (Fig 16.3). This position is undignified and exhausting to maintain for any length of time so that repositioning to the Sims' lateral position, with a pillow under one hip and the bed or trolley in Trendelenburg position is more practical (Fig 16.4). If the baby is viable, and delivery by immediate caesarean section is feasible, these manoeuvres are maintained while the patient is transferred to the operating theatre for delivery.

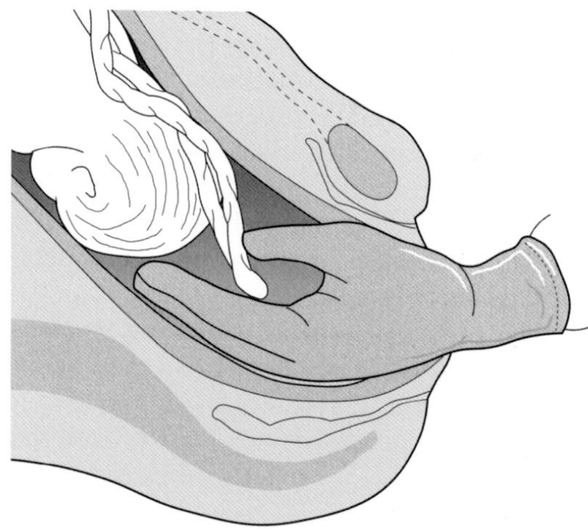

Figure 16.2 Manual relief of cord compression.

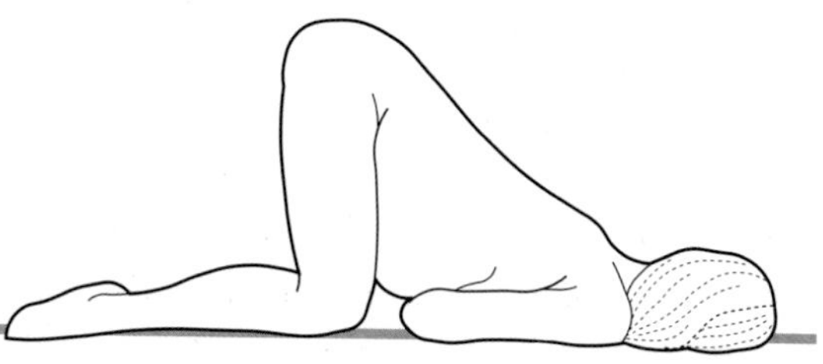

Figure 16.3 Knee–chest position for immediate relief of cord compression.

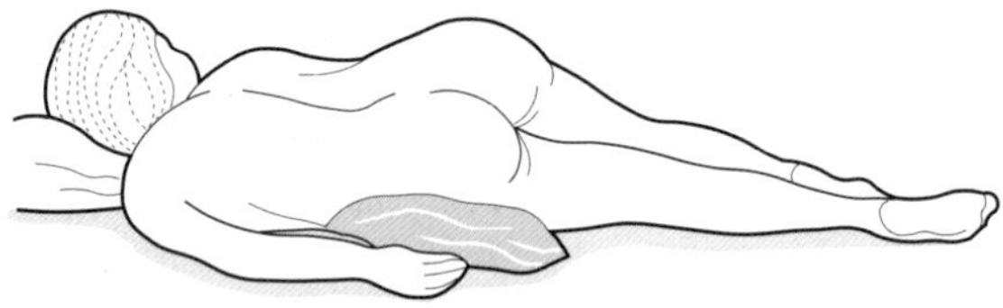

Figure 16.4 Sims' lateral position.

Fetal assessment

Once cord compression has been relieved one must decide whether the fetus is viable. If the fetus is dead, too immature to survive, or has a lethal anomaly then intervention for fetal reasons is contraindicated and labour should be allowed to continue to vaginal delivery.

In most cases one can be reassured that the fetus is alive by palpating the pulsations in the prolapsed cord. This can be done by feeling the loop between two fingers or gently palpating it against the vaginal wall or presenting part. Take care to palpate in between contractions when any cord compression is released. If available a scalp electrode can be applied which, if it produces a normal tracing, allows a more orderly approach. An ultrasound transducer may also be used for this purpose. Even if cord pulsations cannot be felt the fetus may still be alive and this should be checked by ultrasound of the fetal thorax.

The gestational age at which the infant is regarded as viable will depend on the level of neonatal care available.

A lethal anomaly may be known from the antenatal record or obvious on examination (e.g. anencephaly).

Delay in transfer of patient for delivery

If umbilical cord prolapse occurs outside hospital or there is delay before the infant can be delivered the following approach can be used. After the initial attempts at cord decompression have been successful, the patient is guided to the Sims' lateral position, a Foley catheter placed and the bladder filled to approximately 500 ml. This should elevate the presenting part and help relieve cord compression. One should check with the vaginal hand that this is the case, and if so the hand can be removed. A case can be made for filling the bladder in most cases at the time of diagnosis in case there is an unpredictable delay or, should the fetal heart be normal and stable, to allow time for spinal anaesthesia as opposed to rapid and more risky general anaesthesia.

Filling the bladder may also help inhibit uterine contractions. However, if uterine contractions start or continue, tocolysis with ritodrine or terbutaline may be indicated (see Chapter 26).

'The late Dr. Mackenzie, than whom I have not known a man more intelligent in conversation, or more excellent in practice, informed me of another method which he has tried. Instead of attempting to replace the descended funis in the common way, he brought down as much more of it as would come with ease, and then enclosed the whole mass in a small bag made of soft leather, gently drawn together with a string, like the mouth of a purse. The whole of the descended funis, inclosed in this bag, was conveniently returned, and remained beyond the head of the child till this was expelled; and the bag containing the funis having escaped compression, the child was born living. But he very ingenuously told me, that he had afterwards made several other trials in the same manner without success.'

Thomas Denman
An Introduction to the Practice of Midwifery. New York: E. Bliss and E. White, 1825, p545–546

'In my experience, the best repositor is a thick roll of gauze. Quantities of this are pushed into the uterus well above the presenting part: the cord is entangled in the gauze. Now the gauze must be thick – thin gauze is of no use. I most strongly recommend this very simple device.'

Munro Kerr
Operative obstetrics. 4th edn. London: Balliere, Tindall and Cox, 1937, p207

Replacement of cord

Before the era of safe caesarean section many ingenious techniques were devised attempting, with varied success, to replace the cord behind the presenting part. In modern obstetrics there are only rare occasions when conditions favour this approach. Should cord prolapse of a minor degree occur with a cephalic presentation it is occasionally feasible to manually replace the cord up above the head to the nuchal area of the fetus. Fetal heart rate monitoring should be carried out to ensure that any cord compression pattern does not recur. This technique is only rarely applicable and, unless successful with minimal handling of the cord, one should not persist.

Delivery

If cord prolapse occurs at full cervical dilatation with the presenting part in a position and station that allows safe vaginal delivery, breech extraction or vacuum/forceps assisted delivery may be undertaken. If not, caesarean section is the method of choice.

In many instances this requires general anaesthesia. However, if the above measures have been successful in relieving cord compression and the fetal heart is stable and monitored continuously, spinal anaesthesia may be feasible with less risk to the mother. If the vaginal hand is elevating the presenting part, a Foley catheter is placed to empty the bladder and, as the uterine incision is made, the hand is removed. If the full bladder technique has been used to elevate the presenting part, the catheter is opened and the bladder drained just before the caesarean section is started.

While decisive speed is of the essence in this classic obstetric emergency, the calm and systematic approach outlined above will usually produce good perinatal results with least risk to the mother.

Bibliography

Barrett JM. Funic reduction for the management of umbilical cord prolapse. Am J Obstet Gynecol 1991; 165:654–657.

Calder AA. Emergencies in operative obstetrics. Best Pract Res Clin Obstet Gynaecol 2000; 14:43–55.

Chetty RM, Moodley J. Umbilical cord prolapse. S Afr Med J 1980; 57:128–129.

Critchlow CW, Leet TL, Benedetti TJ, Daling JR. Risk factors and infant outcomes associated with umbilical cord prolapse: a population-based case-control study among births in Washington State. Am J Obstet Gynecol 1994; 170:613–618.

Dare FO, Owolabi AT, Fasubaa OB, Ezechi OC. Umbilical cord prolapse: a clinical study of 60 cases seen at Obafemi Awolowo University Teaching Hospital. East Afr Med J 1998; 75:308–310.

Driscoll JA, Sadan O, Van Gelderen CJ, Holloway GA. Cord prolapse – can we save more babies? Br J Obstet Gynaecol 1987; 94:594–595.

Jones G, Grenier S, Gruslin A. Sonographic diagnosis of funic presentation: implications for delivery. Br J Obstet Gynaecol 2000; 107:1055–1057.

Kahana B, Sheiver E, Levy A. Umbilical cord prolapse and perinatal outcomes. Int J Gynaecol Obstet 2004; 84:127–132.

Katz Z, Shoham Z, Lancet M, Blickstein J, Mogilner BM, Zalel Y. Management of labor with umbilical cord prolapse. A 5-year study. Obstet Gynecol 1988; 72:278–280.

Koonings PP, Paul RH, Campbell K. Umbilical cord prolapse: a contemporary look. J Reprod Med 1990; 35:690–692.

Lin MG Umbilical cord prolapse. Obstet Gynecol Surv 2006; 61:269–277.

Murphy DJ, Mackenzie IZ. The mortality and morbidity associated with umbilical cord prolapse. Br J Obstet Gynaecol 1995; 102:826–830.

Prabulos AM, Philipson EH. Umbilical cord prolapse: is the time from diagnosis to delivery critical? J Reprod Med 1998; 43:129–132.

Qureshi NS, Taylor DJ, Tomlinson AJ. Umbilical cord prolapse. Int J Gynaecol Obstet 2004; 86:29–30.

Roberts WE, Martin RW, Roach HH, Perry KG, Martin JN, Morrison JC. Are obstetric interventions such as cervical ripening, induction of labor, amnioinfusion or amniotomy associated with umbilical cord prolapse? Am J Obstet Gynecol 1997; 176:1181–1183.

Runnenbaum IB, Katz M. Intrauterine resuscitation by rapid urinary bladder installation in a case of occult prolapse of excessively long umbilical cord. Eur J Obstet Gynecol Reprod Biol 1999; 84:101–102.

Usta IM, Mercer BM, Sibai BM. Current obstetrical practice and umbilical cord prolapse. Am J Perinatol 1999; 16:479–484.

Yla-Outinen A, Heinonen PK, Tuimala R. Predisposing and risk factors of umbilical cord prolapse. Acta Obstet Gynecol Scand 1985; 64:567–570.

17

Antepartum haemorrhage

In the past antepartum haemorrhage (APH) was defined as bleeding from the genital tract after 28 weeks of gestation – regarded then as the lower limit of fetal viability – and before the onset of labour and delivery. As the age of fetal viability has steadily reduced it has become necessary to redefine antepartum haemorrhage and we consider that it is now sensible to define it as bleeding occurring in the second half of pregnancy, ≥ *20* weeks; earlier bleeding falling into the realm of miscarriage. The causes of antepartum haemorrhage include placenta praevia, abruptio placentae, unclassified APH (sometimes called APH of unknown origin), and bleeding from lower genital tract lesions.

Lower tract genital lesions include cervical ectropion, cervical polyp, vulvovaginal varices, vaginitis and, rarely, cervical carcinoma. While it is important to confirm or exclude these local conditions they will not be discussed in detail in this chapter. It is also important to stress, however, that the presence of these lower genital tract conditions does not preclude the concomitant possibility of the more serious uterine causes of APH.

Although unclassified antepartum haemorrhage is the most common type of APH, it is placenta praevia and abruptio placentae that carry the greatest risk to the mother and infant. The evolving terminology of these conditions is of interest. It was Paul Portal (1630–1703), a physician in Paris, who first clearly described the attachment of the placenta to the lower uterine segment in cases of placenta praevia.[1] In 1775 Edward Rigby (1747–1821) of Norwich made the first clinical differentiation between placenta praevia, which he called 'unavoidable haemorrhage,' and abruptio placentae which he termed 'accidental haemorrhage'. Unavoidable haemorrhage has been replaced with placenta praevia and in the United States the terms ablatio placentae and abruptio placentae, the latter holding sway, came into common use.[1] Recently abruptio placentae has been replaced with 'placental abruption' by many physicians as they become less familiar with the Latin and Greek origins of medical terminology.

Placenta praevia

By definition placenta praevia occurs when part or all of the placenta is implanted in the lower uterine segment. The incidence varies in different populations but is usually about 1 in 200 to 1 in 300 deliveries. The incidence is increased with advanced maternal age, high parity, and previous delivery by caesarean section. Other predisposing factors are surgical termination of early pregnancy, and women who have had a placenta praevia before (the recurrence risk is approximately 5%). Thus, the incidence of placenta praevia will depend on the frequency of the above factors in the obstetric population. An abnormally large surface will also predispose to placenta praevia, such as placenta membranacia, bipartita and succenturiata. However, the placenta of twin pregnancy is not more likely to be praevia compared with singleton pregnancies.[2]

Classification

Classification systems usually include four types or degrees of placenta praevia with additional descriptive terminology, as illustrated in Figure 17.1 and outlined below:

First description of placenta praevia

'I put my fingers into the orifice and felt the after birth which covered the orifice of the matrix from all sides and adhered in all its parts with the exception of the middle.'

Paul Portal
La Pratique des Accouchements Soutenue d'un Grand Nombre d'Observations. Paris: G. Martin, 1685

- Type 1 (lateral or low-lying): the edge of the placenta encroaches on the lower uterine segment but not down as far as the internal cervical os
- Type 2 (marginal): the lower edge of the placenta extends to but not across the internal os
- Type 3 (partial): the placental edge extends asymmetrically across the lower segment and internal os but does not cover it completely after cervical dilatation
- Type 4 (complete or central): the placenta is almost centrally placed over the internal os and likely to cover it even at full dilatation.

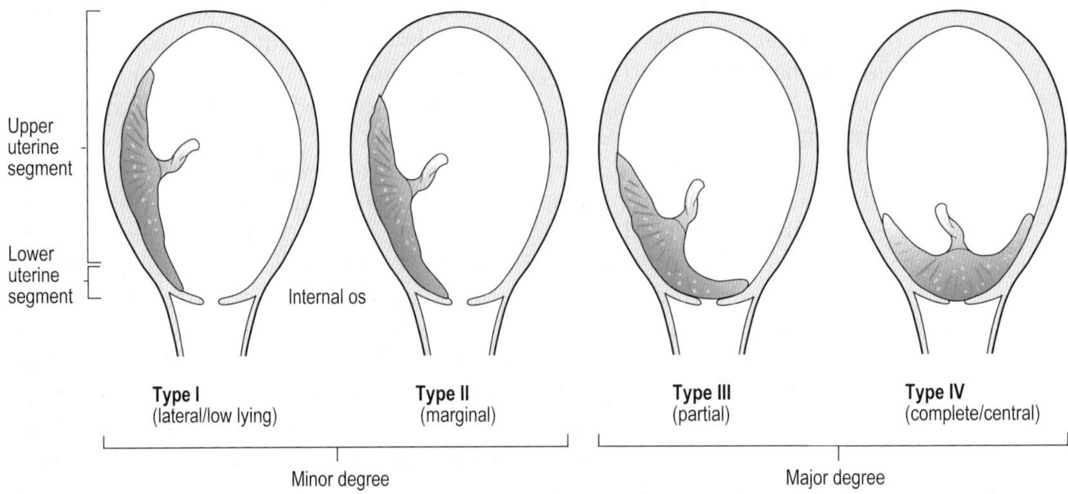

Figure 17.1 Classification of placenta praevia.

There is a tendency, with modern ultrasound diagnosis, to group the types of placenta praevia into minor (types 1 & 2), and major (types 3 & 4) degrees. Approximately half of all cases of placenta praevia are major and half are minor degrees.

Pathophysiology

In the first and early second trimesters the lower uterine segment is not formed and only extends 0.5–1.0 cm from the internal cervical os. Ultrasound procedures define placenta praevia as reaching within 0.5 cm of the internal os. Thus, in the second trimester approximately 5% of all placentas appear this close to the internal os and are judged to be 'low-lying'. As the lower uterine segment develops, ultimately to occupy approximately one-third of the uterine volume, the placenta attached to the upper uterine segment appears to move up and away from the internal os: so-called 'placental migration'. Thus, by term only 1 in 200–300 placentas remain low-lying as a true placenta praevia.

Physiologically the lower uterine segment is that part of the uterus which passively stretches during labour and has no expulsive function. Anatomically it is that portion of the uterus below the reflection of utero-vesical peritoneum. This is the anatomical landmark that defines the upper limit of the lower uterine segment at caesarean section and can be surprisingly high up on the uterine wall in cases of obstructed labour. Clinically, at term, the lower uterine segment is that part of the uterus approximately 6–8 cm from the internal os – the area that can be explored by the examining finger.

With placenta praevia the lower edge may become detached, leading to bleeding as the lower segment forms in the late second and early third trimester. About 80% of all women with placenta praevia bleed before the onset of labour. Major degrees of placenta praevia tend to bleed earlier in gestation, more frequently, and more heavily than minor degrees. However, there are exceptions and on occasions a complete placenta praevia may not bleed until the onset of labour. The fact that the placenta attached to the developing and stretching lower uterine segment would ultimately result in bleeding, if only during labour, led to the original classification of placenta praevia as 'unavoidable' or ' inevitable' antepartum haemorrhage.

It may be appropriate to revisit the question of how the conventional view of a 'lower uterine segment' came about. Anatomy textbooks describe the non-pregnant uterus as having three parts: corpus, isthmus and cervix. The definition of the isthmus may now be considered unsatisfactory since its boundaries were defined as the *anatomical* internal os and the *histological* internal os; being the point at which the lining of the lumen changed from endometrium to endocervical columnar epithelium. Both these landmarks are lumenal and have no identifiable analogues in either the stroma or the serosal surface of the uterus. The lower uterine segment is considered to be the equivalent of the isthmus in late pregnancy and it may have served a useful purpose to accept this concept.

An alternative view would be to consider the uterus as comprising only two parts: corpus and cervix, the boundary between which is what Danforth[3] described as the fibro-muscular junction between the muscular corpus and the predominately fibrous cervix. This junction lies at the internal os of the non-pregnant cervix and migrates up the wall of the uterine cavity in the latter months of pregnancy as the cervix effaces as a prelude to dilatation. This concept more logically explains why so many low-lying placentas are nothing of the sort, and certainly not praevia by the end of pregnancy. Despite the above we are prepared to accept the concept of a 'lower uterine segment' because it is so firmly established in obstetric teaching. We will therefore, for the purposes of this topic, continue to refer to the lower uterine segment and its formation during pregnancy. In doing so we acknowledge that one of the major difficulties we face in regard to this subject is that of defining either clinically or by imaging the upper boundary of the 'lower uterine segment'.

Clinical features

In the later weeks of pregnancy, as the lower uterine segment is formed, the edge of the placenta attached to this area may become detached, producing bleeding. As the blood has little distance to travel, and minimal resistance as it tracks down between the membranes and cervix, this bleeding is usually painless. Unless the woman is in labour the first bleed is often light and usually stops. This may be followed by recurrent bleeds which can be heavy. The first bleed is often referred to as the 'warning bleed'. It is very rare for the first bleed to be severe or life threatening to either the mother or the fetus. Thus, the principle of the 'warning bleed' as something that must be heeded by both the woman and her attendants has been established. If this is ignored and dismissed, subsequent bleeds may be life threatening. Munro Kerr dramatically illustrated this point in an earlier edition:

> *'I arrived one morning on my wards to learn that a patient with placenta praevia had died. She had had one or two slight haemorrhages to which the family physician had not attached much importance; then a severe one occurred, and he sent her into hospital. On her admission the house surgeon examined her vaginally; a most profuse bleeding occurred which neither he nor the more senior resident could control. Before a senior member of the staff arrived by taxi-cab the patient was moribund and could not be rescued. Here the family doctor was to blame for not sending the patient in after the first haemorrhage, but still more to blame was the house surgeon for having examined the patient; a senior member of staff should have been summoned immediately.'*

Although the majority of cases bleed before the onset of labour, surprisingly, some cases of complete placenta praevia may have no bleeding until the onset of labour. It is possible that a placenta so situated is less likely to be dislodged by the formation of the lower uterine segment in the last few weeks of pregnancy than is one which is situated partly in the upper and partly in the lower uterine segment.

Because there is little resistance to the blood tracking down from the lower part of the uterus to the cervix there is usually no myometrial irritation and thus no increased uterine tone, uterine contractions or uterine tenderness. Similarly, there is no occult blood loss so the degree of anaemia and shock correspond to the clinically apparent blood loss. With the presence of part or all of the placenta in the lower uterine segment the presenting part is usually displaced upwards so that malpresentations are common and cephalic presentations are often high and free at the pelvic brim.

The main clinical features differentiating placenta praevia from abruptio placentae are summarized in Table 17.1. It must be emphasized, however, that cases of mild abruptio placentae may present in a similar fashion to placenta praevia, while in some cases of placenta praevia blood may extravasate into the myometrium leading to a degree of uterine irritability and tenderness. Thus, the milder forms of each condition may blend in their clinical presentation.

Management

Women who have an antepartum bleed should be transferred to an appropriate level hospital as soon as possible. Other than assessment of vital signs and abdominal appraisal no pelvic examination should be undertaken and, if appropriate, an intravenous drip should be established with crystalloid and the patient transferred by the quickest and safest route.

Once admitted to hospital the amount of bleeding is quickly assessed to see if treatment of hypovolaemia is urgently needed. Blood tests, including complete blood count, blood type and antibody screen, are performed and at least two units of blood cross-matched. If the clinical appraisal suggests placenta praevia (Table 17.1), and the bleeding settles, or is mild, the woman will be treated expectantly. As soon as possible placental localization by ultrasound should be performed. Despite the

Table 17.1 Differential diagnosis

Placenta praevia	Abruptio placentae
History of 'warning' bleed(s)	Less likely to be preceded by 'warning bleed'
Apparently causeless	May be associated with hypertensive disorders, trauma, etc
Shock and anaemia correspond to apparent blood loss	Shock and anaemia may be out of proportion to apparent blood loss
Uterus has normal tone and is not tender	Increased uterine tone and tenderness
Malpresentation and/or high presenting part	Normal presenting part
Normal fetal heart rate and fetal assessment	More likely absent or abnormal fetal heart rate and fetal growth restriction

admonition not to perform a full pelvic examination before the placenta has been localized it is permissible and safe to use transvaginal ultrasound to localize the placenta. This has been shown to be more accurate than transabdominal ultrasound in delineating the relationship of the lower border of the placenta to the cervix.[4]

Depending on the clinical circumstances there are two broad approaches to the management of placenta praevia – expectant treatment and active treatment.

Expectant treatment

If the patient is less than 37 weeks gestation, not in labour, and the bleeding has settled or is settling, expectant treatment is undertaken in order to gain time for fetal maturation. The main elements of this treatment are as follows:

- The patient is admitted and kept on bed rest with bathroom privileges for at least 3 days following the cessation of bleeding.
- If the ultrasound examination confirms placenta praevia there is no need to perform a speculum examination, provided the patient is up-to-date with cervical cytology and there are no clinical features to suggest a lower genital lesion that requires treatment. If a speculum examination is undertaken then it should not be accompanied by digital examination.
- Cross-matched blood should be available at all times. Anaemia should be sought and treated. If the patient is Rhesus negative Rh immune globulin should be given and a Kleihauer test performed to ensure that the standard dose of Rh immune globulin is adequate.
- If the gestation is less than 34 weeks consider giving corticosteroids to accelerate fetal pulmonary maturity.
- If the ultrasound confirms placenta praevia, the safest course is for the woman to remain in hospital until delivery. In cases with a minor degree of placenta praevia in which the bleeding has settled there is often pressure both from the woman, her family, and hospital accountants to discharge the woman home. This may be considered in the woman who lives nearby, with a telephone, and with readily available transportation. However, there is some evidence that the perinatal outcome is worse, due to fetal growth restriction and premature labour, in women with placenta praevia who manifest this by bleeding before the onset of labour.[5] There are no large series or trials to support or refute the longstanding teaching that the woman with a placenta praevia that bleeds should remain in hospital until delivery. However, even minor degrees of placenta praevia can, after the initial light warning bleed, present with very heavy bleeding. Thus, the safest course is for the woman to remain in hospital until delivery, although local circumstances may dictate otherwise.[4]

- In some women with an APH in the late second and early third trimester the ultrasound on admission may suggest a minor degree of placenta praevia but, as the lower segment continues to develop, the placenta may ultimately be shown not to be implanted in the lower segment. In these cases, it is reasonable to repeat the ultrasound in 2 weeks and, if the placenta is no longer considered praevia, and the bleeding has settled and not recurred, the woman can be discharged from hospital and treated as an unclassified APH (see below).
- As the pregnancy progresses ultrasound assessment of fetal growth and biophysical assessment of fetal wellbeing should be performed.

Provided the clinical course has been satisfactory the move to active treatment at 37–38 weeks should be considered. In this context the role of amniocentesis to assess fetal pulmonary maturity before elective caesarean has to be considered. The advantage of confirming fetal pulmonary maturity must be weighed against the fact that amniocentesis is followed by uterine contractions, albeit mild, which could precipitate bleeding. If the pregnancy can be continued until 38 weeks amniocentesis should be unnecessary.

Active treatment

This is considered when the patient reaches 37–38 weeks gestation, or if there is heavy and sustained bleeding, or if labour starts. In most modern hospitals the accuracy of transvaginal ultrasound is such that the diagnosis of placenta praevia can be made with certainty. Thus, delivery by caesarean section can be planned. Occasionally the ultrasound result may be equivocal and in such cases there is still a role for the double set-up examination which, in the days before ultrasound, was the standard first step in active management.

In the double set-up examination the patient is kept fasting and prepared for immediate general anaesthesia if required. She is examined in the operating theatre with the anaesthetist present, a nurse and assistant scrubbed, and the instruments ready to move immediately to caesarean section. The patient is examined vaginally and initially a finger palpates the fornices to see if there is thick placental tissue between the fornix and the presenting part. If no placenta is suspected the examining finger is gently pushed through the cervix and digital exploration of the lower uterine segment performed. It can be difficult to distinguish between blood clot and placental tissue. The most important distinguishing feature is that placental tissue tends to have a firmer, rubbery and gritty consistency. If no placenta is found upon digital exploration of the lower uterine segment then labour can be safely induced with amniotomy and oxytocin infusion. If placenta praevia is confirmed, or if there is active bleeding, then one moves straight to caesarean section.

Vaginal delivery for placenta praevia

In individual cases, if a minor degree of placenta praevia is felt but the fetal head is settling past the edge and there is no active bleeding, it may be permissible to consider amniotomy and oxytocin induction. Such labours should be monitored very carefully and if there is bleeding there should be no hesitation in moving to caesarean section.

Other than the above exception all cases of placenta praevia with a viable infant should be delivered by caesarean section. There are, however, rare circumstances when the fetus is dead, has a lethal anomaly, or is pre-viable in which the older technique of assisted vaginal delivery by Braxton Hicks bipolar podalic version, perfected almost 150 years ago, may be appropriate.[6] This may also apply in remote areas with limited or unsafe facilities for caesarean section.

Technique of bipolar podalic version

The technique involves the minimum of internal manipulation with 1–2 fingers so that disruption and separation of the low-lying placenta is kept to a minimum. The cervix needs to be partially dilated (> 2 cm) and the placenta praevia should not completely cover the internal os.

The head is pushed up with the fingers and the external hand manipulates the breech down into the pelvis (Fig 17.2). The fingers through the cervix then grasp the foot of the fetus (Fig 17.3) and bring the leg down through the cervix so that the breech creates tamponade by direct pressure on the placenta and uterine wall (Fig 17.4).

It is important not to try and forcibly pull the breech through the cervix. Rather, enough pressure is exerted just to keep the breech firmly against the placenta and lower uterine segment and then await uterine contractions to dilate the cervix and deliver the fetus. A bandage can be tied to the fetal ankle and a small weight, for example a bag of saline, is attached to this to provide the appropriate gentle but sustained traction. If the foot cannot be grasped with the fingers sponge forceps can be used for this purpose, particularly if the fetus is very immature.

It is emphasized that the indications for this potentially dangerous type of version are very few. However, the degree of haemostasis produced by this technique can be impressive and, on the rare occasions it is necessary, life-saving.

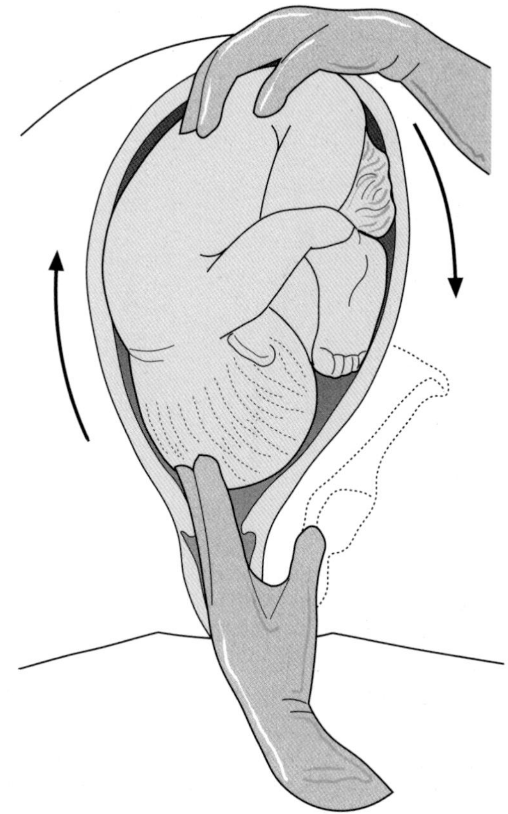

Figure 17.2 Bipolar version: the fetal head is pushed up with the internal finger(s) and the external hand manipulates the breech down to the pelvis.

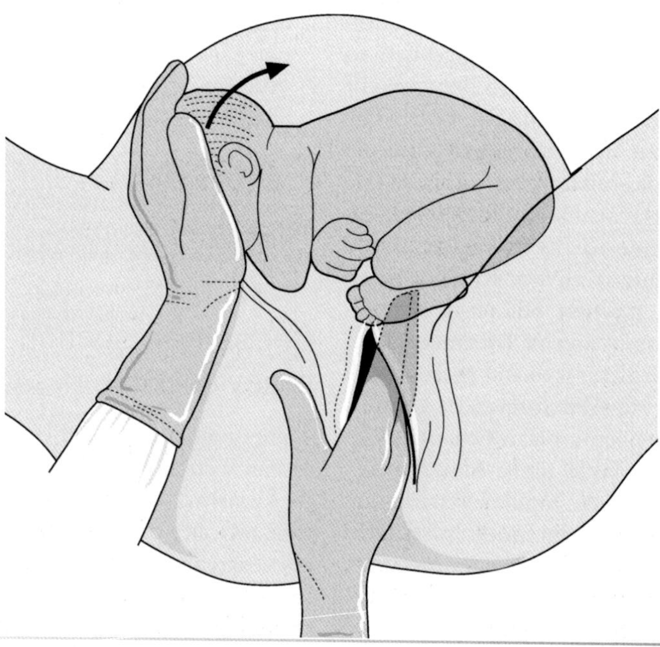

Figure 17.3 Bipolar version: the fetus is turned by combined manipulation and the foot is grasped.

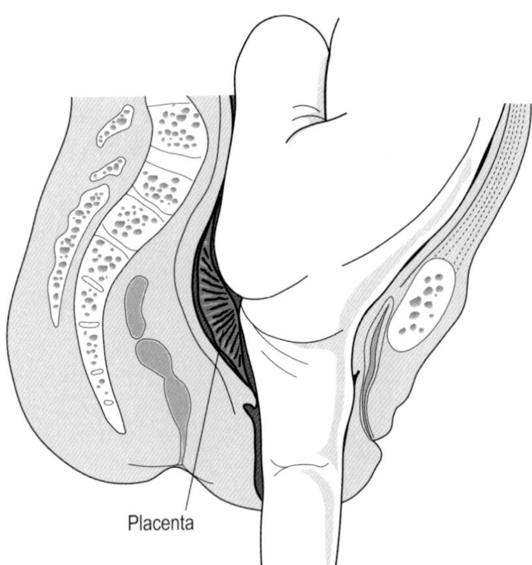

Figure 17.4 Bipolar version: the leg of the fetus is pulled through the cervix so that the breech produces tamponade against the placenta and the lower uterine segment.

An alternative technique for cephalic presentations was described by John Willett using a specially designed T-forceps to grasp the scalp of the fetus and apply cephalic tamponade to the placenta and lower uterus.[7] Having passed the forceps through the cervix and grasped the scalp, gentle traction was applied by means of a bandage tied to the handles of the forceps with a light weight hung over the end of the bed (Fig 17.5). The principle was that the subsequent uterine contractions would dilate the cervix while the traction on the scalp would apply haemostatic tamponade to the lower separated edge of the placenta. Delivery was not to be forced by strong traction but to be accomplished by the normal uterine contractions. It is unlikely that Willett's specific forceps will now be available but Allis forceps or a multi-toothed cervical tenaculum can be used effectively for the non-viable fetus. Haemostasis with both Braxton Hicks bipolar version and Willett's scalp forcep techniques is remarkably efficient and, for the rare circumstances described above, still has an occasional role in modern obstetrics.[1]

BRAXTON HICKS BIPOLAR VERSION

'Introduce the left hand, with the usual precautions, into the vagina, so far as to fairly touch the foetal head, even should it recede an inch ... Having passed one or two fingers (if only one, let it be the middle finger) within the cervix, and resting them on the head, place the right hand on the left side of the breech at the fundus ... Employ gentle pressure and slight impulsive movements on the fundus towards the left iliac fossa. In a very short time it will be found that the head is rising and at the same time the breech is descending ... The foetus is now transverse; the knee will be opposite the os, and the membranes being ruptured it can be seized and brought into the vagina.'

BRAXTON HICKS BIPOLAR VERSION: USE IN PLACENTA PRAEVIA

'Anything which gave the practitioner some power of action was to be earnestly welcomed ... Turn, and if you employ the child as a plug the danger is over. Then wait for the pains, rally the powers in the interval, and let nature, gently assisted, complete the delivery.'

John Braxton Hicks
On a new method of version in abnormal labour. Lancet 1860; 2:28–30

Caesarean section for placenta praevia

The potential for rapid blood loss during caesarean section for placenta praevia is such that these cases cannot be delegated to junior medical staff. In addition to the surgical principles of caesarean section outlined in Chapter 11 the following technical aspects of caesarean section for placenta praevia should be considered.

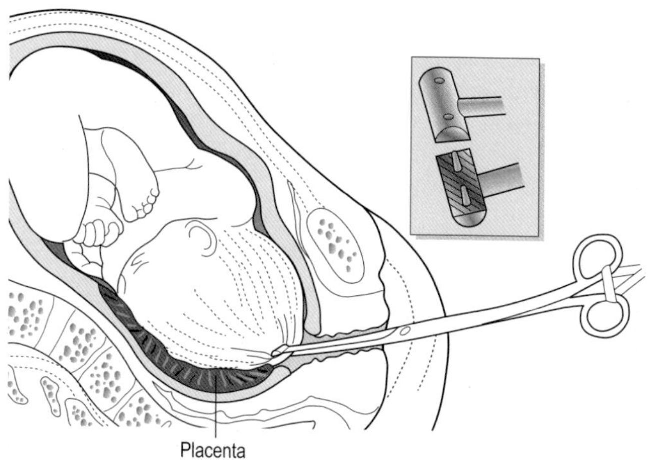

Figure 17.5 Application of Willett's scalp forceps.

WILLETT'S SCALP FORCEPS

'The application of the forceps is easy and they can be applied to the scalp as soon as the os will admit a finger, thus ensuring early treatment ... a weight varying from 1 lb to 2 lb, hanging over the end of the bed, is applied to the handles by a tape. Nothing further is done until the head is in the vagina, when the forceps are removed and the patient is allowed to deliver herself without further interference.'

John Willett
The treatment of placenta praevia by continuous weight traction - a report of seven cases. Proc R Soc Med 1925; 18:90–94

Unless there is already severe haemorrhage at the start of the caesarean section, necessitating critical speed of entry, a Pfannenstiel incision should be adequate for all potential additional manoeuvres required.

In most cases with placenta praevia near term the lower uterine segment is sufficiently developed to allow the standard transverse lower segment incision to be performed. There are, however, a number of situations in which this may not be so. If delivery has to be done early in the third trimester, before adequate formation of the lower uterine segment and compounded by a high presenting part, it may be best to perform a vertical incision, starting in the lower segment and extending into the upper uterine segment as needed. On rare occasions there are huge vessels over the lower uterine segment which extend into the broad ligaments. In such cases, which are rare, a vertical incision may be the most prudent. It may also be worth ligating such large vessels on either side if they transverse the proposed line of uterine incision.

If the placenta praevia is anterior or complete it is inevitable that placental tissue will be encountered immediately after incising the uterine muscle. It is best not to cut through the placenta but to use the hand to separate the placenta either upwards or lateral to the nearest edge, rupture the membranes, deliver the baby and promptly clamp the cord.[8] Careful assessment of the ultrasound images before delivery may help delineate the anterior area covered by the placenta and help guide the site of the uterine incision and the direction of the hand so that the shortest route to the placental edge is achieved.

After delivery of the infant and placenta the usual oxytocic infusion should cause contraction of the upper uterine segment. The site of the placental implantation in the non-contractile lower uterine segment may continue to ooze and can bleed alarmingly. Having secured any bleeding sinuses from the cut edges of the uterine muscle with Green–Armytage clamps, the entire 'bowl' of the lower uterine segment should be tightly packed and pressure applied for 4 minutes timed 'by the clock'. When the pack is removed some discrete points of bleeding may be identified and can be oversewn with figure-of-eight sutures. Another option, which has varying degrees of success, is multiple sub-endomyometrial injections of 1–2 ml solution of vasopressin (5 units in 20 ml saline).[9]

If bleeding continues, uterine and ovarian artery ligation are easily undertaken (see Chapter 26) but are often not successful for bleeding in the lower uterine segment.

If the above measures fail to achieve haemostasis in the lower uterine segment, but the upper uterine segment is well contracted, a balloon device can be inserted and run down through the cervix and the balloon inflated sufficient to tamponade the lower segment. If this is successful, the lower segment incision is then closed in routine fashion over the balloon. Continued haemostasis is ascertained by observing the suture line and looking for bleeding through the cervix, before closing the abdomen. The balloon can be deflated and removed in 12–24 hours (see Chapter 26).

An alternative is to use full thickness horizontal or square compression sutures to oppose the anterior and posterior walls across the lower uterine segment. Make sure you leave a portal in the middle to allow efflux of lochia (see Chapter 26).

If the above procedures are unsuccessful, and preservation of the uterus is desired, embolisation of the anterior branch of the internal iliac artery can be performed provided radiological facilities for this exist. If not, either surgical ligation of the internal iliac arteries or hysterectomy will have to be performed (see Chapter 26). In the vast majority of cases careful and sustained packing of the lower uterine segment as the first move will usually provide adequate haemostasis, and the appropriate duration of this simple manoeuvre is emphasized.

Placenta praevia accreta

This is a rare complication which occurs in about 1 in 3000–5000 deliveries. However, the incidence is rising related to the increased number of women delivered by caesarean section. Both placenta praevia and placenta praevia accreta rise in frequency with the number of previous deliveries by caesarean section. There are three degrees of pathological placental adherence:

- *accreta* – in which there is no plane between the decidua compacta and decidua spongiosa
- *increta* – in which the chorionic villi invade the myometrium
- *percreta* – in which the whole thickness of the myometrium is invaded through to the serosal surface of the uterus.

Diagnosis before delivery can now be made, or at least highly suspected, with the newer imaging techniques including colour Doppler, power amplitude ultrasonic angiography and MRI.[10,11]

These cases must be managed by senior and experienced obstetricians. The haemorrhage at the time of caesarean section can be rapid, massive and unrelenting. In most cases hysterectomy is required. This usually needs to be a total hysterectomy as the lower uterine segment and cervix itself may be involved.[4] Others have used a variety of compression sutures to stem the haemorrhage.[12] If the diagnosis is made before delivery a classical caesarean section can be performed away from the site of implantation and the infant delivered and the cord clamped. Provided the placenta is not separated or does not spontaneously partially separate there should be

Placenta Praevia Accreta

'But when I endeavored to extract the placenta it had adhered so strongly to the cervix uteri that it was near an hour and half before I could remove it; nor then without separating the adhering part with my hands.'

Edward Rigby
An Essay on the Uterine Haemorrhage which Precedes the Delivery of the Full Grown Fetus: Illustrated with Cases. 6th ed. London: Hunter, 1822

no haemorrhage. The caesarean can then be completed and degeneration and sloughing of the placenta awaited. There are those who advocate methotrexate treatment to accelerate this process.[13] However, this conservative treatment is fraught with the risk of potential sepsis and haemorrhage in the weeks following delivery and would only be considered when the desire to retain the uterus for further child-bearing is paramount.[14]

Another rare but difficult variation of placenta praevia accreta is that in which previous delivery was by transverse lower caesarean incision and placenta percreta has developed with invasion of the bladder wall adherent to the previous lower segment incision. Depending on the area of bladder involvement it can be opened and an ellipse of the posterior bladder wall containing the percreta can be excised and the bladder sutured. Obviously this requires careful identification of the ureteric orifices. The other alternative is to retain that portion of the uterine wall that is adherent to the bladder and perform hysterectomy, leaving that area with over-sewing on the uterine side to achieve haemostasis of the remnant of uterine wall. Cases of percreta with bladder involvement are among the most suitable in which to consider conservative management.

In cases of placenta praevia accreta that are known or highly suspected before delivery preoperative acute normovolaemic haemodilution may be advisable. This technique entails removing about 1000 ml maternal blood to a closed circuit storage bag approximately 1 hour before planned delivery. At the same time about 3 litres of intravenous crystalloid are given to replace the litre of withdrawn blood. At the time of the surgery the previously withdrawn litre of blood is autotranfused. The acute blood loss that occurs at the time of surgery is therefore of haemodiluted blood and is replaced by the transfusion of the woman's whole blood.[15] In addition, there is increasing use of red cell salvage techniques at the time of caesarean section which can have application in these cases if the facilities and equipment have been established beforehand.[16] Another potential pre-emptive manoeuvre in these cases is the preoperative placement of vascular catheters in the internal iliac arteries by interventional radiology. If necessary these can be used for immediate postdelivery major vessel embolisation and reduce the potential need for blood transfusion and hysterectomy.[17]

Vasa praevia

On rare occasions the blood loss is fetal and not maternal – an infant can be born 'bled white' from rupture of an umbilical vessel in a velamentous insertion of the umbilical cord. Velamentous insertion occurs in about 1% of singleton and 5% of multiple pregnancies when the umbilical cord is inserted into the membranes with the vessels branching out and running between the chorion and amnion before reaching the placenta. These vessels are not protected by Wharton's jelly and are thus vulnerable to compression and rupture. This is particularly so when the vessels run across the lower segment and cervix in front of the presenting part – vasa praevia – as is the case in about 1 in 5000 pregnancies. This may cause fetal bradycardia during uterine contractions as the vessels are compressed by the presenting part. The other main risk, of course, is tearing of the vessels during spontaneous or artificial rupture of the membranes. The alert obstetrician may be able to palpate the vessels in the membranes, either as part of the investigation of the cause of fetal bradycardia or just before planned amniotomy.

If bleeding occurs after rupture of the membranes, and particularly if there is fetal tachycardia, this diagnosis should be considered. One rapid bedside test to detect the presence of fetal haemoglobin is based on its resistance to denaturation by alkali compared with adult haemoglobin. A few drops of the vaginal blood are added to 10 ml of 0.1% sodium hydroxide. Adult haemoglobin will turn brown in the solution within 30 seconds but fetal haemoglobin, resisting denaturation by alkali, remains pink.[18] If the diagnosis is confirmed, or strongly suspected because of the relationship of the fetal heart rate changes to rupture of the membranes, then delivery by immediate caesarean section is indicated.

Unfortunately the fetus will often succumb rapidly before diagnosis and intervention is possible. Some of the newer techniques of ultrasound Doppler colour flow may allow antenatal diagnosis.[19]

Abruptio placentae

Abruptio placentae is the premature separation of the normally situated placenta. It occurs in about 1 in 100–200 deliveries. In modern obstetric units maternal death is rare, although it is still five times the overall maternal mortality rate.[2] However, the maternal morbidity associated with the complications and management of haemorrhage can be considerable. Perinatal mortality is approximately 10–20%.[20,21] Overall the incidence of placental abruption is increasing, and is dependent on the frequency of the predisposing factors in the obstetric population.

Predisposing factors

There are a variety of social, medical and obstetrical risk factors for abruptio placentae which include:[22–24]

- hypertensive disorders, particularly severe pre-eclampsia and eclampsia
- advanced maternal age is a factor in some but not all studies
- increasing parity is a factor in most reviews
- smoking and cocaine use have been consistently and independently shown to be significant risk factors for abruptio placentae
- prolonged prelabour rupture of the membranes
- multiple pregnancy has approximately twice the incidence of abruptio placentae as singleton pregnancies
- sudden decompression of an over-distended uterus, such as follows uncontrolled rupture of the membranes with polyhydramnios or after delivery of the first twin
- trauma: a fall, domestic violence, car accident, amniocentesis or version; overall these are uncommon contributors
- circumvallate placenta
- thrombophilias have a variable and unconfirmed association.

Classification

There are three types of abruptio placentae (Fig 17.6):

- In *revealed haemorrhage* the edge of the placenta separates and the blood tracks down between the membranes and the uterine wall to escape through the cervix with minimal resistance.
- In 5–10% of cases the bleeding is retroplacental and the blood remains trapped between the placenta and the uterus, often with extensive extravasation of blood into the myometrium but none emerging at the vagina – *concealed haemorrhage*.
- In many cases there is a combination of the two – *mixed haemorrhage*, in which some blood remains retroplacental and some tracks down to be externally revealed.

Cases are sometimes divided into three clinical categories of mild, moderate or severe, depending on the severity of the signs and symptoms of occult or overt blood loss.

Pathophysiology

Placental separation is initiated by haemorrhage into the decidua basalis with subsequent haematoma formation which depresses and adheres to the maternal surface of the placenta. It is this latter feature, seen on examination of the placenta after delivery, which confirms the diagnosis of abruptio placentae. The exact reasons for the haemorrhage into the decidua basalis are unknown but are thought to be caused by vascular fragility, vascular malformations or placental abnormalities associated with the predisposing factors.

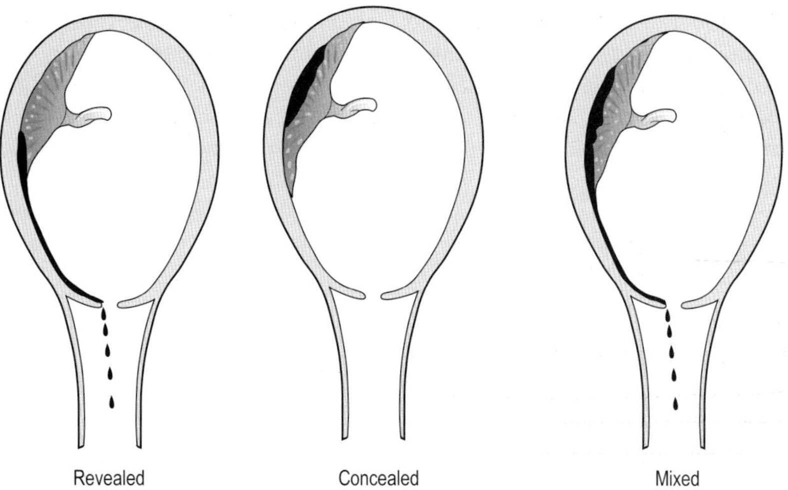

Figure 17.6 Classification of abruptio placentae.

If the lower edge of the placenta separates there is little resistance to the blood tracking down between the membranes and uterine wall and appearing externally. On rare occasions the blood may rupture through the membranes into the amniotic fluid sac. If the haemorrhage is more centrally placed behind the placenta the resistance to its flow is considerable so that much of the blood will be extravasated into the myometrium. In 5–10% of cases there is no vaginal bleeding – the classical concealed abruptio placentae. This extravasation of blood into the myometrium separates and disrupts the myometrial fibres leading to prostaglandin release which causes pain, uterine tenderness, increased uterine tone and contractility. Labour often ensues. In addition, the extravasation of blood releases thromboplastins into the maternal circulation which may initiate disseminated intravascular coagulation (DIC).

In rare cases of concealed or mixed haemorrhage the retroplacental extravasation of blood through the myometrium may be so extensive as to reach the serosal surface, causing bruising and discoloration. This is apparent at the time of caesarean section and is known as the Couvelaire uterus, after Alexandre Couvelaire (1873–1948) of Paris who first described this as 'utero-placental apoplexy'. In the past a Couvelaire uterus was often blamed as the cause of uterine atony and postpartum haemorrhage. In fact, in most cases this is due to the associated DIC, which reflects the severity of the process. The degree of arteriolar spasm that accompanies the hypovolaemic shock of severe abruptio placentae seems to be preferentially intense in the renal vessels, and prolonged renal arteriolar spasm may lead to tubular and cortical necrosis with subsequent renal failure.

Clinical features

The most common clinical presentation is of the mild revealed haemorrhage. These cases can present like placenta praevia with recurrent, mild, painless haemorrhage. However,

Couvelaire uterus

'The uterine wall, in the zone of membranous insertion as well as the zone of placental insertion, was the site of a tremendous bloody infiltration separating the muscle bundles ... The ovaries were peppered with a punctiform bloody suffusion. The broad ligaments were infiltrated with blood. This was indeed a true case of uteroplacental apoplexy.'

Alexandre Couvelaire
Traitement chirurgical des hémorrhagies utéro-placentaires avec décollement du placenta normalement inséré. Ann Gynécol 1911; 8:591–608

usually some blood is extravasated into the myometrium causing pain and an irritable tender uterus. In the mildest cases the fetal heart rate is usually normal.

At the other end of the clinical spectrum is the severe concealed haemorrhage. These patients present with acute, severe and unrelenting abdominal pain and profound hypovolaemic shock. The uterus is hard and tender. The fetus is frequently dead. Labour is often established by the time the patient reaches hospital. In the more severe cases DIC develops along with oliguria and proteinuria secondary to the renal arteriolar spasm.

In the mixed type of haemorrhage the clinical presentation may range anywhere along the spectrum between the mild revealed and severe concealed type of haemorrhage.

Ultrasound is unreliable in the diagnosis of abruptio placentae and may be negative even in the face of clinically significant abruption.

Management

Initial assessment should establish the severity and type of haemorrhage. If the uterus has increased tone, is irritable and tender, and the fetus is viable and alive, arrangements should be made for delivery by caesarean section – unless labour is already well established and vaginal delivery imminent. In such cases with a florid clinical picture of abruption the infant is at imminent risk of death due to further placental separation, and enough to justify caesarean section provided the maternal condition is satisfactory. It must be remembered that in most cases of moderate to severe abruptio placentae, under-transfusion is common. Blood should be taken for complete blood count, group and cross-match at least four units, along with the appropriate coagulation studies (see Chapter 22). These patients require immediate intravenous crystalloid and blood transfusion to maintain tissue perfusion, especially renal perfusion, and to possibly lessen the chance of DIC.

If the fetus is not viable or is dead, amniotomy should be performed, either to induce or to accelerate labour. In many of these cases the patient is already in a rapidly progressive labour. Amniotomy should, at least in theory, help reduce the intrauterine pressure and possibly limit the extravasation of blood and thromboplastins into the myometrium and maternal circulation. As a guide to the transfusion requirements the 'rule of 30s' is worthwhile: the woman may lose up to 30% of her blood volume without alteration in her vital signs – keep the urinary output greater than 30 ml/h and the haematocrit greater than 30%. In severe cases central venous monitoring may be a useful guide (see Chapter 22).

If the case is mild with limited uterine tenderness and bleeding, and normal fetal heart rate, vaginal delivery may be considered. If the patient is in early labour, amniotomy should be performed and the fetal heart rate monitored. If not in labour but the cervix is favourable (which is often the case), amniotomy followed (if needed) by oxytocin is a reasonable choice. These cases should be monitored very carefully and unless progress is steady caesarean section should be chosen. The main problem with this course of action is that if there is further placental separation the oxygenation to the fetus may be suddenly and critically diminished. Even in a relatively mild, but definite, case of abruptio placentae at term, with an unfavorable cervix, caesarean section is the safest course for the fetus.

Many women present with light bleeding and minimal uterine irritability and tenderness and with normal fetal assessment. In these cases ultrasound is required to differentiate the case from one of placenta praevia. If this is done and the pregnancy is preterm then it is permissible to pursue a conservative and expectant course. Provided the bleeding settles and the clinical signs of uterine tenderness and irritability abate, the woman can remain in hospital to gain time for fetal maturity. If the gestation is less than 34 weeks, corticosteroids should be administered. The role of tocolysis in an attempt to suppress uterine contractions is controversial. In most women with abruptio placentae, tocolysis is contraindicated as well as ineffective. However, in very mild cases it may be permissible for 24–48 hours to allow the effective use of corticosteroids for fetal pulmonary maturation. A number of these very preterm cases will settle completely and some may be discharged and managed as an outpatient. This requires careful monitoring of fetal growth and wellbeing, and induction of labour should be considered at 38–39 weeks.

Unclassified antepartum haemorrhage

The diagnosis of unclassified APH can really only be made with certainty after the pregnancy is over and the placenta has been shown not to be praevia and there is no evidence of retroplacental depression or clot, ruling out abruptio placentae. About two-thirds of all cases of APH are, in fact, unclassified. Some of these may be due to very minor degrees of praevia or abruption that cannot be confirmed. Others are probably due to the rupture of small vessels in the cervix as the lower uterine segment develops in the late second and third trimesters. These are usually cases of mild APH that are managed expectantly, with placenta praevia and abruptio placentae ruled out by ultrasound and clinical assessment. After the initial bleed they can be followed on an outpatient basis with careful monitoring of fetal growth and wellbeing. The perinatal loss is slightly increased in this group so induction between 38–40 weeks should be considered.

References

1. Baskett TF. Of violent floodings in pregnancy: evolution of the management of placenta praevia. In: Sturdee D, Olah K, Keane D, eds. The yearbook of obstetrics and gynaecology. Vol 9. London: RCOG Press, 2001:1–14.
2. Hall MH, Wagaarachchi P. Antepartum haemorrhage. In: Maclean AB, Nielson JP, eds. Maternal morbidity and mortality. London: RCOG Press, 2002:227–240.
3. Danforth DN, Ivy AC. The lower uterine segment: its derivation and physiologic behaviour. Am J Obstet Gynecol 1949; 57:831–838.
4. Royal College of Obstetricians and Gynaecologists. Guideline No. 27. Placenta praevia and placenta praevia accreta: diagnosis and management. London: RCOG Press, 2005.
5. Lam CM, Wong SF, Chow KM, Ho LC. Women with placenta praevia and antepartum haemorrhage have a worse outcome than those who do not bleed before delivery. J Obstet Gynaecol 2000; 20:27–31.
6. Hicks JB. On a new method of version in abnormal labour. Lancet 1860; 2:28–30.
7. Willett JA. The treatment of placenta praevia by continuous weight traction – a report of seven cases. Proc R Soc Med 1925; 18:90–94.
8. Ward CR. Avoiding an incision through the anterior previa at cesarean delivery. Obstet Gynecol 2003; 102:552–554.
9. Lurie S, Appelman Z, Katz Z. Intractable postpartum bleeding due to placenta accreta: local vasopressin may save the uterus. Br J Obstet Gynaecol 1996; 103:1164.
10. Moodley J, Ngambu NF, Corr P. Imaging techniques to identify morbidly adherent placenta praevia: a prospective study. J Obstet Gynaecol 2004; 24:742–744.
11. Bhide A, Thilaganathan B. Recent advances in the management of placenta previa. Curr Opin Obstet Gynecol 2004; 16:447–451.
12. Bennich G, Longhoff-Roos J. Placenta percreta treated using a new surgical technique. Eur J Obstet Gynecol Reprod Biol 2005; 122:122–125.
13. Arulkumaran S, Ng CS, Ingemarson I, Ratnan SS. Medical treatment of placenta accreta with methotrexate. Acta Obstet Gynaecol Scand 1986; 65:285–286.
14. Courbiere B, Bretelle F, Porcu G, Gamerre M, Blanc B. Conservative treatment of placenta accreta. J Gynecol Obstet Biol Reprod 2003; 32:549–554.
15. Estella NM, Berry DL, Baker BW, Wali A, Belfort MA. Normovolemic hemodilution before cesarean hysterectomy for placenta percreta. Obstet Gynecol 1997; 90:669–670.
16. DeSouza A, Permezel M, Anderson M, Ross A, McMillan J, Walker S. Antenatal erythropoietin and intra-operative cell salvage in a Jehovah's witness with placenta praevia. Br J Obstet Gynaecol 2003; 110:524–526.
17. Hansch E, Chitkara V, McAlpine J, El-Sayed Y, Dake MD, Razavi MK. Pelvic artery embolization for control of obstetric hemorrhage: a five year experience. Am J Obstet Gynecol 1999; 180:1454–1459.

18. Loendersloot EW. Vasa previa. Am J Obstet Gynecol 1979; 135:702–703.

19. Oyelese Y, Catanzarite V, Prefumo F, et al. Vasa previa: the impact of prenatal diagnosis on outcomes. Obstet Gynecol 2004; 103:937–942.

20. Kayani SI, Walkinshaw SA, Preston C. Pregnancy outcome in severe placental abruption. Br J Obstet Gynaecol 2003; 110:679–683.

21. Matsuda Y, Maeda T, Kouno S. Comparison of neonatal outcome including cerebral palsy between abruptio placentae and placenta praevia. Eur J Obstet Gynaecol Reprod Biol 2003; 106:125–129.

22. Rasmussen S, Irgens LM, Bergsjo P, Dalaker K The occurrence of placental abruption in Norway 1967–1991. Acta Obstet Gynecol Scand 1996; 75:222–228.

23. Hladky K, Yankowitz J, Hansen WF. Placental abruption. Obstet Gynecol Surv 2002; 57:299–305.

24. Ananth CV, Oyelese Y, Yeo L, Prandhan A, Vintzileos AM. Placental abruption in the United States, 1979 through 2001:temporal trends and potential determinants. Am J Obstet Gynecol 2005; 192:191–198.

Bibliography

American College of Obstetricians and Gynecologists. Committee Opinion No. 266. Placenta accreta. Obstet Gynecol 2002; 99:169–170.

Baskett TF. Edward Rigby (1747–1821) of Norwich and his essay on the uterine haemorrhage. J R Soc Med 2002;95:618–622.

Butt K, Gagnon A, Delisle MF. Failure of methotrexate and internal iliac balloon catheterization to manage placenta percreta. Obstet Gynecol 2002; 99:981–982.

Clement D, Kayem G, Cabrol D. Conservative treatment of placenta percreta: a safe alternative. Eur J Obstet Gynecol Reprod Biol 2004; 114:108–109.

Getahun D, Oyelese Y, Salihu HM, Anath CV. Previous cesarean delivery and risks of placenta previa and placental abruption. Obstet Gynecol 2006;107:771–778.

Jain A, Sepulveda W, Patterson-Brown S. Conservative management of major placenta praevia accreta: three case reports. J Obstet Gynaecol 2004; 24(Suppl 1):S63.

Kayem G, Davy C, Goffinet F, Thomas C, Clément D, Cabrol D. Conservative versus extirpative management in cases of placenta accreta. Obstet Gynecol 2004; 104:531–536.

Kayem G, Pannier E, Goffinet F, Grange G, Cabrol D. Fertility after conservative treatment of placenta accreta. Fertil Steril 2002; 78:637–638.

Matsaeng T, Bagratee JS, Moodley J. Pregnancy outcomes in patients with previous history of abruptio placentae. Int J Gynecol Obstet 2006; 92:253–254.

Ononeze BO, Ononeze VN, Hollohan M. Management of women with major placenta praevie without haemorrhage: a questionnaire-based survey of Irish obstetricians. J Obstet Gynecol 2006; 26:620–623.

Oyelese Y, Ananth CV. Placental abruption. Obstet Gynecol 2006; 108:1005–1016.

Oyelese Y, Smulian JC. Placenta previa, placenta accreta, and vasa previa. Obstet Gynecol 2006; 107:927–941.

Royal Australian and New Zealand College of Obstetricians and Gynaecologists. Statement No C-Obs 20. Placenta accreta. [www.ranzcog.edu.au/publications/statements/c-obs20.pdf]

Warshak CR, Eskander R, Hull AD, Scioscia AL, Mattrey RF, Benirschke K, Resnik R. Accuracy of ultrasonography and magnetic resonance imaging in the diagnosis of placenta accreta. Obstet Gynecol 2006; 108:573–581.

18

Postpartum haemorrhage

'The dangerous efflux is occasioned by everything that hinders the emptied uterus from contracting ... in these cases such things must be used as will assist the contractile power of the uterus and hinder the blood from flowing so fast into it and the neighboring vessels.'

William Smellie
Treatise on the Theory and Practice of Midwifery. London: D. Wilson, 1752, p402–404

Every day about 1600 women die in childbirth and of these approximately 500 bleed to death.[1] Most of these are due to atonic postpartum haemorrhage (PPH) and more than 99% are in the developing world. The deaths are caused by the 'Three Delays': delay in seeking care, delay in reaching care, and delay in receiving care. While these 'delays' are most common in the developing world they are not unknown in countries with developed health services. The *United Kingdom Confidential Enquiry into Maternal Deaths* continues to emphasize that deaths due to PPH are often associated with treatment that is 'too little, too late'.[1] While haemorrhage is only fifth or sixth among the leading causes of maternal death in developed countries, it accounts for the majority of cases that result in severe maternal or 'near-miss' obstetric morbidity.[2–4]

This chapter will outline the causes and medical management of postpartum haemorrhage. Other aspects, including surgical management, are covered in separate chapters: retained placenta (Chapter 19); uterine inversion (Chapter 20); lower genital tract trauma (Chapter 21); uterine tamponade, uterine compression sutures, pelvic vessel ligation and embolisation, and obstetric hysterectomy (Chapter 26).

Primary postpartum haemorrhage

Primary PPH is defined as bleeding from the genital tract in excess of 500 ml in the first 24 hours after delivery. In most instances this haemorrhage occurs within the first few hours of delivery. Because the diagnosis is subjective the reported incidence varies widely from 2% to 10%.[5] Blood volume studies have shown that the normal woman loses about 500 ml at the time of spontaneous vaginal delivery, more with assisted vaginal delivery, and up to 1000 ml at caesarean section. In general, medical attendants tend to underestimate blood loss and patients overestimate it. Thus, when the attendant has estimated the blood loss to be more than 500 ml it is usually closer to 1 L, so the clinical definition is reasonable. However, it is important to remember that blood volume is related to body weight. Thus, the small, low-weight woman, particularly if she is anaemic, may tolerate poorly quite small blood losses (see Chapter 22).

Physiology of the third stage of labour

Before discussing the causes and management of primary PPH it is necessary to understand the physiology of the third stage of labour, which lasts from delivery of the infant to delivery of the placenta. While this is the shortest of the three stages of labour it carries the greatest risk to the mother.

During pregnancy the myometrial fibres have been stretched considerably to accommodate the enlarged uterus and its contents. When the infant delivers the uterus continues to contract, leading to a dramatic shortening of these elongated fibres. The permanent shortening of the muscle fibres is achieved by retraction, a unique property of uterine muscle which, in contrast to contraction, requires no energy.

Placental separation is caused by the uterine contraction and retraction greatly reducing the site of placental implantation. The placenta is thus sheared from the uterine wall: analogous to a postage stamp stuck to the surface of an inflated balloon becoming detached when the balloon is deflated. When the placenta is completely separated from the implantation site the contractions continue its descent to the lower uterine segment, through the cervix and into the vagina.

Clinical signs of placenta separation

The triad of clinical signs associated with placenta separation is as follows:

1. The uterus will be felt to contract and, as the placenta is sheared off the uterine wall and descends to the lower uterine segment, the uterine fundus changes from a broad and flat discoid shape to a more elevated, narrow and globular shape. This change from the discoid to globular configuration can be quite difficult to appreciate clinically except in the very thin. However, the uterus will be felt to harden as it contracts, rises in the abdomen and becomes ballotable.
2. A gush of blood often accompanies separation of the placenta from the uterine wall. This can be unreliable as bleeding may occur with only partial separation of the placenta and, even with complete separation of the placenta from the uterine wall, the blood may be contained behind the membranes and not be clinically apparent.
3. When the placenta has separated and descends to the lower uterine segment and through the cervix there is cord lengthening (8–15 cm) at the introitus. This is the most reliable sign.

The *mechanism of haemostasis* at the placental site is one of the physiological and anatomical marvels of nature. The muscle fibres of the myometrium are arranged in a criss-cross pattern and through this lattice-work of muscle fibres the blood vessels pass to supply the placental bed. When the uterine muscle contracts this lattice-work of fibres effectively compresses the blood vessels (Fig 18.1). This myometrial architecture is sometimes appropriately referred to as the 'living ligatures' or 'physiological sutures' of the uterus.

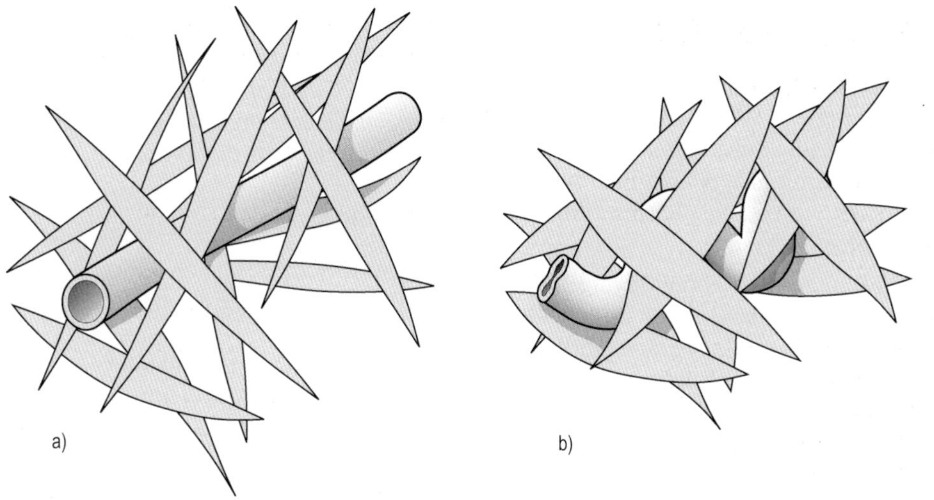

Figure 18.1 Haemostatic mechanism after placental separation. The 'living ligatures' or 'physiological sutures' of the myometrium.

Management of the third stage of labour

After the infant has been delivered the cord is clamped, divided and the necessary cord blood samples taken. Put very light tension on the cord to ensure there are no loops free in the vagina and then place the clamp on the cord at the level of the introitus, ensuring that real cord lengthening becomes clinically apparent. One hand cradles and 'guards the fundus' so that the changes associated with placental separation can be appreciated or to detect an atonic enlarging uterus filling with blood. The uterine hand should not manipulate or massage the fundus as this may cause premature partial placental separation and increased blood loss, or a contraction ring leading to retained placenta. When the clinical signs of placental separation are evident, assist delivery of the placenta by controlled cord traction. The abdominal hand moves to the lower part of the uterus just above the pubic symphysis and gently pushes the uterus upwards and backwards while the other hand exerts steady downward traction on the cord. The distance between the suprapubic hand and the sacral promontory should be such as to prevent the possibility of uterine inversion (Fig 18.2).

There are two approaches, expectant and active, to the routine management of the third stage of labour:

- *Expectant management* involves observation while awaiting the physiological changes that bring about placental separation. This usually takes 10–20 minutes and is favoured by those who prefer limited intervention

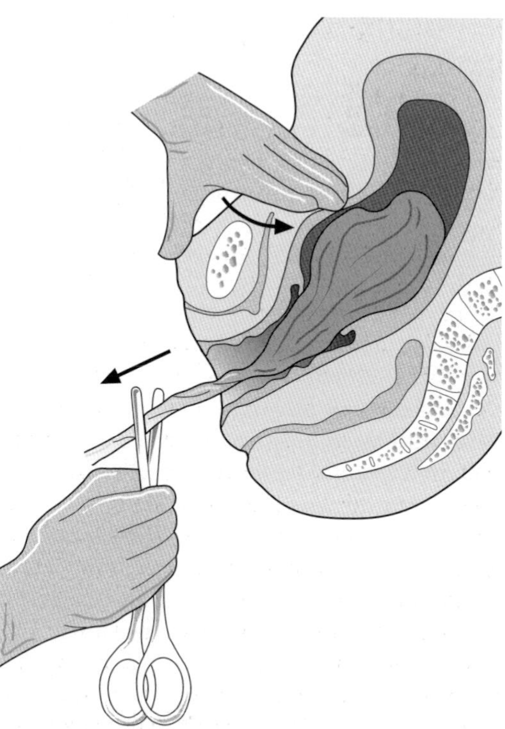

Figure 18.2 Delivery of separated placenta by controlled cord traction.

in the management of labour. Some will encourage suckling immediately after delivery to stimulate physiological oxytocin release.[6] Unfortunately, this physiologically attractive approach is not as effective at reducing PPH when compared with active pharmacological management.[7]

- *Active management* entails giving an oxytocic drug during or just after delivery of the infant in order to consistently cause the uterine contractions that lead to placental separation and haemostasis. Active management of the third stage of labour has evolved over the past half century and several randomized controlled trials have shown that it effectively reduces blood loss, need for therapeutic doses of oxytocic drugs, PPH, and blood transfusion by 50–70% when compared with expectant management.[8] The evidence and experience with active management is such that this has become the standard of care.[9,10] Expectant management is only followed at the express and informed request of the woman.

The choice of oxytocic for routine active management is usually between the cheaper injectable drugs, oxytocin and ergometrine, or a combination of both in the compound Syntometrine. Of these, oxytocin is the cheapest, has the fewest side-effects and does not cause retained placenta. It is, however, shorter-acting (15–30 min). Ergometrine is effective but has more side-effects (see below), has a longer duration of action (60–120 min), and a slightly higher risk of causing retained placenta. Thus, oxytocin is the drug of first choice and is given as a dose of either 5 units intravenously or 10 units by intramuscular injection with delivery of the anterior shoulder or as soon thereafter as feasible.

'In patients liable to haemorrhage, immediately after delivery … ergot may be given as a preventive a few minutes before the termination of the labour.'

John Stearns
Observations on the secale cornutum or ergot, with directions for its use in parturition. Med Rec 1822; 5:90

The risk of atonic postpartum haemorrhage is greatest in the hour following delivery. However, the woman is susceptible to atonic haemorrhage over the next 2–3 hours. Thus, if oxytocin has been used for active management its short duration of action may necessitate the addition of oxytocin to the intravenous infusion for the next 2–3 hours. If ergometrine or Syntometrine have been used the longer duration of action will usually suffice. In women with risk factors for more prolonged postpartum uterine atony (e.g. multiple pregnancy) longer-acting oxytocic drugs such as a prolonged oxytocin infusion and, in selected cases, prostaglandins may be necessary for adequate prophylaxis.

'The uniform operation of the ergot to restrain uterine haemorrhage … has frequently been prescribed, a little previous to the birth of the child, or immediately after, to the patients who have been accustomed to flow immoderately, at such times, and it has always proved an effectual preventive.'

Oliver Prescott
A Dissertation on the Natural History and Medical Effects of Secale Cornutum or Ergot. Andover: Flagg & Gould, 1813, p14

Oxytocic drugs

It is important to know the characteristics and side-effects of the available oxytocic drugs, each of which has application in a variety of clinical circumstances (Table 18.1).

Oxytocin

Oxytocin is the cheapest and safest of the injectable oxytocic drugs. It induces the rapid onset of strong rhythmic uterine contractions which last for 15–30 minutes. The effect is mainly on the upper uterine segment. Oxytocin also produces

Table 18.1 Characteristics of oxytocic drugs

Drug	Dose and route	Duration of action	Adverse effects	Contraindication
Oxytocin	5 units IV 10 units IM 20 units in 500 ml infusion	15–30 minutes	Insignificant hypotension and flushing. Water intoxication in high doses (> 200 units)	None
Ergometrine	0.2–0.25 mg IV or IM	1–2 hours	Nausea, vomiting, hypertension, vasospasm	Pre-eclampsia/ hypertension, cardiovascular disease
Syntometrine (5 units oxytocin, 0.5 mg ergometrine)	1 ampoule IM	1–2 hours	Nausea, vomiting, hypertension, vasospasm	Pre-eclampsia/ hypertension, cardiovascular disease
15-methyl $PGF_{2\alpha}$	0.25 mg IM or IMM 0.25 mg in 500 ml infusion	4–6 hours	Vomiting, diarrhoea, flushing, shivering, vasospasm, bronchospasm	Cardiovascular disease, asthma
Misoprostol	400–600 μg oral, sublingual 800–1000 μg rectal	1–2 hours	Nausea, diarrhoea, shivering, pyrexia	None
Carbetocin	100 μg IM or IV	1–2 hours	Flushing	None

IM = intramuscular, IMM = intramyometrial; IV = intravenous.
Reproduced with permission from: Baskett TF. Essential management of obstetric emergencies. 4th ed. Clinical Press: Bristol, 2004

a transient vascular smooth muscle relaxant effect which may lead to a mild, brief reduction in blood pressure because of the reduced total peripheral resistance. This hypotension is mild and clinically insignificant except in cases of cardiovascular instability.[11] The dose is 5 units intravenously by slow intravenous bolus, 10 units intramuscularly, or 20 units in 500 ml crystalloid by intravenous infusion.

Ergometrine

Ergometrine was the first of the injectable oxytocics and has been in use for 70 years. It produces prolonged uterine contractions involving the upper and lower uterine segments with a duration of 60–120 minutes. Ergometrine produces contraction of smooth muscle throughout the body and this is particularly relevant in the vascular tree. Peripheral vasoconstriction which, in the normal woman is not clinically significant, can produce a severe rise in blood pressure in the hypertensive or pre-eclamptic woman. In such cases it is contraindicated. Ergometrine can also induce coronary artery spasm which is also of no significance in the healthy woman, but has been incriminated in very rare cases of myocardial infarction in susceptible women. Ergometrine-induced vasospasm is responsive to glyceryl trinitrate.

Because of its prolonged effect, ergometrine causes a slight increase in uterine entrapment of the separated placenta.[12] Compared with oxytocin this amounts to about an additional 1 in 200 cases requiring manual removal. Nausea and/or vomiting occur in 20–25% of women who receive ergometrine. The dose of

Ergometrine

'Reckoned in the saving of human life, places it among the enduring achievements of medical science'

Chassar Moir
The obstetrician bids, and the uterus contracts. BMJ 1964; 110:1029

ergometrine is 0.2–0.25 mg by intramuscular injection. Because of the vasopressor effect it is better not given intravenously, although if the indication is urgent it can be given as a slow intravenous bolus of 0.2 mg. The higher dose of 0.5 mg should not be given initially as the side-effect profile is increased, without a concomitant improvement in the uterotonic effect.

Syntometrine

Syntometrine comes in an ampoule combining oxytocin 5 units and ergometrine 0.5 mg. Given intramuscularly, oxytocin has its effect within 2–3 minutes while ergometrine takes 4–5 minutes. The side-effect profile of both drugs is combined and this may have the beneficial effect of the vasodilatation effect of oxytocin ameliorating, to some extent, the vasoconstricting effect of ergometrine. This combination provides the benefit of the short-acting oxytocin along with the more sustained uterotonic effect of ergometrine. It has the benefit, therefore, of providing more sustained oxytocic prophylaxis in the first 2 hours following delivery, thereby obviating the need for an intravenous infusion.[13]

15-methyl prostaglandin F2α

15-methyl $PGF_{2\alpha}$ or carboprost (Hemabate) is the 15-methyl analogue of the parent compound $PGF_{2\alpha}$. This is the most expensive of the injectable oxytocics. Its advantage is that, at a comparable dose, it has a strong uterotonic effect and less of the undesirable smooth muscle stimulation effects including nausea, vomiting, diarrhoea, vasospasm and bronchospasm. As a result it has supplanted the parent compound for this oxytocic indication. Other side-effects which are usually not clinically significant are shivering, pyrexia and flushing. The duration of action is up to 6 hours and while, on the basis of cost and side-effects, it is not recommended for routine prophylaxis it is a very useful agent when a prolonged oxytocic effect is required.

The dose is 0.25 mg and it can be given intramuscularly, intramyometrially or as a dilute intravenous infusion of 0.25 mg in 500 ml saline.[14] The quickest effect is usually attained by the intramyometrial route in which the 1 ml ampoule of 0.25 mg is diluted in 5 ml saline and injected transabdominally at two sites into the uterine fundus. 15-methyl $PGF_{2\alpha}$ can be given in cases of hypertension and asthma, although these are relative contraindications. It is an excellent second line uterotonic agent if oxytocin and ergometrine have failed or if a long-term oxytocic effect is required.

Misoprostol

An analogue of prostaglandin E1, misoprostol is the cheapest oxytocic and the only one that can be given by the non-parenteral route. Misoprostol is used off-label as an oxytocic drug but has the endorsement of many national societies of obstetrics and gynaecology. It has a long shelf life and is stable at extremes of temperature. This is in contrast with oxytocin and ergometrine which lose their potency unless stored in the dark at cool temperatures (0–8°C). Misoprostol can be given orally, sublingually, vaginally or rectally depending on the clinical situation. It has a low side-effect profile with shivering, mild pyrexia and diarrhoea being the main associations. It has been shown to be more effective than placebo in the prevention of PPH but is probably slightly less effective than the injectable oxytocics.[15–17] However, the features mentioned above make it a drug of enormous potential for use in the developing world where obstetric facilities are limited, and where the majority of deaths occur.[18–21] It also has use as a second line oxytocic drug when oxytocin and/or ergometrine have failed. The usual dose is 400–600 µg orally or sublingually, and in the case of haemorrhage, 800–1000 µg rectally.[22] The duration of effect is about 2 hours.

Carbetocin

Carbetocin is a long-acting synthetic analogue of oxytocin. The duration of action is 60–120 minutes. It is given as a single dose of 100 µg by intramuscular or intravenous injection. The side-effects are similar to those of oxytocin, namely flushing and mild hypotension. Its purported advantage is that it provides a prolonged oxytocic effect compared with the parent compound oxytocin, obviating the need for an intravenous infusion of oxytocin for the 2 hours following initial active management of the third stage of labour.[23,24] It is more expensive than oxytocin but less so than 15-methyl $PGF_{2\alpha}$.

Causes of primary PPH

Uterine atony

This is caused by anything that interferes with the ability of the uterus to contract and retract. It is the most common cause (80–85%). Although it can occur in low risk cases, interference with uterine contraction and retraction is most likely in the following:

- Multiparity
- Prolonged labour, particularly if it is associated with chorioamniotitis. The exhausted and infected uterus is vulnerable to uterine atony and may be unresponsive to oxytocic agents.
- Precipitate labour. In the other extreme of uterine action, the very rapid and efficient first and second stages of labour may be followed by uterine atony.
- Uterine over-distension: multiple pregnancy, macrosomnia and polyhydramnios.

HISTORICAL BACKGROUND

The development of modern oxytocic drugs is of interest. Building on the observations by midwives and doctors in the previous four centuries that powdered ergot caused strong uterine contractions, Chassar Moir and the research chemist Harold Dudley set out to discover the active oxytocic component. In 1935, after 3 years of research, during which Moir tested many compounds for their oxytocic effect on the postpartum uterus, they isolated ergometrine – the active oxytocic alkaloid of ergot. Independently, and almost simultaneously, it was discovered in Chicago, Baltimore, and Switzerland. Working under Sir Henry Dale's guidance in London, and recognizing the clinical importance of this first reliable and injectable oxytocic, Moir and Dudley published the full formula and method of production so that no patent or proprietary interest would be served.

In 1952 Vincent DuVigneaud at Cornell University, New York, identified and synthesized pure oxytocin. After the identification of the individual prostaglandins by Sune Bergstrom and his colleagues at the Karolinska Institute in Stockholm, the 15-methyl analogue of $PGF_{2\alpha}$ was applied to the treatment of PPH in the 1970s. By the 1990s misoprostol was being used for the prevention and management of PPH due to uterine atony. Thus, the modern era of oxytocic drug development started with the discovery of ergometrine in 1935, and has moved forward in approximately 20-year epochs over the last 70 years.[25,26]

- Retained placenta or placental fragments.
- Retained blood clots. After delivery of the placenta the uterine fundus should be firmly massaged and an oxytocin drip kept running for 2–3 hours if there is any tendency for uterine relaxation. If not, a small amount of oozing from the placental site may occur, leading to clots in the uterus. As these accumulate they interfere with the ability of the uterus to contract and retract, leading to an insidious filling of the uterus with clots and blood, establishing a vicious cycle.
- Tocolytic drugs, such as glyceryl trinitrate or terbutaline and deep general anaesthesia, particularly with fluorinated hydrocarbons.
- Structural abnormalities of the uterus, including uterine anomalies and fibroids.
- Placenta praevia: the implantation site of the placenta is on the lower uterine segment which has limited ability to contract and retract.
- Inappropriate management of the third stage of labour with premature manipulation of the fundus and cord traction may lead to partial separation of the placenta and increased blood loss.

Genital tract trauma

See Chapter 21. This is the next most common cause accounting for the majority of the remaining 10–15% of cases and includes:

- lacerations of the perineum, vagina and cervix
- episiotomy
- uterine rupture
- vulvo-vaginal and broad ligament haematomas.

Other causes

Other causes of primary PPH are uterine inversion (see Chapter 20) and coagulation disorders (see Chapter 23).

Prevention of primary PPH

Women with risk factors for PPH should be delivered in hospitals with appropriate anaesthetic and obstetric personnel and available blood transfusion. In all women careful attention should be directed to details of safe management of the third stage of labour, including:

- Oxytocin is given with or shortly after delivery of the anterior shoulder.
- Avoid inappropriate manipulation of the uterine fundus ('fundus fiddling') and/or premature traction on the umbilical cord before clear signs of placental separation are present.
- When the placenta is delivered, inspect it closely for completeness.
- Firmly massage the uterus to expel all clots that might interfere with contraction and retraction.
- Keep the uterus well contracted with an oxytocic for the next 2 hours, and longer in high-risk cases.
- Close surveillance, including attention to keeping the bladder empty and the uterine fundus well contracted for 2–3 hours following delivery.

Management of primary PPH

The medical management of uterine atony will be covered here. The other causes and the surgical management of uterine atony are covered in other chapters. The immediate management of atonic postpartum haemorrhage is to enlist the normal physiological mechanism of uterine haemostasis – namely initiate uterine contraction and retraction. While getting the appropriate oxytocic drugs ready the hand should be used to apply firm but gentle fundal massage.

Oxytocic drugs

It should be remembered that oxytocin administration down-regulates oxytocin receptors.

Thus, if labour is augmented by oxytocin during the first and second stages of labour the receptors may be less responsive to oxytocin in the third stage of labour. In normal labour, oxytocin levels do not change in the third stage, but endogenous prostaglandin production increases. The myometrium has different receptors for each of the oxytocic drugs, so that if one drug is ineffective move quickly to the next choice. The following application and sequence of oxytocic drugs is recommended:

- Intravenous oxytocin 5 units and establish an infusion with 40 units of oxytocin in 500 ml crystalloid running rapidly enough to initiate and sustain uterine contractions.
- If this fails give ergometrine 0.2 mg intravenously (provided there are no contraindications).
- The doses of oxytocin and ergometrine can be repeated. If oxytocin and ergometrine are ineffective do not delay in moving to the prostaglandins.
- 15-methyl prostaglandin $F_{2\alpha}$ 0.25 mg can be given by intramuscular or preferably by intramyometrial injection. This can be repeated up to four times if necessary. An alternative is an infusion of 0.25 mg in 500 ml crystalloid.
- In the presence of active haemorrhage the oral and vaginal routes for misoprostol are less appropriate – the latter because the tablets are washed away by the haemorrhage. The preferred route is the rectal administration of 1000 μg. Because it is cheap and simple to administer many will move to misoprostol earlier in the sequence.
- Treat hypovolaemia. Hypovolaemia should be actively treated with intravenous crystalloid, colloid, blood and blood products as required (see Chapter 22).

If uterine atony is unresponsive to fundal massage and the available oxytocic drugs, surgical techniques including uterine tamponade, uterine compression sutures, major vessel ligation and embolisation, and even hysterectomy will have to be considered. These are all outlined in Chapter 26.

While preparations are being made for the surgical techniques *bimanual uterine compression* may be undertaken as a stop-gap measure. The vaginal hand forms a fist in the anterior fornix while the abdominal hand cups the postero-fundal aspect of the uterus pulling it down against the vaginal fist. The vaginal hand also elevates the uterus. In this way the uterine vessels may be attenuated and compressed to reduce the bleeding. The hands may also provide rotary massage to try and stimulate uterine contraction (Fig 18.3).

In desperate circumstances, while awaiting the muster of surgical instruments, *external aortic compression* can be tried. This involves the two hands lifting the fundus of the uterus up out of the pelvis; the lower hand then pushes upwards and backwards on the lower uterine segment while the other hand pushes the fundus firmly down onto the aorta. This may be of limited value if the uterus is very atonic, as it may not provide a firm enough compression pad. An alternative technique is to use the fist applied directly in the midline, just above the umbilicus and uterus with the heel of the hand pressing down on the aorta.[27] This may be feasible due to the stretched abdominal muscles and separation of the rectus muscles, but is obviously a short-term measure.

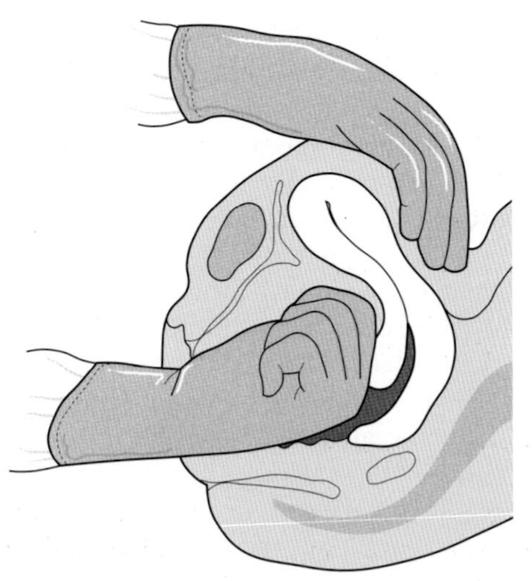

Figure 18.3 Bimanual uterine compression.

Secondary PPH

This is defined as abnormal bleeding from the genital tract between 24 hours and 6 weeks postpartum. It is much less common than primary PPH, occurring in about 1% of deliveries. The majority of cases occur within 3 weeks of delivery.

Causes

- Retained placental tissue is found in about one-third of cases.
- Intrauterine infection often co-exists with retained tissue. In many cases neither can be clearly demonstrated but the patient will have a history of primary PPH and/or manual removal of the placenta at this delivery.
- Extremely rare causes also have to be considered, including: trophoblastic disease, chronic uterine inversion and the development of a false aneurysm or arteriovenous fistula at the site of a healing caesarean section scar.

Management

If the bleeding is mild and settling, the uterus is not tender, is appropriately involuted, and there are no other signs of sepsis, initial observation is justified. Ultrasound may help this decision if it suggests that the uterus is empty and without retained placental tissue.[28]

Those patients with heavy bleeding, with signs of intrauterine sepsis and a subinvoluted uterus suggesting infected retained placental tissue, should have uterine exploration under anaesthesia. Ultrasound may help confirm this decision but it is not always accurate so that it should be over-ruled by clinical considerations. These cases require intravenous crystalloid, cross-match blood and broad-spectrum intravenous antibiotics to cover Gram-positive, Gram-negative and anaerobic organisms. Occasionally these patients can bleed severely and require transfusion.

Under anaesthesia the lower genital tract and cervix should be carefully inspected in case there is a laceration or discharging haematoma. Usually the cervix is open enough that the finger can enter and explore the uterine cavity. One may be able to detect and detach placental tissue from the uterine wall. This may be removed with sponge forceps followed by gentle suction curettage.

The tissue removed should be sent for histopathology to rule out trophoblastic disease. In septic cases a portion may be sent for culture and antibiotic sensitivity testing.[29]

The recently puerperal uterus is soft and very prone to perforation. One should be particularly cautious in cases delivered by caesarean section and avoid curetting the incised part of the uterus. Quite severe haemorrhage can be induced by curettage as organized portions of placental tissue, some of which may be areas of partial accreta, are removed from the uterine wall opening up the partially thrombosed vessels. This bleeding is usually not responsive to oxytocic agents. On occasions, surgical management has to be considered including uterine tamponade, major vessel embolisation and hysterectomy (see Chapter 26).

References

1. Confidential Enquiry into Maternal and Child Health. Why Mothers Die 2000–2002. London: RCOG Press, 2004.
2. Drife JO. Maternal 'near-miss' reports? BMJ 1993; 307:1087–1088.
3. Baskett TF, Sternadel J. Maternal intensive care and near-miss mortality in obstetrics. Br J Obstet Gynaecol 1998; 105:981–984.
4. Baskett TF, O'Connell CM. Severe obstetric maternal morbidity: a 15-year population-based study. J Obstet Gynaecol 2005; 25:7–9.
5. Dildy GA, Paine AR, George NC, Velasco C. Estimating blood loss: can teaching significantly improve visual estimation? Obstet Gynecol 2004; 104:601–606.
6. Chua S, Arulkumaran S, Lim I, Selamat N, Ratnam SS. Influence of breast-feeding and nipple stimulation on postpartum uterine activity. Br J Obstet Gynaecol 1994; 101:804–805.
7. Bullough CHW, Msuku RS, Karonde L. Early suckling and postpartum haemorrhage: controlled trial in deliveries by traditional birth attendants. Lancet 1989; 2:522–525.

8. Baskett TF. A flux of the reds: evolution of active management of the third stage of labour. J R Soc Med 2000; 93:489–493.

9. Elbourne D, Prendiville W, Chalmers I. Choice of oxytocic preparation for routine use in the management of the third stage of labour: an overview of the evidence from controlled clinical trials. Br J Obstet Gynaecol 1988; 95:17–30.

10. Nordstrom L, Fogelstam K, Fridman G, Larsson A, Rydhestroem PH. Routine oxytocin in the third stage of labour: a placebo controlled randomised trial. Br J Obstet Gynaecol 1997; 104:781–786.

11. Davies GAL, Tessier JL, Woodman MC, Lipson A, Hahn PM. Maternal hemodynamics after oxytocin bolus compared with infusion in the third stage of labor: a randomized controlled trial. Obstet Gynecol 2005; 105:294–299.

12. Hammar M, Bostrom K, Borgvall B. Comparison between the influence of methyergometrine and oxytocin on the incidence of retained placenta in the third stage of labour. Gynecol Obstet Invest 1990; 30:91–94.

13. Choy CMY, Lau WC, Tam WH, Yuen PM. A randomised controlled trial of intramuscular Syntometrine and intravenous oxytocin in the management of the third stage of labour. Br J Obstet Gynaecol 2002; 109:173–177.

14. Granstrom L, Ekinan G, Ulmsten U. Intravenous infusion of 15 methyl prostaglandin F2 alpha in women with heavy postpartum haemorrhage. Acta Obstet Gynecol Scand 1989; 68:365–367.

15. Gülmezoglu AM, Villar J, Ngoc NT, et al. WHO multicentre randomised trial of misoprostol in the management of the third stage of labour. Lancet 2001; 358:689–695.

16. Surbek DV, Fehr PM, Hosli I, Holzgreve W. Oral misoprostol for third stage of labour: a randomized placebo-controlled trial. Obstet Gynecol 1999; 94:255–258.

17. Walraven G, Blum J, Dampha Y, et al. Misoprostol in the management of the third stage of labour in the home delivery setting in rural Gambia: a randomised controlled trial. Br J Obstet Gynaecol 2005; 112:1277–1283.

18. El-Rafaey H, O'Brien P, Morafa W, Walder J, Rodeck C. Use of oral misoprostol in the prevention of postpartum haemorrhage. Br J Obstet Gynaecol 1997; 104:336–369.

19. Sharma S, El-Rafaey H. Prostaglandins in the prevention and management of postpartum haemorrhage. Best Pract Res Clin Obstet Gynaecol 2003; 17:811–823.

20. Derman RJ, Kodkany BS, Goudar SS, Geller SE, Niak VA, Bellad MB, et al. Oral misoprostol in preventing postpartum haemorrhage in resource-poor communities: a randomised controlled trial. Lancet 2006; 368:1248–1253.

21. Prata N, Hamza S, Gypson R, Nada K, Vahidnia F, Potts M. Misoprostol in active management of the third stage of labor. Int J Gynecol Obstet 2006; 94:149–155.

22. O'Brien P, El-Rafaey H, Gordon A, Geary M. Rodeck CH. Rectally administered misoprostol for the treatment of postpartum hemorrhage unresponsive to oxytocin and ergometrine: a descriptive study. Obstet Gynecol 1998; 92:212–214.

23. Boucher M, Harbay GL, Griffin P. Double-blind randomised comparison of the effect of carbetocin and oxytocin on intraoperative blood loss and uterine tone of patients undergoing cesarean section. J Perinatol 1998; 18:202–207.

24. Leung SW, Ng PS, Wong WY, Cheung TH. A randomized trial of carbetocin versus syntometrine in the management of the third stage of labour. Br J Obstet Gynaecol 2006; 113:1459–1464.

25. Baskett TF. The development of prostaglandins. Best Pract Res Clin Obstet Gynaecol 2003; 17:703–706.

26. Baskett TF. The development of oxytocic drugs in the management of postpartum haemorrhage. Ulster Med J 2004; 73:2–6.

27. Riley DP, Burgess RW. External abdominal aortic compression: a study of a resuscitation manoeuvre for postpartum haemorrhage. Anaesth Intens Care 1994; 22:571–575.

28. Skinner J, Turner MJ. Postpartum exploration of the genital tract under general anaesthesia reviewed. J Obstet Gynaecol 1997; 17:273.

29. Hoveyda F, Mackenzie IZ. Secondary postpartum haemorrhage: incidence, morbidity and current management. Br J Obstet Gynaecol 2001; 108:927–930.

19

Retained placenta

'Since it is a verity indubitable, that the after-birth remaining behind after the child is born, becomes a useless mass, capable of destroying the woman, we must take care that it be never left, if possible.'

Francois Mauriceau
The Diseases of Women With Child, and in Child-Bed. London: John Darby, 1683, p212

With traditional or expectant management of the third stage of labour the placenta usually delivers within 10–20 minutes. With active management the placenta is commonly delivered within 5–10 minutes. In general, 90% of placentas deliver within 15 minutes, 96% within 30 minutes and 98% within 60 minutes. The definition and incidence of retained placenta, therefore, depends on the time chosen.[1–3]

Once the infant has delivered and as time passes without placental separation and delivery, the risk of haemorrhage increases and the chance of spontaneous delivery of the placenta decreases.[4] The time at which one declares the placenta retained and takes active steps for its removal depends on the facilities and personnel available for safe anaesthesia, as well as the presence or absence of haemorrhage. These considerations are illustrated in Figure 19.1.

Types of retained placenta

- The placenta has separated from the uterine wall but is retained in the uterus because of atony or, more commonly, a contraction ring between the lower and upper uterine segments or in one uterine cornu.

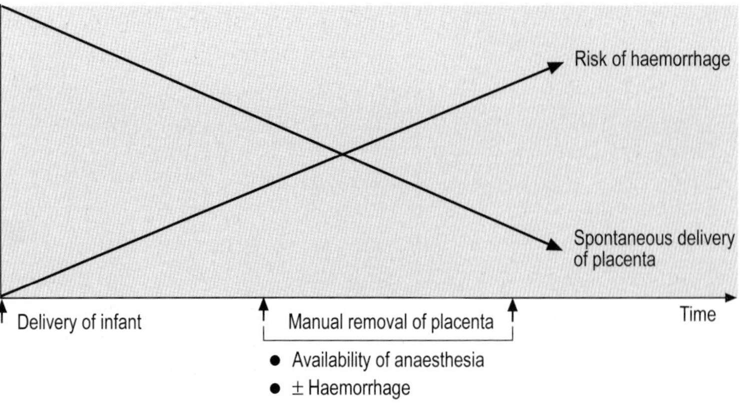

Figure 19.1 Factors in decision and timing of manual removal of retained placenta.

- Ordinary adherence of the placenta is due to failure of the normal separation through the decidua spongiosa layer. Until separation occurs, either partially or completely, these cases do not bleed excessively.
- Pathological adherence of the placenta may be of three degrees: *placenta accreta* – invasion of the decidua basalis and adherence to the myometrium; *placenta increta* – invading the myometrium; *placenta percreta* – invasion through the myometrium to the serosal layer. Placenta accreta is much more likely when the site of implantation is the lower uterine segment, due to the poor decidual response in this area. Thus, women with placenta praevia are more prone to pathological adherence. Women with previous caesarean section, particularly repeated caesarean sections, are more likely to have placenta praevia and for this to be associated with accreta. The more invasive degree of placenta praevia percreta represents one of the most hazardous haemorrhagic conditions in obstetrics.[5]

Pathological adherence of the placenta in the upper uterine segment is quite rare and almost never complete. However, during manual removal of the placenta, small accretic areas may be encountered (see later). The management of placenta praevia accreta is discussed in Chapter 17.

Predisposing factors

- Retained placenta in previous pregnancy.
- Preterm labour. The earlier the gestation the longer the duration of the third stage of labour.
- Long-acting oxytocic agents, such as ergometrine or the combination of oxytocin and ergometrine (Syntometrine). The increased risk of retained placenta with the longer-acting oxytocics is small and often overstated.[6]
- Uterine fibroids.
- Uterine anomaly, such as bicornuate uterus.
- Uterine scar – previous caesarean section, myomectomy, hysteroscopic surgery, curettage.
- Placenta praevia (placenta accreta).

Management

In most cases of retained placenta, management consists of manual removal. However, as outlined in the introduction, the timing of this procedure depends on the availability of safe anaesthesia and also on the presence or absence of haemorrhage. If there is little or no bleeding most will delay for 30 minutes and then marshal the resources needed for anaesthesia and manual removal. This usually takes about another 30 minutes so that 1 hour after delivery of the infant, manual removal is undertaken. Just before induction of anaesthesia a pelvic examination should be carried out, as in a number of cases the placenta will deliver spontaneously while the resources for anaesthesia are being mustered. With this approach, manual removal is required in about 2% of all vaginal deliveries.[7]

If the woman has delivered with an existing regional anaesthetic in place this delay is not necessary as the risks of anaesthesia have already been undertaken. On balance, waiting about 15 minutes in the absence of haemorrhage is reasonable.

In any case in which haemorrhage supervenes, manual removal should be carried out at once.

Technique of manual removal

General anaesthesia has the advantage of speed and will also assist by providing uterine relaxation. However, the additional risks of general anaesthesia to the mother make the choice of spinal anaesthesia better, provided there is no haemorrhage. With spinal anaesthesia, uterine relaxation may not occur and this can be provided by intravenous nitroglycerine if necessary (see Chapter 26).

With the patient in the dorsal lithotomy position and appropriate asepsis, one hand is placed on the abdomen to steady the fundus and push the uterus downwards. The well lubricated other hand follows the cord into the vagina and through the cervix. The lower uterine segment can be very thin and ballooned out, above which is a thick contraction ring at the junction of the upper and lower uterine segments (Fig 19.2). For the unwary operator this ballooned out lower uterine segment may be mistaken for the uterine cavity proper. In some instances the contraction ring provides such an obstruction that the hand may be pushed through the thinned-out lower uterine segment. To avoid uterine rupture with the exploring hand, press down on the fundus of the uterus with the external hand and extend the internal hand as a cone and slowly pass it upwards through the contraction ring. Uterine relaxation either by general anaesthesia or intravenous nitroglycerine may be necessary to allow the hand into the upper part of the uterine cavity.

'I find it both amongst the ancients and moderns there have been different opinions and directions about delivering the placenta; some alleging that it should be delivered slowly, or left to come, of itself; others, that the hand should be immediately introduced into the uterus, to separate and bring it away ... So in my opinion we ought to go the middle way, never to assist but when we find it necessary: on the one hand, not to torture nature when it is self-sufficient, nor delay too long, because it is possible that the placenta should be sometimes, though seldom, retained several days.'

William Smellie
Treatise on the Theory and Practice of Midwifery. London: D Wilson, 1752, p239

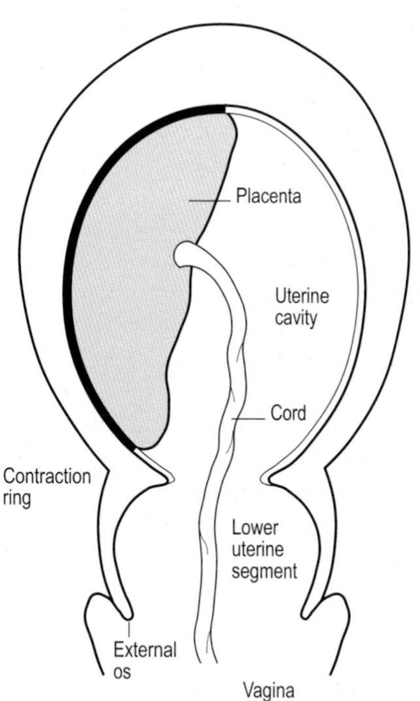

Figure 19.2 A contraction ring has formed below the placenta at the junction of the upper and lower uterine segments. The thin, ballooned lower segment is vulnerable to perforation by the exploring hand during manual removal.

The fingers and thumb of the uterine hand should be kept extended and used as one unit to advance to the lower margin of the placenta and begin to detach it by sweeping the hand from side to side within a plane of cleavage between the placenta and uterine wall. The external hand steadies the fundus to facilitate these internal manipulations (Fig 19.3).

Once the placenta is felt to be completely separated it is grasped between the fingers and thumb and the external hand is moved down to apply traction to the cord to help move the placenta into the grasp of the uterine hand. The placenta is then removed slowly as it is not uncommon for a small portion of the placenta to remain adherent to the uterine wall and this, along with the uterine relaxation, can lead to uterine inversion.

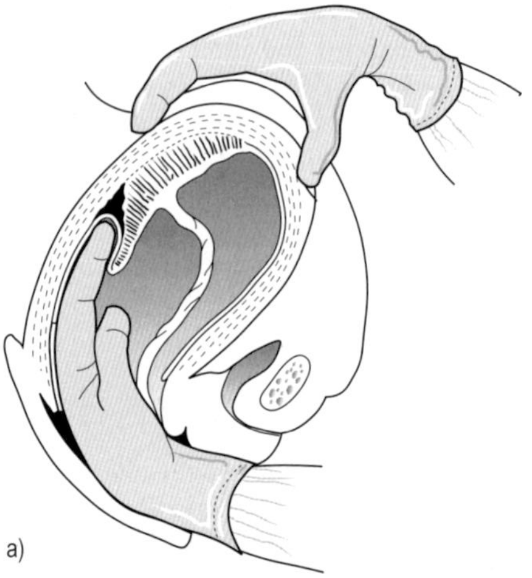

Once the placenta has been removed the uterus is re-explored to ensure that there are no placental fragments remaining and that the uterine wall is intact.

In the first edition (1908) of this book, written shortly after the introduction of rubber surgical gloves, Munro Kerr made this observation:

> *'In removing the whole placenta adherent or retained, I advise using a rubber glove. I have found, however, that it is quite impossible to remove small portions of the placenta or membranes with the gloved hand'.*

a)

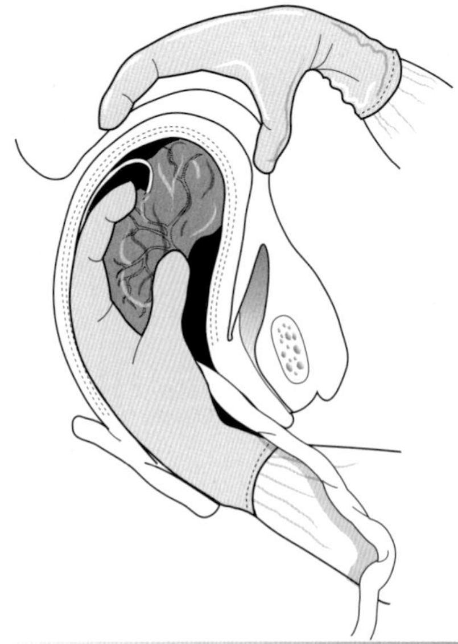

b)

Figure 19.3 (a) A sweeping movement separates the placenta. (b) The detached placenta is grasped and removed.

On rare occasions one will encounter small accretic areas of placenta. Usually these are so small that they can be removed piecemeal as best as possible and will not interfere with contraction and retraction of the uterus.

The cervix and vagina are examined and any lacerations sutured. An intravenous injection of 5 units of oxytocin followed by an infusion of 40 units in 1 L is established to initiate and maintain uterine contraction and retraction. A broad-spectrum antibiotic is given for 12–24 hours to prevent infection.

Intraumbilical vein injection of oxytocics

There is increasing, but still inconclusive, experience with intraumbilical vein injection of oxytocic drugs.[8–10] In most series this has been shown to aid spontaneous delivery of the placenta and reduce the need for manual removal. Both oxytocin and prostaglandins have been used, but there is more experience with the former.[11] Usually 20 units of oxytocin are mixed in 20 ml saline and injected up the umbilical vein. The effect is probably due to a combination of distension of chorionic villi and local oxytocic effect on the myometrium. The maternal plasma oxytocin levels are not increased with this technique, confirming the local action. Although the results of this technique are not fully endorsed by a suitable randomized controlled trial, it is cheap and there are no complications.[12] Thus, it may have a role before resorting to anaesthesia or in areas where anaesthesia is not available. A multicentre randomized trial is underway.[13]

Tocolysis

In those cases in which the placenta is felt to be retained by a contraction ring the use of acute tocolysis is logical, although extensive experience with this is lacking and it carries the increased possibility of atonic haemorrhage.[14] The technique of administration of intravenous nitroglycerin for this purpose is covered in Chapter 26.

References

1. Adelusi B, Soltan MH, Chowdhury N, Kanjave D. Risk of retained placenta: multivariate approach. Acta Obstet Gynaecol Scand 1997; 76:414–418.
2. Dombrowski MP, Bottoms SF, Salah AAA, Hurd WW, Romero R. Third stage of labor: an analysis of duration and clinical practice. Am J Obstet Gynecol 1995; 172:1279–1284.
3. Soltan MH, Khashoggi T. Retained placenta and associated risk factors. J Obstet Gynaecol 1997; 17:245–247.
4. Magann EF, Evans S, Chauhan SP, Lanneau G, Fisk AD, Morrison JC. The length of the third stage of labour and the risk of postpartum hemorrhage. Obstet Gynecol 2005; 105:290–293.
5. Stones RW, Paterson CM, Saunders NJ. Risk factors for major obstetric haemorrhage. Eur J Obstet Gynaecol Reprod Biol 1993; 48:15–18.
6. Hammar M, Bostrom K, Borgvall B. Comparison between the influence of methylergometrine and oxytocin on the incidence of retained placenta in the third stage of labor. Gynecol Obstet Invest 1990; 30:91–94.
7. Johanson RB, Cox C, Grady K, Howell C, eds. Retained placenta. In: Managing obstetric emergencies and trauma. London: RCOG Press, 2003:189–192.
8. Selinger M, MacKenzie I, Dunlop P. James D. Intra-umbilical vein oxytocin in the management of retained placenta. A double blind controlled study. J Obstet Gynaecol 1986; 7:115–117.
9. Carroli G, Belizan JM, Grant A, Gonzalez L, Campodonico L, Bergel E. Intra-umbilical vein injection and retained placenta: evidence from a collaborative large randomised controlled trial. Grupo Argentino de Estudio de Placenta Retenida. Br J Obstet Gynaecol 1998; 105:178–185.
10. Gazvani MR, Luckas MJM, Drakeley AJ, Emery SJ, Alfirevic Z, Walkinshaw SA. Intraumbilical oxytocin for the management of retained placenta: a randomized controlled trial. Obstet Gynecol 1998; 91:203–207.
11. Bider D, Dulitzky M, Goldenberg M, Lipitz S, Mashiach S. Intra-umbilical vein injection of prostaglandin F2alpha in retained placenta. Eur J Obstet Gynaecol Reprod Biol 1996; 64:59–61.
12. Weeks AD, Mirembe FM. The retained placenta – new insights into an old problem. Eur J Obstet Gynecol Reprod Biol 2002; 102:109–110.
13. Weeks A, Mirembe F, Alfirevic Z. The release trial: a randomised controlled trial of umbilical vein oxytocin versus placebo for the treatment of retained placenta. Br J Obstet Gynaecol 2005; 112:1458.
14. DeSimone CA, Norris MC, Leighton BL. Intravenous nitroglycerine aids manual extraction of a retained placenta. Anesthesiology 1990; 73:787–789.

20

Acute uterine inversion

'The child was born about an hour before I came, and the midwife in attempting to bring away the placenta, had inverted the uterus; for upon examination, I found the whole body of the uterus with the placenta, adhering to the fundus, hanging out beyond the labia; there was a great profusion of blood, and the woman was dead before I came ... This case should be a caution to all practitioners how they attempt to bring away the placenta, and not to pull the string too rudely, lest they invert and draw out the uterus, by which the woman dies a martyr to their temerity and ignorance, as was too plainly the case in the precedent observation.'

William Giffard
Cases in Midwifry. London: Motte, 1734, p421–422

Acute uterine inversion is a rare but life-threatening complication of the third stage of labour. The incidence varies widely between 1 in 2000 to 1 in 50 000 deliveries, largely dependent upon the standard of management of the third stage of labour. Acute uterine inversion occurs within 24 hours of delivery; subacute between 24 hours and 4 weeks of delivery; and chronic uterine inversion presents after 4 weeks or in the non-pregnant state. Cases of subacute and chronic uterine inversion require surgical management and in this chapter we are concerned only with acute uterine inversion.

Types

- *Incomplete inversion* occurs when the fundus of the uterus has turned inside out, rather like the toe of a sock, but the inverted fundus has not descended through the cervix.
- *Complete inversion* occurs when the inverted fundus has passed completely through the cervix to lie within the vagina or, less often, outside the introitus.

Uterine inversion is sometimes described in degrees:

- 1st degree = incomplete inversion
- 2nd degree = complete inversion in the vagina
- 3rd degree = complete inversion outside the introitus (Fig 20.1).

Causes

For the uterus to be inverted it must be relaxed and this, along with fundal insertion of the placenta, are important predisposing conditions. Additional factors are as follows:[1]

- Mismanagement of the third stage of labour involving fundal pressure and/or cord traction before placental separation and while the uterus is still relaxed. This can be implicated in the majority of cases, despite the manifest surprise of the accoucheur. When reviewing a series of cases of acute uterine inversion to establish the causes Munro Kerr (1908) wrote:

  'In examining them it is very evident that in the majority of cases the occurrence has followed pressure from above or traction from below … In looking over the series I was not a little surprised at the large proportion of cases in which traction on the cord was the cause'.

- Abnormally short umbilical cord, or functionally shortened by being wrapped around the fetal body, can, in theory, cause the fundus of the uterus to be pulled

> *'A contracted uterus can be no more inverted than a stiff jackboot, but when it is soft and relaxed you may invert it.'*
>
> **William Hunter**
> *In: Andrews H R. William Hunter and his work in midwifery. BMJ 1915; 1:277–282*

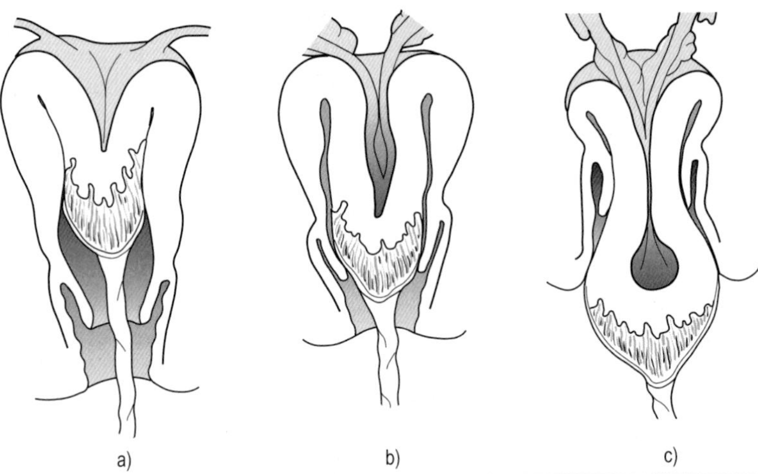

Figure 20.1 Types of uterine inversion: (a) incomplete (1st degree), (b) complete (2nd degree), (c) complete (3rd degree).

inside-out by traction on the cord as the fetus delivers. This is extremely rare but plausible cases have been described.

- Sudden rise in intra-abdominal pressure due to maternal coughing or vomiting. This may occur in a vulnerable situation with the uterus relaxed and fundal insertion of the placenta followed by sudden and strong propulsion on the uterine fundus caused by the acute rise in intra-abdominal pressure.
- Morbid adherence of a fundally implanted placenta.
- Manual removal of the placenta. When separating a retained placenta from the uterine wall a portion may remain attached and as the placenta is withdrawn so too is the fundus of the uterus. This can occur with those who routinely undertake manual removal of the placenta at the time of caesarean section before the uterus has contracted.
- Connective tissue disorders, such as Marfan's syndrome, can predispose to acute uterine inversion.[2]

Clinical presentation

The diagnosis may be obvious and dramatic with a large boggy mass appearing at the introitus, with or without the placenta attached. While this is the most dramatic presentation it is also the least common. Other signs and symptoms are as follows:[3,4]

- Severe and sustained hypogastric pain in the third stage of labour.
- Shock that is initially out of proportion with apparent blood loss, due to the infundibulo-pelvic and round ligaments, ovaries and associated nerves being pulled into the crater of the inversion which provides a strong vaso-vagal stimulus. Thus, the woman often becomes pallid and sweaty, with bradycardia, profound hypotension and even, on rare occasions, cardiac arrest. Within a short time, in the majority of cases, there is also marked haemorrhage and hypovolaemic shock.
- With complete inversion the uterus is not palpable per abdomen and the inverted fundus is either obvious at the introitus or on vaginal examination. In cases of incomplete uterine inversion, however, the fundus of the uterus may appear to be normal and only in thin women is it possible to feel the fundal dimple of the partial inversion.

Management

For acute uterine inversion to occur the myometrium and cervix must be relaxed. If the diagnosis is made immediately after it occurs, then that same degree of relaxation may allow immediate uterine replacement. Thus, if one is on the spot when the inversion happens, try immediate manual replacement. However, usually within 1–2 minutes the cervix and lower uterine segment clamp down and, along with increasing congestion, oedema and contraction of the inverted uterine fundus, this makes manual replacement without anaesthesia difficult, painful and usually impossible. If one attempt at immediate manual replacement of the uterus fails, move to the following sequence:

- Summon assistance (anaesthesia, nursing, obstetrician).
- Although the initial shock in these cases is usually of the neurogenic type, it is wise to be prepared for the haemorrhage and hypovolaemia that will follow in many cases. Therefore, establish two wide-bore intravenous cannulae, rapidly run in 1–2 L of crystalloid, take blood for cross match of 4 units, and place a Foley catheter in the bladder.

> *'Much of your success will depend upon your promptidude: the uterus should be returned quickly; but if there be much delay or violence, it may become impossible to do so.'*
>
> **Edward W. Murphy**
> *London Medical Gazette 1849; 8:751*

- If pain is a dominant symptom, small doses of intravenous morphine may be given.
- *Anaesthesia* should be administered depending on the facilities and appraisal by the anaesthetist. If an epidural anaesthetic is already in place this may provide adequate analgesia. In those rare cases in which the patient is stable, not bleeding, and with normal vital signs some anaesthetists may give a spinal anaesthetic. In most patients, however, cardiovascular instability and shock make regional anaesthesia inappropriate. Thus, general anaesthesia is usually chosen using one of the fluorinated hydrocarbons (sevoflurane or isoflurane) to aid uterine relaxation. In the past halothane was used effectively for this purpose, but it has been replaced because of its association with rare cases of myocardial irritability/arrhythmia and hepatotoxicity.
- If general anaesthesia does not produce adequate uterine relaxation, or if a regional anaesthetic has been used, tocolysis will be necessary.[5,6] The available drugs and technique are outlined in Chapter 26.
- *Manual replacement of the uterus* should be undertaken once anaesthesia and tocolysis have been established. If the placenta is still attached to the fundus do not remove it, as this will increase the blood loss. If the placenta is partially attached to the fundus it should be peeled off.

The uterine fundus, with or without the attached placenta, is cupped in the palm of the hand, the fingers and thumb of which are extended to feel the utero-cervical junction (Fig 20.2). The whole uterus is lifted up towards and beyond the umbilicus. Additional pressure is exerted with the fingertips to systematically and sequentially push and squeeze the uterine wall back through the cervix. This pressure may have to be sustained for 3–5 minutes to achieve complete replacement. Once the fundus has been replaced, keep the hand in the uterus while a rapid infusion of oxytocin is given to contract the uterus. When the uterus is felt to contract the hand is slowly withdrawn.

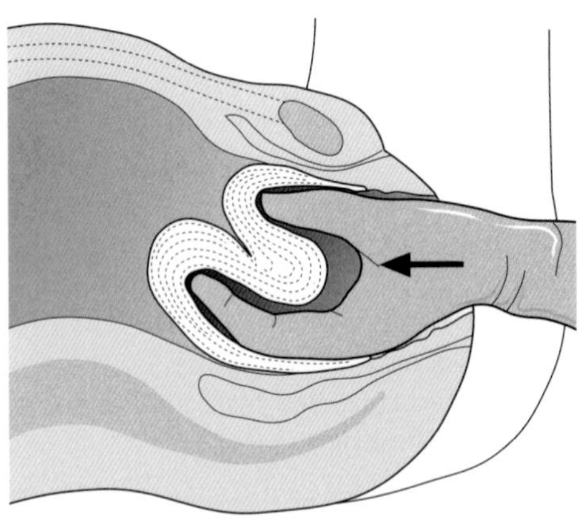

Figure 20.2 Manual replacement of inverted uterus.

The sooner manual replacement is undertaken the more likely it is to succeed with relative ease. With suitable anaesthesia and tocolysis within 2 hours of the diagnosis, it is usually successful.

- If there is delay and/or manual replacement is unsuccessful try *O'Sullivan's hydrostatic replacement* technique.[7] Before using this procedure it is important to make sure that the uterus and vagina have no lacerations, and if these are found they should be sutured. The principle of this technique is to instill a large volume of fluid (3–5 L) into the upper vagina, thus distending the fornices, which serves to pull open the cervical ring, allowing replacement of the uterine fundus. Use 1 L bags of warmed saline with a pressure infuser. The intravenous tubing is guided into the posterior fornix by one hand which also cups the fundus. The other hand seals the introitus around the wrist so that there is no egress of fluid (Fig 20.3). Alternatively, the tubing can be attached to a silastic vacuum extractor cup which is placed inside the introitus and may help provide a better seal.[8,9] For cases in which manual replacement has failed, O'Sullivan's technique can be remarkably and gratifyingly effective.[10]
- In rare delayed cases, manual replacement, with or without the hydrostatic technique, may be unsuccessful. In such cases

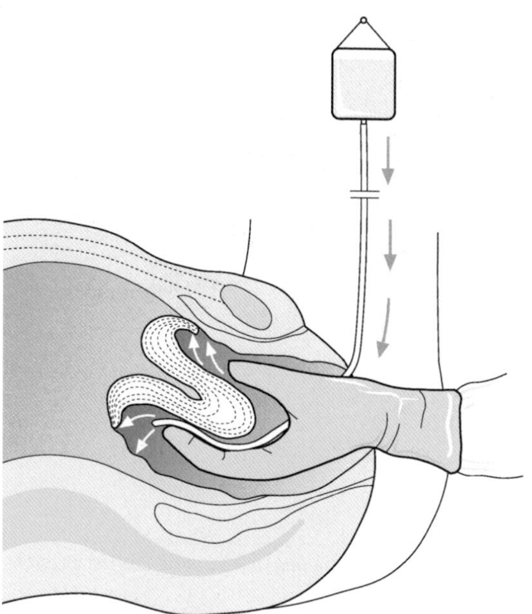
Figure 20.3 Hydrostatic replacement of inverted uterus.

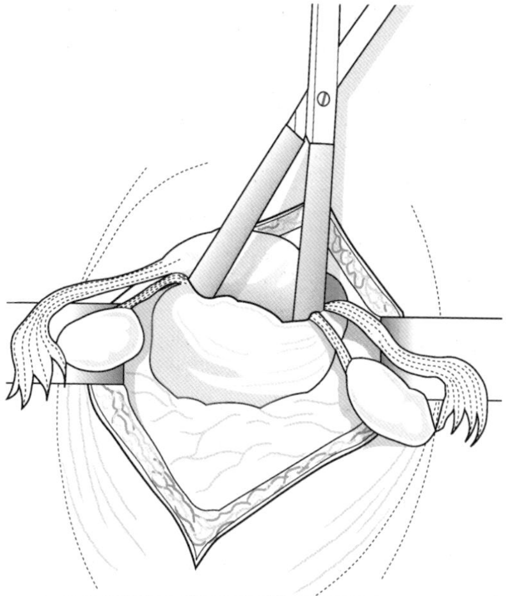
Figure 20.4 Stretching the constriction ring.

surgical replacement will have to be undertaken. This involves laparotomy and *Huntington's operation* in which Allis or similar forceps are used to grasp the myometrium just inside the dimple of the inverted fundus.[11] Before using the Allis forceps the cervical ring may be stretched, either with the fingers or by opening the blades of a large forceps (Fig 20.4). Systematically and sequentially, using forceps on both sides, the inverted fundus is then withdrawn from the crater to fully correct the inversion (Fig 20.5).

On occasions the cervical ring is so tight that Huntington's technique is unsuccessful and merely causes tearing of the uterine muscle. In such cases *Haultain's operation* should be used.[12] This involves incision of the posterior cervical ring followed by withdrawal of the fundus using Allis forceps as described in the Huntington procedure. Once the fundus has been replaced the incision is sutured (Fig 20.6)

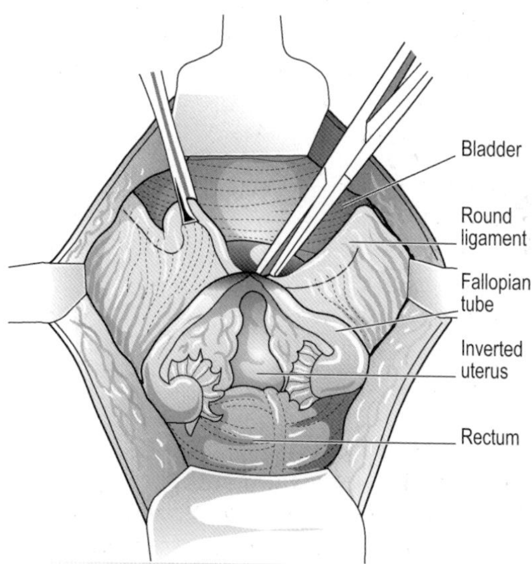

Figure 20.5 Huntington's operation.

- Whatever method of uterine replacement is used it should be followed by an oxytocic to keep the uterus well contracted for 8–12 hours. After the initial use of intravenous oxytocin to contract the uterus there is much to be said for using the longer-acting prostaglandins, such as 15-methyl $PGF_{2\alpha}$ or misoprostol for this purpose (see Chapter 18).
- A broad-spectrum antibiotic should be given for 24–48 hours because of the manipulation and the large uterine surface area which is traumatized and exposed to the vaginal bacterial flora.

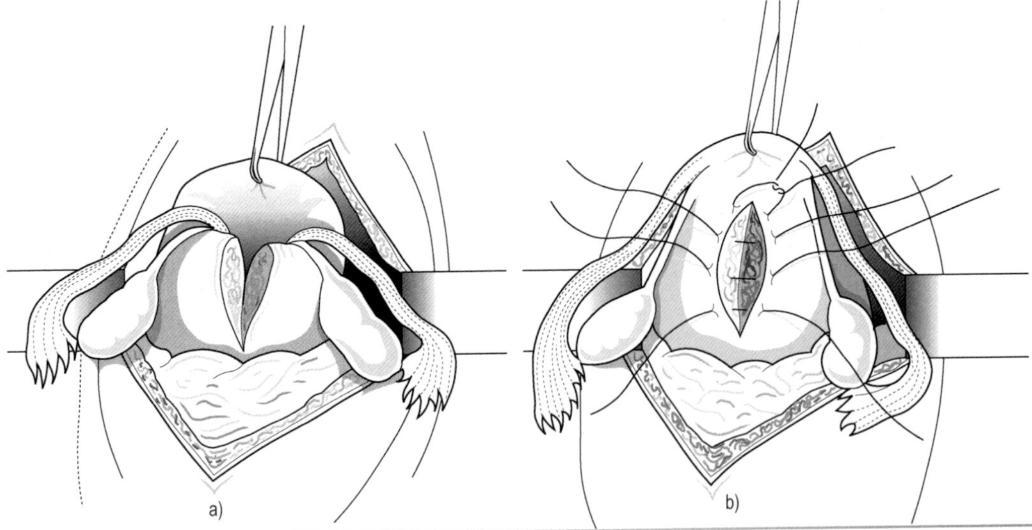

Figure 20.6 Haultain's operation. (a) Incision of the posterior part of constricting ring. (b) Suturing uterine incision after reduction of the inversion.

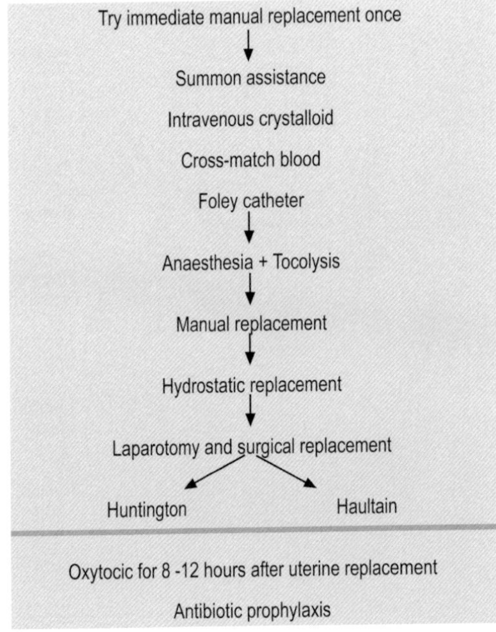

Figure 20.7 Management of acute uterine inversion.

The management of acute uterine inversion is summarized in Figure 20.7.

Should acute uterine inversion occur in a setting without anaesthetic facilities, replacement will have to be undertaken with a combination of intravenous narcotic, inhalation analgesia, and combined pudendal and paracervical block, as available and feasible (see Chapter 25). If manual replacement cannot be achieved O'Sullivan's hydrostatic technique should be used.

Acute uterine inversion presents a distinct risk of maternal death, particularly if facilities for anaesthesia and replacement are not available. It is almost completely preventable with careful and appropriate management of the third stage of labour.

References

1. Baskett TF. Acute uterine inversion. A review of 40 cases. J Obstet Gynaecol Can 2002; 24:953–956.
2. Quinn RJ, Mukerjee B. Spontaneous uterine inversion in association with Marfan's syndrome. Aust NZ J Obstet Gynaecol 1982; 22:163–164.
3. Wendell PJ, Cox SM. Emergent obstetric management of uterine inversion. Obstet Gynecol Clin North Am 1995; 22:261–274.
4. Rachagan S P, Sivanesaratnam V, Cock KP, Raman S. Acute puerperal inversion of the uterus – an obstetric emergency. Aust NZ J Obstet Gynecol 1988; 28:29–32.
5. Brar HS, Greenspoon JS, Platt LD, Paul RH. Acute puerperal uterine inversion: new approaches to management. J Reprod Med 1989; 34:173–177.
6. Dommisse B. Uterine inversion revisited. S Afr Med J 1998; 88:849–853.

7. O'Sullivan JV. Acute inversion of the uterus. BMJ 1945; 2:282–284.
8. Ogueh O, Ayida G. Acute uterine inversion: a new technique of hydrostatic replacement. Br J Obstet Gynaecol 1997; 104:951–952.
9. Antonelli E, Irion O, Tolck P, Morales M. Subacute uterine inversion: description of a novel replacement technique using the obstetric ventouse. Br J Obstet Gynaecol 2006; 113:846–847.
10. Mamani AW, Hassan A. Treatment of puerperal uterine inversion by the hydrostatic method. Report of five cases. Eur J Obstet Gynecol Reprod Biol 1989; 32:281–285.
11. Huntington JL. Acute inversion of the uterus. Boston Med J 1921; 184:376–380.
12. Haultain FWN. Treatment of chronic uterine inversion by abdominal hysterotomy, with a successful case. BMJ 1901; 2:74–76.

21

Lower genital tract trauma

Varying degrees of trauma to the lower genital tract (cervix, vagina, perineum) are common in vaginal delivery, particularly in nulliparous women. It is now recognized that the long-term sequelae of pelvic floor damage during childbirth can be considerable. Excessive stretching and tearing of the pelvic floor musculature and branches of the pudendal nerve can lead to long-term utero-vaginal prolapse and associated urinary and faecal incontinence.[1] Thus, measures to reduce trauma to the lower genital tract, knowledge of anatomy of the pelvic floor and perineum, and techniques to repair trauma are integral components of obstetric care.

Anatomy

The muscles of the pelvic floor and perineum are shown in Figure 21.1. The perineal body is composed of dense connective tissue to which is attached the bulbocavernosus muscle anteriorly, the superficial transverse perineal muscles laterally and the anal sphincter complex posteriorly. Also attached to the perineal body is the recto-vaginal septum and fascia. The puborectalis component of the levator ani muscle forms a sling around the whole anal sphincter complex.

The anal sphincter complex is shown in Figure 21.2. The internal anal sphincter is a thickened continuum of the muscularis layer of the rectum.

Principles of surgical repair

- The tissues of the lower genital tract are very vascular and heal well. The principles of repair involve haemostasis and tissue approximation. The tissue should be brought together firmly but lightly, otherwise subsequent

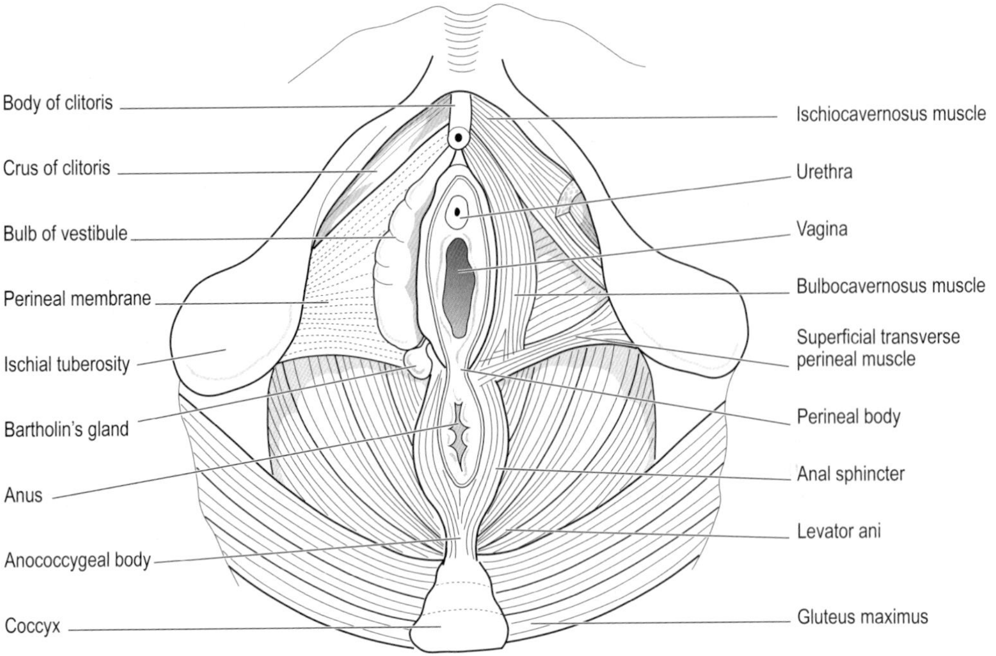

Figure 21.1 Muscles of the perineum and pelvic floor.

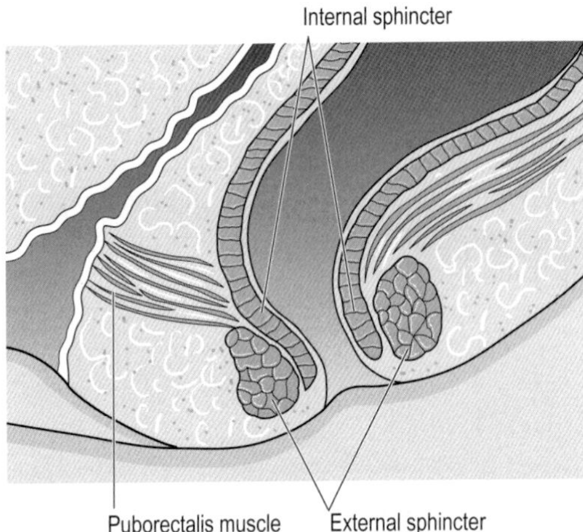

Figure 21.2 Anal sphincter complex.

oedema may cause excessive tension on the sutured tissues with increased pain and necrosis.

- Tissue reaction is related to the gauge and type of suture material and the knot size. Three throws on the knot are adequate. Use continuous suture technique when feasible and limit the number of individual stitches to reduce the number of knots and thereby diminish the foreign body and tissue reaction.
- The use of absorbable synthetic suture material – polyglycolic acid (Dexon) and polyglactin 910 (Vicryl) – is associated with less perineal pain and dehiscence compared with catgut.[2] The only problem with these materials is their delayed absorption and the increased need for removal of residual sutures. This has been largely overcome by the use of the more rapidly absorbed form of polyglactin 910 (Vicryl rapide).[3] Since 2002, catgut as a suture material has been withdrawn from the market in Europe and the United Kingdom.
- In general, large bites of tissue with firm but gentle approximation of tissues are better than multiple small individual stitches.
- If discreet bleeding points are identified, they should be clamped and ligated individually. Generalized oozing from tissues is usually dealt with successfully by a continuous suture. Firm pressure on the area with a swab for 1–2 minutes before suturing will often greatly reduce the amount of oozing and allow a more precise and gentle suturing technique.

- To produce a clear field it may be necessary to place a pack higher in the vagina. If so, this must be tagged. All episiotomy and other lower genital tract trauma repairs should have a formal swab and needle count at the end of the procedure. This is justified by the potential clinical and medicolegal sequelae of leaving a swab in the upper vagina.

Episiotomy

The traditional teaching that episiotomy was protective against more severe perineal lacerations has not been substantiated.[4] Thus, the liberal use of 'prophylactic' episiotomy is no longer recommended. However, there are still valid reasons for the performance of episiotomy:

- To shorten the second stage in cases of fetal distress.
- In selected cases of assisted vaginal delivery with forceps and, less frequently, for vacuum assisted delivery.
- To obtain more room for obstetrical manoeuvres such as those associated with shoulder dystocia, assisted breech delivery, and delivery of the second twin.

> **FIRST DESCRIPTION OF EPISIOTOMY**
>
> *'It sometimes happens … that the head of the child … cannot however come forward by reason of the extraordinary constriction of the external orifice of the vagina … wherefore it must be dilated if possible by the fingers … if this cannot be accomplished, there must be an incision made towards the anus with a pair of crooked probe-scissors, introducing one blade between the head and the vagina, as far as shall be thought necessary for the present purpose and the business is done at one pinch, by which the whole body will easily come forth.'*
>
> **Fielding Ould**
> *A Treatise of Midwifery in Three Parts. Dublin: Nelson and Connor, 1742, p145*

There are two types of episiotomy:

- *Midline episiotomy*. Two fingers are placed in the vagina between the fetal head and the perineum and, using straight scissors, the incision is made from the fourchette through the perineal body up to but not including the external anal sphincter. Advantages of the midline episiotomy are that it does not cut through the belly of the muscle, the two sides of the incised area are anatomically balanced making surgical repair easier, and blood loss is less than with medio-lateral episiotomy. A major drawback is the propensity for extension through the external anal sphincter and into the rectum. For this reason many practitioners avoid the midline technique.
- *Medio-lateral episiotomy*. The incision is made starting at the midline of the posterior fourchette and aimed towards the ischial tuberosity to avoid the anal sphincter. The incision is usually about 4 cm long. In addition to the skin and subcutaneous tissues the bulbocavernosus, transverse perineal, and puborectalis muscles are cut. Whether the incision is to the right or left depends on operator preference.

Repair of episiotomy

The principles involved in repairing both midline and medio-lateral episiotomies are similar. First, it is essential to assess the extent of damage and, unless this careful appraisal is carried out, partial or complete tears of the anal sphincter can be missed. This may include a rectal examination.

Using 2/0 or 3/0 rapidly absorbed polyglactin 910 (Vicryl rapide) the vagina and underlying fascia are closed in one continuous suture, starting 1 cm above the apex to ensure haemostasis. If the tissues are very vascular a locking suture is used. This suture is continued to the fourchette and held (Fig 21.3a). Beneath the lower end of this suture a separate 'crown suture' may be placed to approximate the bulbocavernosus muscle (Fig 21.3b). The deep transverse perineal and puborectalis muscles are brought together with individual sutures. It is important to place the finger into the incision to appreciate the full depth of the wound, particularly in the medial-lateral episiotomy. This is necessary to ensure that the deep muscle fibres are carefully brought together. On occasions, two layers of individual sutures are required to bring these muscle fibres together: otherwise a single continuous layer will suffice (Fig 21.3c).

The end of the continuous vaginal suture is then directed through the vagina to the deeper tissues and run down in a continuous manner approximately 1 cm from the edges of the perineal skin to the apex of the episiotomy. The same needle is then used to carry a continuous subcuticular suture just beneath the skin back up to the fourchette where it is tied (Fig 21.3d). In some cases the depth of tissue separation is small (particularly in the midline episiotomy) and a single run of the suture in subcuticular fashion from the fourchette to the apex may be all that is required. The subcuticular technique should be used and sutures should not be placed through the skin as this is more painful and the stitches have to be removed.

Repair of episiotomy dehiscence

Breakdown of episiotomy repair occurs due to poor technique and/or infection. Small areas of breakdown, provided there is adequate drainage, can be treated by antibiotics and sitz baths. These minor breakdowns will then granulate and heal-in nicely in the ensuing days and weeks. More extensive breakdown of episiotomy repair can be treated initially with antibiotics and sitz baths and, when signs of active infection have subsided, a secondary repair can be undertaken.[5,6] This will require regional anaesthesia and careful surgical debridement of the wound. With a third/fourth degree tear breakdown, bowel preparation should be carried out before secondary repair. The principles of repair involve using the minimum number of sutures and knots. Subcuticular and external skin sutures should not be placed. Repair of the underlying tissues should allow the skin edges to gape slightly to promote drainage. The skin edges will come together well during the subsequent weeks of healing.

Perineal tears

Anatomically the perineum encompasses the area between the coccyx and the pubic arch. The anterior perineum includes the clitoris,

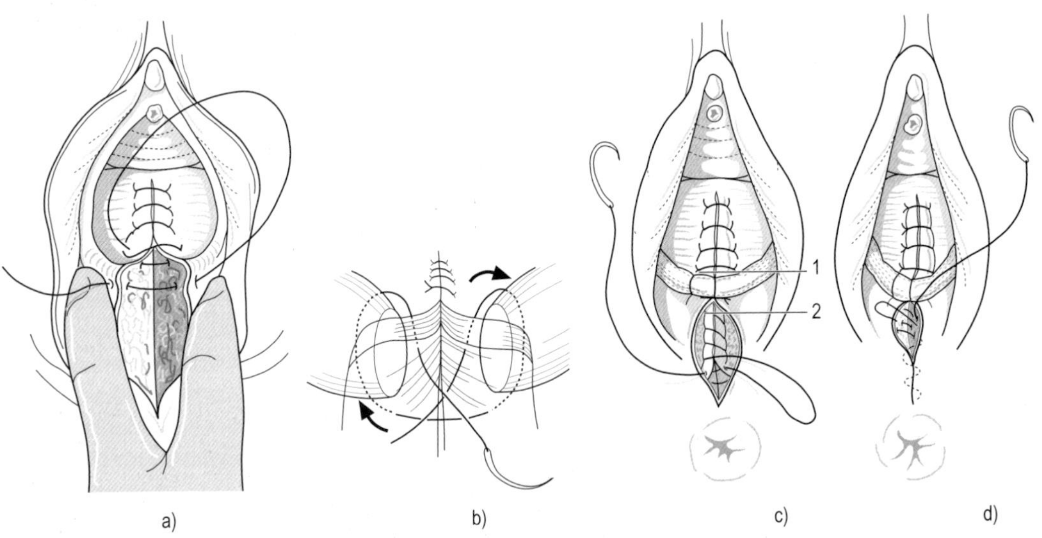

Figure 21.3 Repair of episiotomy.

REPAIR OF PERINEAL TEAR

'But sometimes it happens by an unlucky and deplorable accident, that the perineum is rent, so that the privity and fundament is all in one ... Let it be strongly stitched together with three or four stitches or more, according to the length of the separation, and taking at each stitch good hold of the flesh, that so it may not break out ...'

Francois Mauriceau
The Diseases of Women with Childbed and in Childbed. Translated by Hugh Chamberlen. London: John Darby, 1683, p316

urethra, labia and anterior vaginal wall. The posterior perineum includes the posterior vaginal wall, the perineal and levator ani muscles, and the anal sphincter complex. In an attempt to get standard definitions of perineal tears that can be correlated with subsequent pelvic floor morbidity, the following classification has been proposed:[7]

- *First degree* – vaginal and perineal skin only
- *Second degree* – separation of the skin and perineal muscles
- *Third degree* – injury involving the anal sphincter complex:
  - 3a – less than 50% of the external anal sphincter
  - 3b – more than 50% of the external anal sphincter
  - 3c – both external and internal anal sphincter
- *Fourth degree* – injury to external and internal anal sphincters and the ano-rectal epithelium.

The reported incidence of third/fourth degree tears usually ranges between 0.5–5.0%.[8,9] Subsequent endo-anal ultrasound shows that up to one-third of women after their first vaginal delivery may develop occult sphincter injury (Fig 21.4). Disruption of the anal sphincter at delivery, therefore, may go unrecognized unless an experienced operator looks carefully in cases of apparent second degree tears.[10–12]

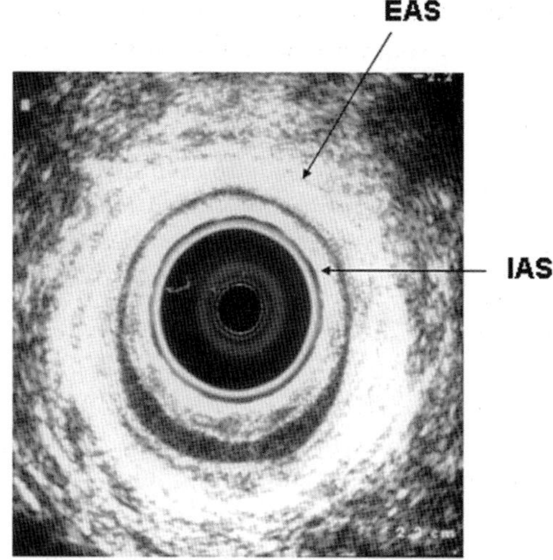

Normal EAS & IAS

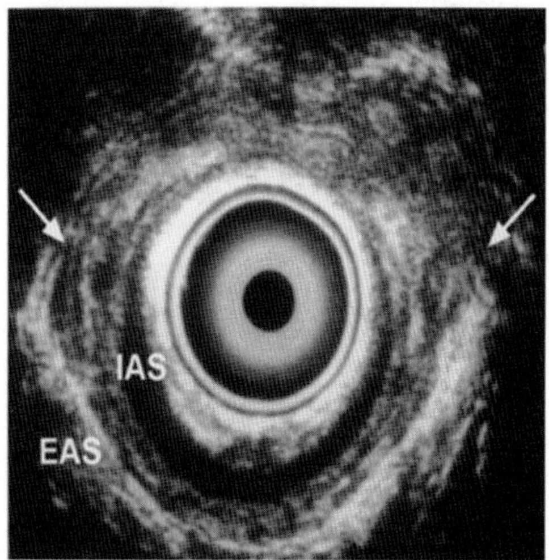

IAS EAS Defect

Figure 21.4 Endo-anal ultrasound demonstrates postpartum disruption of external and internal anal sphincters.

The principles involved in the suture and repair of first and second degree tears are similar to those for episiotomy. A skillful initial repair of third and fourth degree tears gives the woman the best chance of a good long-term outcome and restoration of anal sphincter function. The following principles should be followed: [13]

- The repair should be performed in a delivery room or operating theatre with appropriate assistance, lighting, equipment and positioning.
- Regional anaesthesia, either spinal or epidural, is optimal as this allows relaxation of the sphincter and better identification and approximation of the separated ends of the muscle.
- The torn ano-rectal epithelium is closed with continuous 3/0 Dexon/Vicryl suture (Fig 21.5a).
- The internal anal sphincter tends to retract so one has to look lateral to the torn anal epithelium for this structure. It should be repaired with interrupted 3/0 polydioxanone (PDS/Maxon) sutures (Figure 21.5b). This suture has a longer half life and greater tensile strength than Dexon and Vicryl.
- Identify and grasp the torn ends of the external anal sphincter with Allis forceps. It is not uncommon for the sphincter to be torn off to the side rather than in the midline. Therefore, one end of the sphincter may have retracted into a recess on one side. Having grasped each end of the torn muscle with Allis forceps, mobilize the muscle ends by carefully dissecting the connective tissue away with Metzembaum scissors.
- There are two accepted techniques for repair of the torn external sphincter muscle:
    1. In the *end-to-end technique* the torn muscle ends are reapproximated with two or three figure-of-eight sutures (Fig 21.5c).
    2. With the *overlapping technique* the torn muscle ends are mobilized such that they can be overlapped by 1–1.5 cm. Two, or if possible three, 3/0 PDS/Maxon sutures are placed using the technique shown in Figure 21.5d. The distal end of the overlapped muscle is then anchored to the underlying muscle with two sutures (Fig 21.5d). For the overlapping technique each of the sutures is placed and held with an artery forcep until the other sutures are placed and then all are tied down together. This ensures accurate placement of all sutures.
- After either technique of repairing the external sphincter the remainder of the tear is closed using the same principles and suture material outlined in the repair of episiotomy.
- Broad-spectrum antibiotics are given for 5–7 days, and stool softeners can be administered for the first 2 weeks postpartum.

There is no proof that either of these techniques is superior.[14] It is likely that careful attention to identification of third/fourth degree tears and meticulous application of either technique will bring good results.[15,16]

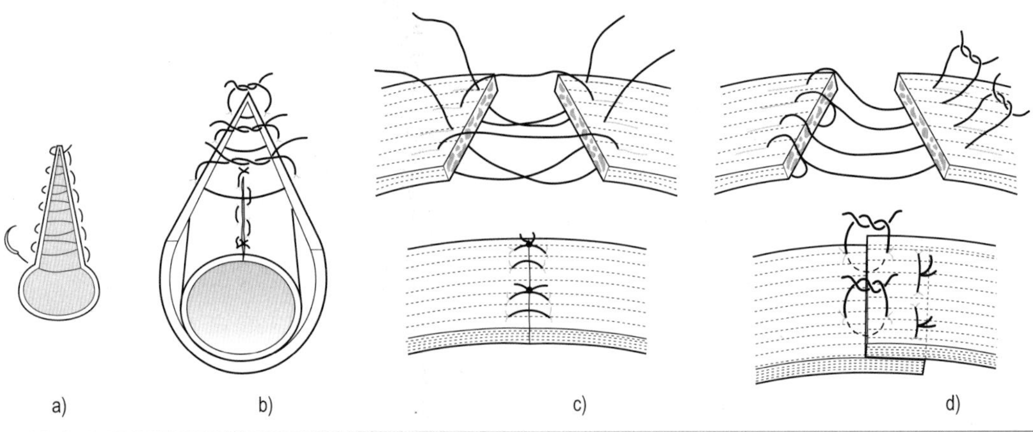

Figure 21.5 Repair of third/fourth degree tear.

Lacerations

In addition to perineal tears, lacerations of the vulva and vagina are common.

Periurethral and periclitoral lacerations

Small periurethral and periclitoral lacerations are common, particularly in the nulliparous woman when episiotomy is not performed and pressure from the delivering head is transferred to the anterior perineum by the intact posterior perineum. However, these lacerations are usually small and the edges come together when the woman's legs are positioned normally following delivery. If there is light bleeding, pressure with a pad for 1–2 minutes will usually arrest the bleeding. If there is significant bleeding these lacerations should be repaired with a fine continuous suture. It may be necessary to place a urethral catheter to guide the placement of sutures.

Vaginal lacerations

Vaginal lacerations are common and usually involve the lower two-thirds of the posterolateral vaginal sulci. They may also occur as an extension of an episiotomy. Lacerations in the anterior sulcus of the vagina are less frequent, but can be associated with a narrow subpubic arch and elevation of the forceps before the occiput has descended completely below the symphysis pubis. Lacerations of the upper third of the vagina are rare and most often associated with forceps rotation delivery. This can produce crescentic lacerations high in the vaginal vault which can be difficult to expose.

The principles of repair of vaginal lacerations are the same as those for episiotomy repair. One of the main problems can be exposure and access. Regional or general anaesthesia may be required. Assistance, retractors, and good light are necessary. If one still cannot see the upper extent of the laceration place a suture as high as you can and use this as a tractor to bring the apex of the laceration into view (Fig 21.6). A continuous or, if very vascular, a continuous locking suture is used. In the case of extensive and high vaginal lacerations it may be necessary to pack the vagina tightly following suture for haemostasis and to avoid haematoma formation. If so, a Foley catheter is placed in the bladder and both this and the pack can be removed in 12–24 hours. In such cases broad-spectrum antibiotic coverage is advisable.

Cervical lacerations

Cervical lacerations are relatively rare and in most cases do not bleed and require no treatment. The cervix can usually be inspected by applying ring (sponge) forceps to the anterior and posterior lips. If the posterior lip is not

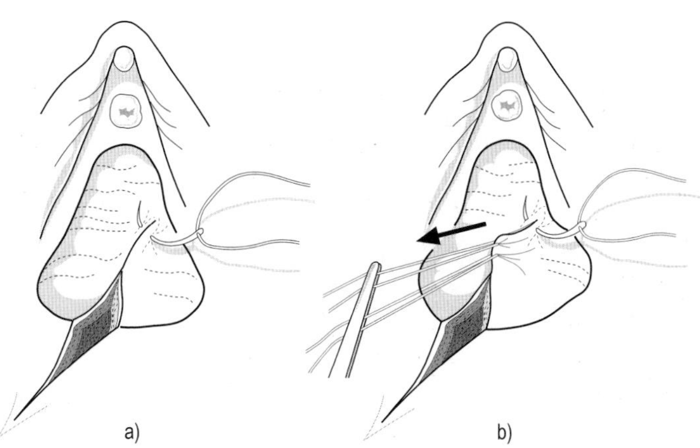

Figure 21.6 Use of first suture as a tractor to expose apex of vaginal laceration.

accessible apply one forcep to the anterior lip and a second one just lateral at the 2 o'clock position. The anterior forcep is then removed and 'leapfrogged' over the other forcep to the 4 o'clock position. In this manner the entire cervix can be closely inspected. Lacerations usually occur laterally and if they are less than 2 cm and not bleeding do not require suture. If they are bleeding or large, place ring forceps on either side of the laceration and repair with a continuous locking suture (Fig 21.7). The cervix is extremely vascular and even with a continuous locking suture oozing may continue, while additional sutures only produce further bleeding points. In these cases apply ring forceps over the oozing areas and leave them in place for 4 hours, after which they can be removed. Surprisingly, this can be done with minimal disruption to the woman in the early postpartum period.

Annular detachment of the cervix

Annular detachment of the cervix is an extremely rare condition associated with cervical dystocia from a rigid or scarred cervix causing an annular detachment of the lower portion of the cervix in its entirety, such that a doughnut-shaped portion of the cervix is detached in front of the fetal head. In an earlier edition of this text Chassar Moir graphically described such a case:

> *'I recall the family doctor who came to the front door to greet the obstetrician. In his outstretched hand he held a detached cervix and in a scared voice he explained, "Just as I was about to put on the forceps this thing came away in my hand". Interestingly, this patient later came under my charge in a future confinement. Her cervix was minutely examined but showed no apparent abnormality.'*

In modern obstetrics annular detachment of the cervix is virtually never seen but small 'bucket-handle' tears and small areas of detachment of the anterior lip of the cervix may occur with prolonged late first stage and second stages of labour. Unless it is bleeding this requires no treatment and, like Chassar Moir's case described above, the postpartum cervix looks normal.

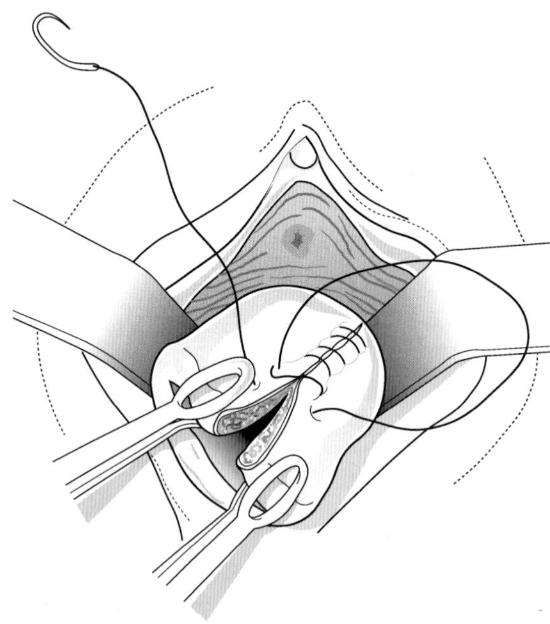

Figure 21.7 Repair of cervical laceration.

Haematomas

Postpartum vulvo-vaginal haematomas can be classified as *vulval*, *paravaginal*, *broad ligament* and *retroperitoneal*. Predisposing causes include prolonged second stage of labour, instrumental delivery, pudendal nerve block and vulval varicosities. Haematomas may be associated with incomplete suturing of vaginal lacerations or episiotomy. In many cases there is no obvious trauma, the delivery is spontaneous and the vaginal epithelium overlying the damaged blood vessel is intact.

Clinical presentation

- *Vulval* haematomas have an obvious clinical presentation with an acutely painful, tender, purple swelling in the area of the labium majus. These may extend into the lower vagina and into the ischiorectal fossa.
- *Paravaginal* haematomas are not visible externally and usually present with a combination of some or all of the following factors – pain, restlessness, inability to void and rectal tenesmus. A gentle one-finger vaginal examination will usually reveal the tender mass bulging into the vagina.
- *Broad ligament* and *retroperitoneal* haematomas occur when a vessel ruptures above the urogenital diaphragm. The bleeding extends into the supravaginal space between the leaves of the broad ligament and may track retroperitoneally, even as high as the kidneys. This type of haematoma may be associated with deep cervical lacerations extending into the lower uterine segment or with an occult rupture of the lateral aspect of the lower uterine segment. Large broad ligament haematomas can be felt on bimanual examination and push the uterus to one side. Extensive broad ligament and retroperitoneal haematomas can cause profound hypovolaemic shock and may rupture into the peritoneal cavity. Diagnosis may be aided, if available, by ultrasound or MRI examination.

Management

Small vulval haematomas (≤ 5 cm) may be treated conservatively with analgesia, observation and ice packs. However, if the pain is not adequately controlled and if there is enlargement they have to be incised and evacuated. Paravaginal haematomas also need incision and evacuation. This requires regional or general anaesthesia. The incision is made over the area of maximum distension and the clot evacuated. Seek and ligate discreet bleeding points, although frequently none are found. Oozing areas may be oversewn with figure-of-eight sutures. Tamponade for 2–3 minutes should help identify any bleeding points or persistently oozing areas that require suture. The vagina is then tightly packed with gauze moistened with lubricating gel or antiseptic cream. A Foley catheter is placed in the bladder and both of these can be removed in 12–24 hours.

Broad ligament and retroperitoneal haematomas may be self-limiting and will absorb in the coming weeks. Provided the patient is stable they may be initially treated conservatively with intravenous crystalloid, cross-matched blood, analgesia and observation. If available, it is wise to muster the personnel and equipment for angiographic embolisation of branches of the internal iliac arteries.[17] Should there be signs of progressive bleeding this can then be implemented and is often very effective. If angiographic embolisation facilities are not available laparotomy is required and the haematoma is evacuated followed by ligation of bleeding points. A careful check should be made to confirm or deny uterine rupture as the source of the haematoma. This may require repair of the uterine rupture, or even hysterectomy.

References

1. Kearney R, Miller JM, Ashton-Miller JA, DeLancey JOL. Obstetric factors associated with levator ani muscle injury after vaginal birth. Obstet Gynecol 2006; 107:144–149.
2. Royal College of Obstetricians and Gynaecologists. Methods and material used in perineal repair. Guideline No. 23. London: RCOG Press, 2004.

3. Dent K, Kettle C, O'Brien S. Repair of perineal trauma. In: Hillard T, Purdie D, eds. The yearbook of obstetrics and gynaecology. Vol 11. London: RCOG Press, 2004:132–141.
4. Renfrew MJ, Hannah W, Albers L, Floyd E. Practices that minimize trauma to the genital tract in childbirth: a systematic review of the literature. Birth 1998; 25:143–160.
5. Ramin SM, Ramus RM, Little BB, Gilstrap LC. Early repair of episiotomy dehiscence associated with infection. Am J Obstet Gynecol 1992; 167:1104–1107.
6. Arona AJ, Al-Marayati L, Grimes DA. Early secondary repair of third and fourth degree perineal lacerations after outpatient wound preparation. Obstet Gynecol 1995; 86:294–296.
7. Sultan AH, Thakar R. Lower genital tract and anal sphincter trauma. Best Pract Res Clin Obstet Gynaecol 2002; 16:99–115.
8. Samuelsson E, Ladfors L, Weinnerholm UB, Gareberg B, Nyberg K, Hagberg H. Anal sphincter tears: prospective study of obstetric risk factors. Br J Obstet Gynaecol 2000; 107:926–931.
9. De Leeu JW, Struijk PC, Vierhout ME, Wallenburg HCS. Risk factors for third degree perineal ruptures during delivery. Br J Obstet Gynaecol 2001; 108:383–387.
10. Sultan AH, Kamm MA, Hudson CN. Anal sphincter disruption during vaginal delivery. N Engl J Med 1993; 329:1905–1911.
11. Andrews V, Thakar R, Sultan AH. Diagnosis of obstetric anal sphincter trauma. In: Hillard T, Purdie D, eds. The yearbook of obstetrics and gynaecology. Vol 11. London: RCOG Press, 2004:12–19.
12. Faltin DL, Boulvain M, Floris LA, Irion O. Diagnosis of anal sphincter tears to prevent fecal incontinence: a randomized controlled trial. Obstet Gynecol 2005; 106:6–13.
13. Royal College of Obstetricians and Gynaecologists. Management of third and fourth-degree perineal tears following vaginal delivery. Guideline No. 29. London: RCOG Press, 2001.
14. Fitzpatrick M, Behan M, O'Connell PR, O'Heirlihy C. A randomized clinical trial comparing primary overlap with approximation of third-degree obstetric tears. Am J Obstet Gynecol 2000; 183:1220–1224.
15. Elfagli I, Ernste BJ, Rydhstroem H. Rupture of the sphincter ani: the recurrence rate in second delivery. Br J Obstet Gynaecol 2004; 111:1361–1364.
16. Fernando RJ, Sultan AH, Kettle C, Radley S, Jones P, O'Brien PMS. Repair techniques for obstetric anal sphincter injuries. Obstet Gynecol 2006; 107:1261–1268.
17. Chiu HG, Scott DR, Resnik R. Angiographic embolization of intractable puerperal hematomas. Am J Obstet Gynecol 1989; 160:434–438.

22

Haemorrhagic shock

'It is clear that when patients are in this condition, trembling upon the very brink of destruction, there is but little time for you to think what ought to be done; these are moments in which it becomes your duty not to reflect, but to act. Think now, therefore, before the moment of difficulty arrives. Be ready with all the rules of practice, which those very dangerous cases require.'

James Blundell
The Principles and Practice of Obstetricy. London: E. Cox, 1834, p336

Obstetric haemorrhage is the leading direct cause of maternal death in the developing world and remains a major cause of death and severe maternal morbidity in the developed world. A number of the complications discussed in this book are associated with obstetric haemorrhage and thus the pathophysiology, clinical features and management of hypovolaemic shock will be discussed here.

Physiological changes in pregnancy

Part of the physiological adaptation to pregnancy includes an increase of about 40% in the circulating blood volume. This accommodates the increased uteroplacental circulation and also prepares the woman, to some extent, to withstand haemorrhage at delivery. This is necessary because the 'normal' blood loss at vaginal delivery and caesarean section is about 500 ml and 1000 ml respectively, and such loss is accommodated well by the normal pregnant woman. However, obstetric haemorrhage is often rapid and may be poorly tolerated by the woman who is anaemic, dehydrated after prolonged labour, or with the reduced blood volume and contracted intravascular space associated with pre-eclampsia/eclampsia.

An additional important consideration is the size of the woman and therefore her circulating blood volume. In the non-pregnant woman the formula to calculate blood volume is about 70 ml/kg or her weight in kilograms divided by 14. Thus, the circulating blood volume of a 50 kg woman and an 80 kg woman would be about 3500 ml and 5600 ml respectively. In pregnancy with the 40% increase in blood volume the formula is approximately 100 ml/kg; so in the same 50 kg and 80 kg weight categories the blood volume would be 5000 ml and 8000 ml respectively – a difference of 3 L. The woman of small stature who is anaemic may withstand poorly even a blood loss of 1000–1500 ml, which the larger, non-anaemic woman would tolerate with relative impunity.

Pathophysiological response to haemorrhage

Severe haemorrhage associated with hypotension causes an increased release of catecholamines and stimulation of the baroreceptors leading to increased sympathetic tone, with the following results:

- Increased cardiac output due to an increase in the rate and force of myocardial contraction.
- Maintenance of blood flow to the critical organs (heart and brain) by selective peripheral arteriolar constriction reducing blood flow to all the other organs.
- Venous constriction causing, in effect, an autotransfusion from these capacitance vessels.
- As a result of the peripheral vasoconstriction the reduced hydrostatic pressure in the capillaries causes them to imbibe extracellular fluid in an attempt to augment the intravascular volume. Increased levels of aldosterone and antidiuretic hormone cause sodium and water retention by the kidneys.

These mechanisms are aimed at improving cardiac output, sustaining the blood pressure, restoring the intravascular volume and maintaining tissue perfusion. At this stage, provided the haemorrhage is arrested and the circulation restored, the shock is completely reversible without sequelae. However, if the blood loss continues, the above mechanisms fail to sustain adequate circulation, leading to reduced tissue perfusion, tissue hypoxia, metabolic acidosis, cell damage and ultimately cell death. The hypoxic metabolites damage the capillary cells leading to more loss of intravascular volume as fluid leaks through the damaged capillary walls. Persistent hypoperfusion of peripheral organs may cause damage to the lung ('shock lung', adult respiratory distress syndrome), the kidney (acute tubular and cortical necrosis), the liver and to the pituitary (Sheehan's syndrome).

As the diastolic blood pressure falls, coronary artery perfusion is compromised, leading to myocardial hypoxia and failure. Such extensive hypoxic tissue damage and release of metabolites may initiate disseminated intravascular coagulation (see Chapter 23).

Clinical features

In the early phase of blood loss, peripheral arteriolar constriction will sustain normal maternal blood pressure but may lead to a reduction in utero-placental perfusion. Thus, abnormalities of the fetal heart rate may serve as an early warning sign of maternal vascular decompensation.

The classic early signs of haemorrhagic shock are changes in the vital signs with tachycardia, hypotension, tachypnoea and air hunger. In addition to these vital signs one can monitor the skin, brain and kidney for clinical manifestations of hypovolaemia as these are end-organs sensitive to reduced perfusion and hypoxia. The clinical manifestations of hypoperfusion and hypoxia in these end-organs are as follows:

- Skin: sweating, cold, pallor, cyanosis. A clinically useful sign of skin perfusion is the capillary refill time. This is easily assessed by compressing a finger nail for 5 seconds; if normal, the colour in the nail bed returns within 2 seconds.
- Brain: alteration in mental state including restlessness, anxiety, aggression, confusion and coma.
- Kidney: oliguria and anuria.

Hypovolaemic shock can be classified into three categories:

- *Mild*: 10–25% loss of blood volume. In cases of mild hypovolaemic shock there is tachycardia and possibly mild hypotension along with decreased perfusion of non-vital organs and tissue such as skin, fat and skeletal muscle. Provided bleeding stops at this stage the circulation is well compensated, will respond to intravenous crystalloid alone, and does not require blood replacement.
- *Moderate*: 25–40% loss of blood volume. With moderate shock there is decreased perfusion to the vital organs due to peripheral vasoconstriction and this is usually manifest by tachycardia, hypotension, tachypnoea, cool skin and oliguria. This requires intravenous crystalloid and blood replacement.
- *Severe*: > 40% loss of blood volume. This is life threatening with all of the clinical manifestations of shock present in their most extreme form. A working guide to the presence of severe haemorrhagic shock is when the radial pulse is impalpable, which means the systolic blood pressure is less than 70 mmHg – at which level perfusion to the vital organs (heart, brain and kidney) is critically reduced. Loss of more than 50% of blood volume results in loss of consciousness. These patients require immediate blood replacement and urgent measures to stop the bleeding.

Management

When excessive blood loss is encountered the first task is to identify the source and stop the bleeding. While it is also important to mobilize blood transfusion, this should not detract from efforts to immediately stem the haemorrhage. The principles of management of haemorrhagic shock are simple – maintain and restore the circulating blood volume to sustain tissue perfusion and oxygenation. The simple 'rule of 30s' is a useful background guide to treatment:

- up to 30% of blood volume can be lost without major haemodynamic changes
- keep the haematocrit above 30%
- keep the urinary output above 30 ml/h.

The individual principles of management are as follows:

Protect the airway and administer oxygen by face mask. In severe shock with an unconscious patient, intubation and ventilation will be necessary.

During resuscitation undelivered pregnant women should be placed in the left lateral tilt (15–30°).

Keep the patient warm and warm all intravenous fluids. Platelet and other coagulation factor functions are inhibited by the cold.

Two portals of venous access in the arms are required. If normal venous access is unsuccessful, cut-down of the antecubital or saphenous vein of the ankle will have to be established. Intravenous cannulae should be of 14 gauge – the flow through a cannula is proportional to the diameter, such that crystalloid can be infused twice as fast through a 14 gauge compared with an 18 gauge cannula.

Intravenous crystalloid is the first choice for fluid resuscitation in hypovolaemia. The crystalloid chosen is one of the isotonic solutions – Ringer's lactate, Hartmann's solution or 0.9% saline. Crystalloids provide short-term expansion of the intravascular space but are soon excreted by the kidneys and rapidly distributed to the extracellular fluid, such that 80% of the volume is lost to the circulation.

The key is rapid transfusion of warmed crystalloid solution at a volume approximately 2–3 × the estimated blood loss. Crystalloid has no powers of coagulation or of oxygenation but is very valuable as a short-term volume expander. As such, it may be all that is required in women with mild hypovolaemic shock in whom the blood loss is promptly arrested. If not, it has value in maintaining the circulating blood volume until blood products are available for transfusion. Better to have an anaemic circulating blood volume perfusing the tissues than no perfusion. It is possible that future trials will show that hypertonic saline may be advantageous in the initial management of acute hypovolaemic shock.

The colloids are an alternative solution to crystalloids. These include the human derivatives, albumin 5% and plasma protein fraction (plasmanate) or the artificial colloids, hydroxyethyl starches (pentaspan) and the gelatins (gelofusine, haemaccel). The previously used dextrans (macrodex, rheomacrodex) are no longer recommended because they adversely affect platelet function, interfere with subsequent blood cross-match tests, and can rarely initiate severe anaphylactoid reactions. The colloids have the advantage of remaining longer in the intravascular space but are also rapidly distributed to the extracellular fluid in large amounts. In the case of crystalloid this fluid is usually reabsorbed quite rapidly, whereas colloid will persist and may, for example, exacerbate pulmonary oedema by drawing further fluid into the extracellular tissues. The combination of pre-eclampsia and hypovolaemic shock renders these women very susceptible to overload with either crystalloid or colloid due to the combination of vasospasm and reduced intravascular capacity, hypoproteinaemia and increased capillary permeability. Thus, women with severe pre-eclampsia/eclampsia and hypovolaemic shock require cautious administration of crystalloid or colloid and may need central venous pressure and pulmonary artery wedge pressure monitoring to guide safe restoration of blood volume.

In general, crystalloid is the initial infusion of choice and 2–3 L should be given rapidly. If blood is still unavailable and more than 3 L of crystalloid is necessary to sustain the circulation then colloid may be given. If albumin is chosen it is very viscous and should be drawn up with a wide bore needle and added to saline so it can be infused rapidly.

In moderate and severe haemorrhage the oxygen-carrying capacity of blood is essential in addition to restoration of the intravascular volume. Packed red blood cells have a haematocrit of 70–80% and these are transfused for their oxygen-carrying capacity, while simultaneously transfused crystalloid or colloid provides the volume. Packed red cells have a high viscosity and it is best to add 50–100 ml isotonic saline to each unit to facilitate rapid transfusion. In an extreme emergency 2 units of O Rh-negative blood (the universal donor blood) can be transfused. However O Rh-negative donors may have anti-A, anti-B antibodies in their plasma which can react with A or B cells of a non-type O recipient. There is almost always time (15 minutes) to ascertain the patient's ABO and Rh type so that type-specific blood can be given without cross-match. In most cases it is possible to both type and screen for irregular antibodies with a short (20 minute) saline cross-match. It is essential that the transfused blood is warmed. There are a number of electric blood warmers with thermostats suitable for this purpose. If these are not available, additional intravenous tubing can be coiled in a basin of water warmed to 37–40°C. It is important that the water should not exceed this temperature otherwise haemolysis of the blood can occur. Thus, the temperature in the basin should be monitored by a thermometer and one usually needs to add warm water frequently as the heat loss to the cold blood is considerable. If equipment is limited the temperature in the water basin can be assessed by the elbow, in the same way that one tests the bath water for a baby. Generally speaking, however, if laboratory facilities exist for blood transfusion the equipment for blood warming is also available.

The avoidance of hypothermia is extremely important. Transfusion of cold intravenous fluids will cause shivering, which increases oxygen consumption. In addition, the activity of coagulation factors, citrate, lactate and potassium metabolism are all negatively affected by hypothermia. At its most extreme, blood transfused at a temperature < 30°C can cause ventricular fibrillation and cardiac arrest.

Dilutional coagulopathy generally begins to operate after 5 units of packed cells have been transfused. Thus, as a working rule, 1–2 units of fresh frozen plasma should be transfused for every 5 units of packed cells. Furthermore, for every 15 units of packed red cells 5 units of platelets should be given.

Monitoring progress

It is important to involve senior staff early on in cases of haemorrhagic shock. In addition, when available, guidance from a haematologist is advisable. Depending on the amount of blood loss and the facilities available the following monitoring may be necessary:

- Vital signs of blood pressure, pulse, respiration and temperature.
- Indwelling urinary catheter to assess oliguria and the desired goal of keeping urinary output > 30 ml/h.
- Haemoglobin, haematocrit, platelets and coagulation profile should be performed at regular intervals, remembering that these do not reflect the acute changes but may be useful to show trends over the longer term.
- Auscultation of the lung bases for signs of pulmonary oedema.
- Pulse oximetry, which provides a useful continuous assessment of pulse rate and oxygen saturation.
- If undelivered, continuous fetal heart rate monitoring is advisable. As mentioned before, in general terms if the fetus is well oxygenated then so is the mother.
- More sophisticated invasive monitoring may be required in selected cases and include arterial blood pressure, central venous pressure and pulmonary artery wedge pressure (Swan–Ganz). This is particularly so in cases of severe pre-eclampsia/eclampsia associated with hypovolaemia.

FIRST SUCCESSFUL HUMAN BLOOD TRANSFUSION BY DR JAMES BLUNDELL, DESCRIBED BY HIS COLLEAGUE, DR WALLER

'The vein in the bend of the arm was laid bare, and an incision of sufficient extent to admit the pipe of the syringe was made into it ... The syringe used by Dr. B. was similar to the common injecting syringe, and contained two ounces ... The blood was drawn from the patient's husband into a tumbler, and Dr. B. stood ready with his syringe to absorb it instantly, in fact, while it was flowing: it was then immediately introduced into the orifice in the vein, and cautiously injected. No effect appeared to be produced by the first injection of two ounces, but towards the end of the second there was an approach to syncope; the pulse fell a little; there was sighing ...'

C Waller
Case of uterine haemorrhage, in which the operation of transfusion was successfully performed. Med Phys J 1825; 54:273–277

'After floodings, women sometimes die in a moment, but more frequently in a gradual manner; and over the victim, death shakes his dart, and to you she stretches out her helpless hands for the assistance which you cannot give, unless by transfusion. I have seen a woman dying for two or three hours together, convinced in my own mind that no known remedy could save her: the sight of these moving cases first lead me to transfusion'

J Blundell
The Principles and Practice of Obstetricy. London: E. Cox, 1834, p337

Stop the bleeding

As already emphasized, in parallel with the above treatment, measures should be taken to arrest the haemorrhage. These are described in the appropriate chapters on haemorrhagic complications elsewhere in this book.

Bibliography

American College of Obstetricians and Gynecologists. Educational Bulletin No. 235. Hemorrhagic shock. Washington DC: ACOG, 1997.

Baskett TF. Preparedness for postpartum haemorrhage: Obstetric haemorrhage equipment tray. In: B-Lynch C, Keith LG, Lalonde AB, Karoshi M (eds). A textbook of postpartum haemorrhage. Duncow: Sapiens Publishing, 2006. pp 179–182.

Bonnar J. Massive obstetric haemorrhage. Clin Obstet Gynaecol 2000; 14:1–18.

Bose P, Regan F, Paterson-Brown S. Improving the accuracy of estimated blood loss at obstetric haemorrhage using clinical reconstructions. Br J Obstet Gynaecol 2006; 113:919–924.

Dildy GA, Scott JR, Saffer CS, Belfort MA. An effective pressure pack for severe pelvic hemorrhage. Obstet Gynecol 2006; 108: 1222–1261.

Grady K, Cox C. Shock. In: Johanson R, Cox C, Grady K, Howell C, eds. Managing obstetric emergencies and trauma. London: RCOG Press, 2003:61–90.

Hofmeyr CJ, Mohala BKF. Hypovolaemic shock. Best Prac Res Clin Obstet Gynaecol 2001; 15:645–662.

Miller S, Hamza S, Bray EH, Lester F, Nada K, Gibson R. First aid for obstetric haemorrhage: the pilot study of the non-pneumatic anti-shock garment in Egypt. Br J Obstet Gynaecol 2006; 113:424–429.

Patel A, Goudar SS, Geller SE. Drape estimation vs. visual assessment for estimating postpartum hemorrhage. Int J Gynecol Obstet 2006; 93:220–224.

Prata N, Mbaruku G, Campbell M. Using the kanga to measure postpartum blood loss. Int J Gynecol Obstet 2005; 89:47–50.

Rees GAD, Willis BA. Resuscitation in late pregnancy. Anaesthesia 1998; 43:347–349.

Santoso JT, Saunders BA, Grosshart K. Massive blood loss and transfusion in obstetrics and gynaecology. Obstet Gynaecol Surv 2005; 60:827–837.

Shevell T, Malone FD. Management of obstetric hemorrhage. Semin Perinatol 2003; 27:86–104.

Skupski DW, Lowenwirt P, Weinbaum FI, Brodsky D, Danek M, Eglinton GS. Improving hospital systems for the care of women with major obstetric hemorrhage. Obstet Gynecol 2006; 107:977–983.

Society of Obstetricians and Gynaecologists of Canada. Clinical Practice Guidelines No 115. Haemorrhagic Shock. J Obstet Gynaecol Can 2002; 24:504–511.

Yazer MH. The blood bank 'black box' debunked: pretransfusion testing explained. Can Med Assoc J 2006; 174:29–32.

Younes RN, Aun F, Ching CT, et al. Prognostic factors to predict outcome following the administration of hypertonic/hyperoncotic solution in hypovolemic patients. Shock 1997; 7:79–83.

Young P, Johanson R. Haemodynamic, invasive and echocardiographic monitoring in the hypertensive parturient. Best Prac Res Clin Obstet Gynaecol 2001; 15:605–622.

23

Disseminated intravascular coagulation

Haemostasis is a dynamic balance between coagulation and fibrinolysis. Normal pregnancy is accompanied by profound changes in both of these systems. In addition to the increased blood volume there is a rise in most of the procoagulant factors and a relative suppression of fibrinolysis.[1] These changes help prepare the woman to restrict blood loss at delivery and to produce haemostasis in the large and vascular uterine 'wound' following placental separation. As a result of these physiological changes the pregnant woman is rendered more vulnerable to the whole spectrum of coagulation disorders, ranging from venous thromboembolism to disseminated intravascular coagulation.

Causes

Disseminated intravascular coagulation (DIC) is always secondary to another condition that provokes clotting within the vascular compartment. There are three main mechanisms by which obstetric conditions may activate the coagulation system:[2]

1. *Release of thromboplastins* from placental and decidual tissue into the maternal circulation. This may happen with dramatic suddenness in cases of amniotic fluid embolism and abruptio placentae. It can occur at the time of surgical intervention for placenta praevia accreta, ruptured uterus and trophoblastic disease. In patients with intrauterine fetal death or missed abortion, release of thromboplastins into the maternal circulation is delayed and less consistent. In such cases about 25% will develop DIC some 5–6 weeks after fetal demise. Fetal death and missed abortion are now rare causes of DIC because, with ultrasound, the diagnosis is usually made early and the pregnancy terminated before DIC can develop.

2 *Endothelial damage* exposes the underlying collagen to plasma and procoagulants. Such endothelial damage may be caused insidiously by pre-eclampsia/eclampsia or by sepsis. Another cause of endothelial hypoxia and damage is haemorrhagic shock with delayed restoration of the circulating intravascular volume. This is now one of the commonest causes of DIC in obstetrics.

3 *Red blood cell/platelet injury* may occur with incompatible blood transfusion reactions leading to the release of phospholipids and initiation of the coagulation cascade.

Pathophysiology

Normal haemostasis is a complex and dynamic balance between coagulation, which leads to fibrin formation, and the fibrinolytic system, which disposes of fibrin once its haemostatic function has been fulfilled. In DIC there is excessive and widespread coagulation which leads to consumption and depletion of the coagulation factors resulting in haemorrhage.[3] In response to this widespread coagulation and deposition of fibrin in the microvasculature the fibrinolytic system is activated. As plasminogen is converted to plasmin it breaks down the fibrin to form fibrin degradation products (FDP). FDP have anticoagulant properties as they inhibit both platelet function and the action of thrombin, serving to aggravate the coagulopathy. While the haemorrhagic diathesis is the dominant pathology in most cases, extensive microvascular thrombosis can also occur, leading to organ ischaemia and infarction. This can be a secondary factor, along with hypovolaemic shock, in the causation of renal cortical necrosis, lung damage and Sheehan's syndrome. The causes and pathophysiological features of DIC are outlined in Figure 23.1.

Clinical presentation

It is common for the main clinical features to be those of the obstetric complication that has triggered the DIC. Clinical manifestations of the DIC per se will depend upon its severity. These will range across the spectrum from no clinical manifestations with only haematological changes of DIC (↓ platelets, ↑ FDP); relatively subtle clinical signs such as bruising, epistaxis, purpuric rash, and oozing from venepuncture sites; to the dramatic torrential postpartum haemorrhage and bleeding from all operative sites.

Diagnosis

Diagnosis is aided by recognition of the obstetric initiating causes of DIC. Certain haematological tests are useful in the diagnosis and

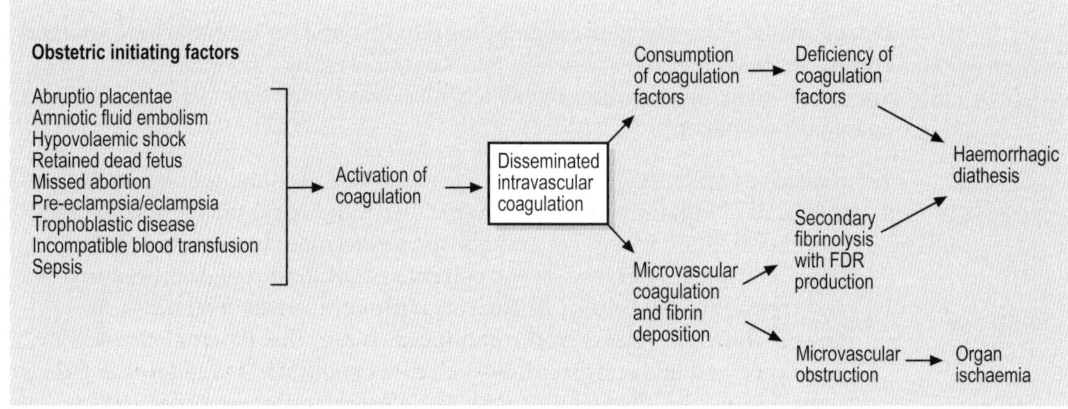

Figure 23.1 Causes and pathophysiology of disseminated intravascular coagulation (adapted from Baskett TF. Essential management of obstetric emergencies. 4th ed. 2004, with permission of Clinical Press Ltd)

if available it is appropriate to enlist the aid of a haematologist. Depending upon the level of sophistication of the hospital laboratory some tests may be unavailable. In addition, the process of DIC is so dynamic that results, as they become available, may not reflect the current status. Bedside whole-blood clotting tests are not helpful as their accuracy is limited unless controlled laboratory conditions are applied.[4]

The most rapid and useful screening tests are the platelet count (low and falling), activated partial thromboplastin time (which is usually prolonged when clotting factors are severely depleted), prothrombin time (usually prolonged), and the thrombin time, which is usually prolonged and is one of the more valuable tests. Fibrinogen levels are increased in normal pregnancy to 400–650 mg/dl; with DIC this level falls but may still be in the normal non-pregnant range. In severe DIC the fibrinogen levels usually fall below 150 mg/dl. FDP levels of > 80 μg/ml confirm the diagnosis of DIC, but these levels may remain elevated for 24–48 hours after the DIC has been controlled.

Management

With awareness of the initiating obstetric causes it may be possible to treat these before there is progression to severe DIC. Obvious examples of this are the evacuation of the uterus in cases of fetal death and missed abortion. Cases of severe pre-eclampsia and/or HELLP syndrome may have haematological changes of mild DIC with low platelets and elevated FDPs. These cases should be stabilized and delivered before the clinical manifestations of DIC become apparent.

In most obstetric situations DIC develops rapidly and prompt treatment is required. The initial treatment of haemorrhage is the same whether DIC is a contributing factor or not. Thus, the principles of managing hypovolaemic shock outlined in the preceding chapter are relevant. While it is important to send the appropriate bloods for haematological testing and to involve the consultant haematologist, the minute-by-minute management will not be influenced by these tests. The principles of management are as follows.

Treat the obstetric cause

As DIC is always secondary to an initiating cause it is obvious that the obstetric trigger must be promptly treated in order to cure the DIC. In most cases this entails emptying the uterus and controlling the surgical or obstetric haemorrhage.

Maintain circulation

While treating the obstetric cause, and therefore removing the trigger and ultimately curing the DIC, it is necessary to sustain the patient's circulation and maintain organ perfusion. These management principles have been outlined in Chapter 22 and include oxygen, rapid infusion of crystalloid, colloid and blood transfusion. An effective circulation is also essential to help clear the FDP, which is largely achieved by the liver. FDP compound the DIC as they interfere with platelet function, have an antithrombin effect, and inhibit the formation of firm fibrin. They also interfere with myometrial function and possibly with myocardial function as well. Thus, the clearance of FDP is a very important part of the recovery from DIC.

Replacement of procoagulants

Because of the risk of infection, fresh whole blood, which would be ideal, is not available. Packed red blood cells are deficient in platelets and other procoagulants, particularly factors V and VIII. Thus, it is essential in cases of severe haemorrhage complicated by DIC to add procoagulants using the following guidelines:

- *Fresh frozen plasma* (FFP) has all of the clotting factors present in the plasma of whole blood, without the platelets. These clotting factors are not in concentrated form however, so it is difficult to raise the circulating levels. The guiding rule is to give 1 unit of fresh frozen plasma after 5 units of blood and thereafter give 1 unit for every 2 units of blood transfused.

- *Cryoprecipitate* is rich in fibrinogen, in addition to von Willebrand factor and factors VIII and XIII. It is usually reserved for cases with severe hypofibrinogenaemia (< 100 mg/dl).
- *Platelets* deteriorate quite rapidly in stored blood and are not present in FFP. In a woman with persistent bleeding and severe thrombocytopaenia (< 30 000) platelet transfusion is indicated. One unit of platelets will raise the count by approximately 5000–10 000.
- *Antithrombin* is rapidly consumed in DIC and, under the guidance of a haematologist, antithrombin concentrate may be given if the levels are low.[5]
- *Recombinant activated factor VIIa* was originally used in haemophilia but has recently been applied to obstetric haemorrhage with DIC. It combines with the local tissue factor at the site of haemorrhage to enhance thrombin generation and stabilize fibrin formation. Experience in obstetric haemorrhage is limited but such treatment looks promising. It is given as an intravenous injection of 60–80 μg/kg. It is expensive and has a short half-life but obstetricians should be aware of its potential for the patient in whom standard blood transfusion and treatment with procoagulants is ineffective.[6–10]

It is emphasized that most cases of obstetric haemorrhage and DIC occur in previously healthy young women. Such women have a great ability to recover rapidly and completely once the initial obstetric cause of haemorrhage and DIC is removed, provided their circulating blood volume can be sustained to ensure adequate tissue perfusion. If this can be achieved the liver will usually remove the harmful FDP and replace most of the other desirable coagulation factors within 24 hours. Platelets may continue to fall in the next 24 hours, but as long as there is no haemorrhage they do not need to be replaced at this stage.

References

1. O'Riordan MN, Higgins JR. Haemostasis in normal and abnormal pregnancy. Best Prac Res Clin Obstet Gynaecol 2003; 17:385–396.
2. Baskett TF. Disseminated intravascular coagulation. In: Essential management of obstetric emergencies. 4th ed. Bristol: Clinical Press Ltd, 2004:242–245.
3. Lurie S, Feinstein M, Mamet Y. Disseminated intravascular coagulation in pregnancy: thorough comprehension of etiology and management reduces obstetricians' stress. Arch Gynecol Obstet 2001; 263:126–130.
4. Letsky EA. Disseminated intravascular coagulation. Best Prac Res Clin Obstet Gynaecol 2001; 15:623–644.
5. Bucur SZ, Levy JH, Despotis GJ. Use of antithrombin III concentrate in congenital and acquired deficiency states. Transfusion 1998; 38:481–498.
6. Hedner V, Erhardsten E. Potential role for r F VIIa in transfusion medicine. Transfusion 2002; 42:114–124.
7. Zupanic SS, Sololic V, Vishovic T, Sanjug J, Simic M, Kastelan M. Successful use of recombinant factor VIIa for massive bleeding after caesarean section due to HELLP syndrome. Acta Haematol 2002; 108:162–163.
8. Branch DW, Rodgers GM. Recombinant activated factor VII: a new weapon in the fight against hemorrhage. Obstet Gynecol 2003; 101:115–116.
9. Bouwmeester FW, Jonkhoff AR, Verheijen RHM, van Geijn HP. Successful treatment of life-threatening hemorrhage with recombinant activated Factor VII. Obstet Gynecol 2003; 101:117–116.
10. Pepas LP, Arif-Adib M, Kadir RA. Factor VIIa in puerperal hemorrhage with disseminated intravascular coagulation. Obstet Gynecol 2006; 108:757–761.

24

Amniotic fluid embolism

'Pulmonary embolism by the particulate matter contained in amniotic fluid which gained entrance to the maternal circulation has been demonstrated by us at autopsy in 8 cases in which it seemed to be the cause of death ... Having gained entrance to the maternal venous system, the emboli would be carried to the first filter bed, in these instances the lungs, and would lodge in vessels corresponding to their size. Sudden showers of foreign particulate material lodging in the lungs may produce severe systemic reactions resembling shock or anaphylactoid reactions.'

C. C. Steiner and P. E. Lushbaugh
Maternal pulmonary embolism by amniotic fluid as a cause of obstetric shock and unexpected death in obstetrics. JAMA 1941; 117:1245–1254, 1340–1345

Amniotic fluid embolism is rare (1 in 20 000–80 000 deliveries) but is a potentially catastrophic complication of pregnancy. Despite its rarity, it has such a high fatality rate (30–80%) that it accounts for 7–10% of direct maternal deaths in the developed world.

There are no consistent risk factors for amniotic fluid embolism (AFE). It can occur in association with termination of early pregnancy, but usually happens in late pregnancy during labour and delivery. In about 10% of cases it occurs immediately postpartum and very rarely the manifestations may be delayed for 1–2 hours after delivery.[1] Amniotic fluid may gain entry into the maternal circulation during spontaneous labour and delivery, at amniotomy, or at caesarean section. There are minor associations with certain risk factors such as induction and augmentation of labour, operative delivery, uterine rupture, amniotomy, abruptio placentae, intrauterine fetal death, intrauterine pressure catheter insertion and amnioinfusion.[2–5]

Pathophysiology

It is not uncommon for amniotic fluid and fetal squames to enter the maternal circulation without ill effect. In certain susceptible women, however, it seems that the presence of fetal cells and/or other components of amniotic fluid may trigger a complex pathophysiological cascade similar to that seen with anaphylaxis and septic shock.[6,7] The initial pathophysiological mechanism is of acute pulmonary vascular obstruction and hypertension leading to cor pulmonale. This is quite transient and soon followed by left ventricular failure leading to profound hypotension and shock. An acute inflammatory response disrupts the pulmonary capillary endothelium and alveoli leading to a ventilation–perfusion imbalance – resulting in severe hypoxia, convulsions and coma.[8] If the patient survives for more than 1 hour it is virtually inevitable that she will develop disseminated intravascular coagulation due to the activation of coagulation factors by the amniotic fluid (which contains tissue factor) and fetal cells, in addition to the profound shock.

Diagnosis

The clinical diagnosis is based on the sudden development of acute respiratory distress and cardiovascular collapse in a patient in labour or recently delivered. In some cases the signs and symptoms occur within minutes of the triggering event, such as amniotomy or caesarean section. The following spectrum of signs and symptoms can occur:[9]

- Occasionally there are premonitory symptoms of restlessness, anxiety and dyspnoea.
- Respiratory collapse with dyspnoea, cyanosis, hypoxia, pulmonary oedema and ultimately respiratory arrest.
- Cardiovascular collapse: tachycardia, hypotension, arrhythmias, cardiac arrest.
- Seizures and coma.
- Uterine hypertonus may occur and this is often following AFE rather than, as was previously thought, a contributing cause.
- Acute fetal hypoxia with corresponding fetal heart rate changes rapidly ensues.
- If the woman survives for more than 30–60 minutes disseminated intravascular coagulation and haemorrhage almost inevitably follow.

The differential diagnosis includes other acute catastrophies that may present with similar features such as: venous pulmonary embolism, acute myocardial infarction, eclampsia, gastric acid aspiration, air embolism and anaphylactic drug reaction.[10] The clinical features and context should help differentiate between these causes but, in any event, the initial management – cardiopulmonary resuscitation – may be required for all of these conditions. The initial clinical diagnosis of AFE, then, is really a combination of the above clinical features without any of the other obvious clinical causes. If the patient survives, it may be possible to take a sample of blood from the right side of the heart via a central venous pressure line and confirm the diagnosis by looking for amniotic fluid debris, along with newer immunohistochemical techniques to identify isoantigens.

Management

Amniotic fluid embolism is one of those 'all hands on deck' situations with, if the patient survives long enough, the need for specialist assistance from anaesthesia, intensive care and haematology. The following management principles may improve survival:[4,9,10]

- Early institution of effective cardiopulmonary resuscitation (CPR).

- If CPR is not effective within 5 minutes the fetus, if not delivered, will die. Unless it is feasible to perform immediate assisted vaginal delivery this will have to be by caesarean section. This is one of the few indications for perimortem caesarean section and should ultimately help the effectiveness of CPR for the mother (see Chapter 11). These efforts on behalf of the fetus should not interrupt the maternal resuscitation.
- If the woman survives the initial onslaught, intensive care guided by experts should improve survival.[11,12] This may include inotropic support with dopamine and, although it is empirical, intravenous hydrocortisone 500 mg IV 6-hourly on the basis of a possible anaphylactic aetiology.
- If the initial resuscitation and treatment is successful be prepared for haemorrhage and disseminated intravascular coagulation that nearly always develops in those who survive the first hour. This is outlined in Chapters 22 and 23.
- Recently, plasma exchange and haemofiltration have been used in isolated cases with some benefit to help clear or 'wash out' the effects of the amniotic fluid in the circulation.[13]

Unfortunately, the initial hypoxic insult may be so profound that a number of the survivors suffer permanent neurological damage. Similarly, the outlook for the fetus undelivered at the time of diagnosis is very poor unless it can be delivered within 5–10 minutes.

References

1. Clark SL, Hankins GDV, Audley DA, Dildy GA, Porter TF. Amniotic fluid embolism: analysis of the national registry. Am J Obstet Gynecol 1995; 172:1158–1169.
2. Burrows A, Khoo SKK. The amniotic fluid embolism syndrome: 10 years experience at a major teaching hospital. Aust NZ J Obstet Gynaecol 1995; 35:245–250.
3. Dorairajan G, Soundararaghaven S. Maternal death after intrapartum saline amnioinfusion – report of two cases. Br J Obstet Gynaecol 2005; 112:1331–1333.
4. Davies S. Amniotic fluid embolus: a review of the literature. Can J Anaesth 2001; 48:88–98.
5. Kramer MS, Rouleau J, Baskett TF, Joseph KS. Amniotic-fluid embolism and medical induction of labour: a retrospective, population-based cohort study. Lancet 2006; 368:1444–1448.
6. Benson MD. Anaphylactoid syndrome of pregnancy. Am J Obstet Gynecol 1996; 175:749.
7. Benson MD, Kobayashi H, Silver RK, Oi H, Greenberger PA, Terao T. Immunologic studies in presumed amniotic fluid embolism. Obstet Gynecol 2001; 95:510–514.
8. Clark SL. New concepts of amniotic fluid embolism: a review. Obstet Gynecol Surv 1990; 45:360–368.
9. Tuffnell DJ. Amniotic fluid embolism. In: MacLean AB, Neilson JP, eds. Maternal mortality and morbidity. London: RCOG Press, 2002:190–200.
10. Goswami K, Young P, Grady K, Cox C. Amniotic fluid embolism. In: Johnston R, Cox C, Grady K, Howell C, eds. Managing obstetric emergencies and trauma. London: RCOG Press, 2003:29–34.
11. Gilbert WM, Danielson B. Amniotic fluid embolism: decreased mortality in a population-based study. Obstet Gynecol 1999; 93:973–977.
12. Tuffnell DJ. United Kingdom Amniotic Fluid Embolism Register. Br J Obstet Gynaecol 2005; 112:1625–1629.
13. Kancko Y, Ogihara T, Tajima H, Mochimaru F. Continuous hemofiltration for disseminated intravascular coagulation and shock due to amniotic fluid embolism: report of a dramatic response. Intern Med 2001; 40:945–947.

25

Analgesia and anaesthesia

Introduction

Labour is an intense and painful experience for most women, many of whom find it worse than they expected. For the woman having her first baby there is often additional fear and anxiety about the unknown. Mothers who have had a bad and painful experience in a previous labour will understandably dread a repeat performance. At its worst, this may lead to the 'never again' syndrome, in which the woman remembers the pain so bitterly that she will absolutely avoid another pregnancy. It may also have a bad effect on the relationship with her husband and child. In most cases the first labour is the longest and most difficult and subsequent labours tend to be shorter and less painful. A woman's experience in her first labour is therefore a sentinel event and it is essential that she does not look back on this with negative and bitter feelings. Thus, if she can be provided with adequate guidance and pain relief to a safe and successful first delivery, within the framework of her own wishes, subsequent labours will be approached with confidence and often require minimal assistance.

It is not appropriate to accept that inadequate pain relief is a natural component of labour. As the American College of Obstetricians and Gynecologists and the American Society of Anesthesiologists states:[1]

> *'There is no other circumstance where it is considered acceptable for a person to experience untreated, severe pain, amenable to safe intervention, while under a physician's care. In the absence of a medical contraindication, maternal request is a sufficient medical indication for pain relief during labour.'*

Although antenatal preparation and education, along with relaxation techniques, are helpful to many mothers, most will request pharmacological methods of pain relief. Every woman's response to the pain of labour is individual but in the majority of cases, nulliparous women have a slower labour with pain over a longer period of time. Thus, while non-pharmacological methods may be helpful they will frequently seek more effective methods of pain relief.[2]

Multiparous women, particularly those in their second labour, are often pleasantly surprised by how far they have advanced in labour before the pain becomes difficult to manage. They tend to get a more rapid onset of intense pain in the later part of the first stage of labour and often there is only about 1 hour between their request for pain relief and full dilatation and/or delivery. Thus, in multiparous women it is often possible to see her through this intense and sometimes overwhelming pain with good one-to-one nursing support, small doses of intravenous narcotics and inhalation analgesia.

Along with the humane and psychological aspects of pain relief in labour there are potential pathophysiological effects of pain and anxiety, leading to increased output of adrenaline, noradrenaline and other stress hormones. In addition there may be maternal hyperventilation, increased oxygen consumption, and vasoconstriction in the utero-placental circulation – these changes can potentially lead to fetal hypoxia and ineffective uterine action.

Pain pathways

In the first stage of labour the origin of pain is from effacement and dilatation of the cervix and formation of the lower uterine segment. These painful impulses pass through the hypogastric plexus to the lumbar sympathetic chain and, via the dorsal horn, to T10, T11, T12 and L1 at the spinal cord level. The nociceptive information passes from the dorsal horn via the spinothalamic tract through the brain stem and medulla to the posterior thalamic nuclei. From here fibres pass to the somatic sensory cortex and thence to the frontal cortex. These pathways help regulate the associated responses to pain, such as anxiety, adverse reaction and learned behaviour.

In the second stage of labour, in addition to the uterine contractions, pain results from stretching of the pelvic floor and perineum. These painful stimuli enter the spinal cord via the somatic pudendal nerves: S2, S3 and S4.

Methods of pain relief

Non-pharmacological methods

Most of these techniques rely on counter-stimulation as the basis for their success.

Prepared childbirth

The so-called 'natural childbirth' movement started in the early part of the 20th century in response to the 'twilight sleep' era at the beginning of the century with its excessive use of narcotics and sedatives. The basis of childbirth preparation is that women who are properly prepared can control the pain of labour themselves and either do without or reduce their need for pharmacological pain

NATURAL CHILDBIRTH

'It is not generally recognized that in childbirth there is an "emotional labour" which is as definite and important as its physical counterpart. This must be understood if parturition is to be conducted as a physiological performance ... Is a woman pained and frightened because her labour is difficult, or is her labour difficult and painful because she is frightened? ... Pain is the mental interpretation of harmful stimulus, and fear the intensifier of stimulus-interpretation. The biological purpose of each is protective. The physiological reaction to each is tension.'

Grantly Dick Read
Natural childbirth. London: Heinemann, 1933

relief. There have been a number of prominent, often consumer-led, movements following the lead of Grantly Dick Reid in Britain, Velvoski in Russia and Lamaze and Le Boyer in France. In addition to these specific techniques many regions and hospitals will provide antenatal classes with information about the various methods of pain relief in labour (both non-pharmacological and pharmacological) as well as infant care classes, with the overall aim of engendering confidence in the couple.

Continuous support

No woman in labour should be left alone. In addition to the trained nurse or midwife many women will have social support in the form of their male partner or other family member and some will choose to have a specially trained lay person (sometimes known as a doula). These personnel can provide reassurance, encouragement and explanation during labour. In addition they may help guide counter-stimulation techniques such as touch, massage, change of position, baths, ambulation, music, etc. Cultural factors may dictate the personnel and techniques used for support to the woman in labour.

Hypnosis

This often requires extensive antenatal training sessions and individual receptivity to hypnosis varies. In some cases the hypnotherapist also needs to be present during labour. When successful, the results of hypnosis are very impressive, however, the time and personnel commitment required are such that this is not practical for the majority of women.

Transcutaneous electrical nerve stimulation (TENS)

This consists of a small, battery-driven pulse generator which is connected to two pairs of electrodes on either side of the spine overlying the dermatomes, T10 to L1, and attached to the skin with adhesive tape. When activated it causes a tingling sensation in the skin under the electrodes. The strength of the stimulus can be adjusted by the control generator. It is said to be most helpful in early labour with back pain and may stimulate the release of endorphins. The woman can remain ambulant but TENS equipment may interfere with electronic fetal heart rate monitoring using a fetal scalp electrode.

Intradermal injection of water

Using a 1 ml syringe and a 25-gauge needle, injections of 0.05–0.1 ml of sterile water are injected into the skin in four sites: one on each side over the posterior iliac spines and one each just medial and below the upper sites. This causes intense stinging for about 30 seconds and may provide amelioration of back pain for 45–90 minutes. It is thought to act by counter-irritation, possible release of endorphins, or, according to the gate-control theory of pain, the intense superficial sensory stimulation may inhibit pain signals in the deeper, slower nerve fibres. In general this technique may give short-term relief from back-ache but rarely influences the total analgesia requirements.

Acupuncture

This and related procedures may have application in societies which have practitioners skilled in this technique and in women who are knowledgeable and receptive to this method.

Inhalation analgesia

The safest and most practical agent for inhalation analgesia is nitrous oxide. The aim is to administer subanaesthetic concentrations of nitrous oxide providing analgesia without loss of consciousness and with retention of protective laryngeal reflexes. Nitrous oxide is absorbed from and excreted by the lungs. It crosses the placenta but is also eliminated efficiently and there are no untoward neonatal effects. It has no effect on uterine contractility. The exact mode of action is unknown but it works at the level of the brain producing analgesia in low doses and anaesthesia with higher and sustained doses.

The advantage of nitrous oxide inhalation analgesia is that it is cheap, safe and simple to administer. In one-third to one-half of women it provides helpful, albeit incomplete, analgesia.

> **First use of nitrous oxide/oxygen inhalation analgesia in labour**
>
> *'The woman should be coached to exhale deeply and then inhale as much gas as possible ... It is important to begin the first anaesthesia early in order to obtain good pain relief; a late start will prevent the deep inhalation and, thus render the effect incomplete ... Thereafter the inhalation is begun at one-half to one minute prior to the anticipated next contraction. Two to five breaths of the gas mixture usually suffice to produce the desired effect.'*
>
> **Stanislav Klikovich**
> *Über das Stickstoffoxydul als Anaestheticum bei Geburten. Arch Gynäk 1881; 18:81–108*

It is most effective for short-term (1–2 hours) pain relief. As such, it is of most benefit in the multiparous woman in the late first stage of labour, in whom analgesia is usually required for the last hour or so before and during the second stage of labour. It is also of benefit as an adjunct to local anaesthetic techniques, such as infiltration of the perineum and pudendal block for instrumental vaginal delivery, assisted breech and twin delivery, and suture of genital tract lacerations.

Technique of administration

There is a variety of equipment for self-administration of nitrous oxide. The simplest and most commonly used is a pre-mixed gas cylinder of 50% nitrous oxide and 50% oxygen (Entonox). An alternative is a blender apparatus that produces the appropriate 50/50 concentration from separate cylinders via hospital gas lines (Nitronox, Midogas).

The breathing circuit is connected to a face mask or mouthpiece – the latter is a useful alternative for women who find the face mask suffocating. Within the breathing circuit is a demand valve which only opens when the user applies negative pressure with strong inhalation. For this to occur the user has to retain enough consciousness to keep the seal of the mouthpiece or face mask intact. If the woman becomes drowsy, and long before protective laryngeal reflexes are lost, her grip on the apparatus will break the seal and not permit further inhalation of gas. This protective mechanism is one of the most important safety features of the self-administered apparatus.

There is a latent period from when the woman starts inhalation until there is sufficient gas tension in the central nervous system to produce analgesia. This time lag is approximately 30–40 seconds. In the first stage of labour, uterine contractions are palpable about 20 seconds before the woman feels pain. The most important point, therefore, for those assisting the woman in labour is to palpate the uterine contraction and get her to start the inhalation so that some concentration of the gas is effective before the pain becomes intense. This is an essential practical point that is often overlooked. An alternative, if the contraction pattern is regular and predictable, is to guide the inhalation of nitrous oxide by the clock so that it starts about 30–40 seconds before the contraction. If nitrous oxide is to be used as an adjunct to local anaesthesia for painful procedures, it can be administered continuously until satisfactory analgesia is provided. Once again, the safeguard of self-administration by the woman should prevent anaesthesia and loss of protective reflexes.

Narcotic analgesia

Over the past century parenteral administration of narcotics has been one of the most frequently used methods of pain relief in labour. For the past 50 years the most commonly used narcotic has been meperidine (demerol, pethidine). In many countries, midwives have autonomous use of meperidine in labour and it is this practical point that has accounted for its widespread use. Unfortunately, narcotics by intramuscular injection are not very effective at providing adequate pain relief in labour. The half-life of meperidine is about 2–3 hours and it rapidly crosses the placenta. The maximum fetal tissue uptake occurs about 2–3 hours after

First use of ether and chloroform inhalation analgesia in labour

'Whilst this agent has been used extensively, and by numerous hands, in the practice of surgery, I am not aware that anyone has hitherto ventured to test its applicability to the practice of midwifery. I am induced, therefore, to hope that the few following hurried and imperfect notes, relative to its employment in obstetric cases may not at the present time prove uninteresting to the profession.'

James Young Simpson
Ether inhalation in parturition. Edinb Mon J Med Sci 1847; 74:639–640

'This new anaesthetic agent is chloroform ... as an inhaled anaesthetic agent, it possesses, I believe, all the advantages of sulphuric ether, without its principle disadvantages ... greatly less quantity of chloroform than of ether is required to produce the anaesthetic affect ... Its action is much more rapid and complete, and generally more persistent ... The inhalation and influence of chloroform ... far more agreeable and pleasant than those of ether.'

James Young Simpson
On a new anaesthetic agent, more efficient than sulphuric ether. Lancet 1847; 2:549–551

maternal administration and the half-life in the neonate is about 12 hours. Thus, the neonate is at greatest risk for respiratory depression 2–3 hours after meperidine administration to the mother. Maternal side-effects include nausea, vomiting, hypotension, pruritis and reduced laryngeal protective reflexes. All narcotics may reduce the baseline variability of the fetal heart rate. In addition to neonatal depression there is altered neonatal behavior for the first 12–24 hours and impairment of breast feeding.

Despite the overall poor rating of narcotic analgesia in labour there are individual circumstances in which the use of narcotic analgesia can be adjusted to the woman's requirements:

- Meperidine can be given by intramuscular or subcutaneous injection (the latter route gives more reliable absorption) in a dose of 50–150 mg depending on the patient's size. This can be useful in the anxious woman early in established labour. The effect is maximal in 45–60 minutes and lasts about 3 hours. Phenothiazine is sometimes administered at the same time to reduce nausea and vomiting.
- Intravenous administration of narcotic can be very useful for the woman who has uncontrolled and distressing pain. By providing quick relief from her pain it reassures her that pain control is available and allows her to make more considered decisions about analgesia for the rest of her labour. Given intravenously, narcotics act within 1 minute, with maximum effect within 2–5 minutes and a total effect for 1–2 hours. Using meperidine, intravenous doses are given in 20–25 mg increments with 3–5 minutes between each dose to assess the effect and avoid hypotension. Satisfactory analgesia is usually achieved with 50–75 mg. Ideally the injection should be given at the start of an uterine contraction, which in theory reduces the transfer of the drug to the fetus because of reduced utero-placental blood flow during the contraction and rapid protein binding of meperidine in maternal plasma. A rational plan for long-term analgesia in the labour can then be established. An alternative to meperidine is fentanyl, which is a highly lipid-soluble synthetic opioid. Its maternal side-effects are similar to meperidine but less pronounced. It has a rapid onset of action and is highly protein bound with a short duration of action – about 30 minutes. It appears to have fewer neonatal respiratory or neurobehavioral depressive effects. The intravenous dose is 50–100 μg.

- Patient controlled intravenous analgesia (PCIA), using fentanyl, can be a useful alternative if epidural analgesia is unavailable, unacceptable to the woman, or contraindicated. Fentanyl is chosen because of its reduced maternal and neonatal side-effects, compared with meperidine. This system is usually established in consultation with anaesthetic colleagues. It entails one-to-one nursing and the provision of pulse oximetry. The woman is usually given a loading dose of about 150 μg and the PCIA machine is set up to allow bolus doses of 50 μg with a variable lock out period – usually 10 minutes. These can be fine-tuned depending on the woman's response and the side-effects. The woman needs to be instructed in the use of the machine and she alone activates the doses. This has the added advantage of giving her some control over the situation and, as with inhalation analgesia, this is an attractive component of this technique.

Local anaesthesia

The use of local anaesthetic for infiltration and regional blocks is of great value for obstetric operative procedures. It is important to know the dose and potential toxicity of local anaesthetics. The most commonly used is lidocaine (lignocaine) and the dose is 3–4 mg/kg plain solution, and 7–8 mg/kg with added epinephrine (adrenaline). A 1% solution of lidocaine contains 10 mg/ml, and the dose for a 70 kg woman should, therefore, not exceed 250 mg or 25 ml.

Another frequently overlooked detail is the fact that like good wine, within reason, local anaesthetics improve with age. Thus, after local infiltration one should wait 3 minutes, and after minor regional blocks 5 minutes, before proceeding.

Local infiltration

The cutaneous nerve supply of the perineum is shown in Figure 25.1. For perineal and lower vaginal lacerations, direct infiltration of the involved areas is performed by advancing the needle and injecting and aspirating, to avoid intravascular injection, as the needle is advanced and withdrawn. Before the performance of episiotomy the site of the proposed incision and the adjacent areas of the fourchette and labia are infiltrated to reduce both the pain of incision and distention of the perineum.

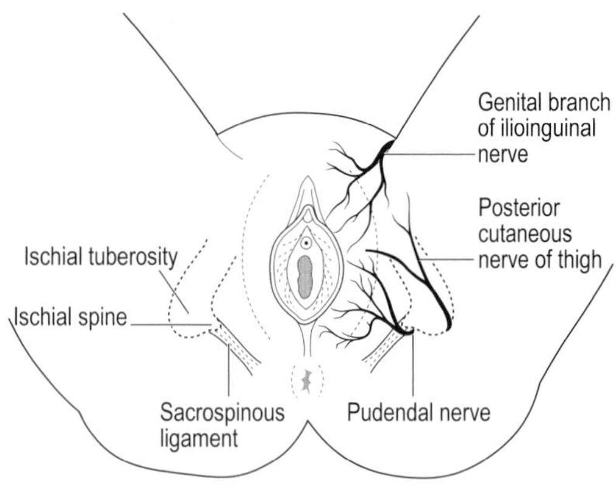

Figure 25.1 Cutaneous nerve supply of the perineum.

As an adjunct to pudendal block the site of the proposed episiotomy can be infiltrated as well as the areas of the lower labia supplied by the posterior cutaneous nerve of the thigh and the genital branch of the ilio-inguinal nerve.

Pudendal block

If epidural or spinal anaesthesia is not available or is contraindicated, pudendal block is a safe and useful technique for low assisted vaginal delivery with forceps or vacuum and for the manipulations necessary for assisted breech delivery and delivery of the second twin. Pudendal block can be performed by two techniques:

- *Transvaginal* – this is the technique of choice as it is less painful and more accurate than the transperineal route. Using a 20 ml syringe with 1% lidocaine the needle guard is guided medial and just below the ischial spine. Use the left index and middle fingers to guide to the left side and the right hand to guide to the right ischial spine (Fig 25.2). If the special needle guard is not available it is possible to guide a bare spinal needle to the spine

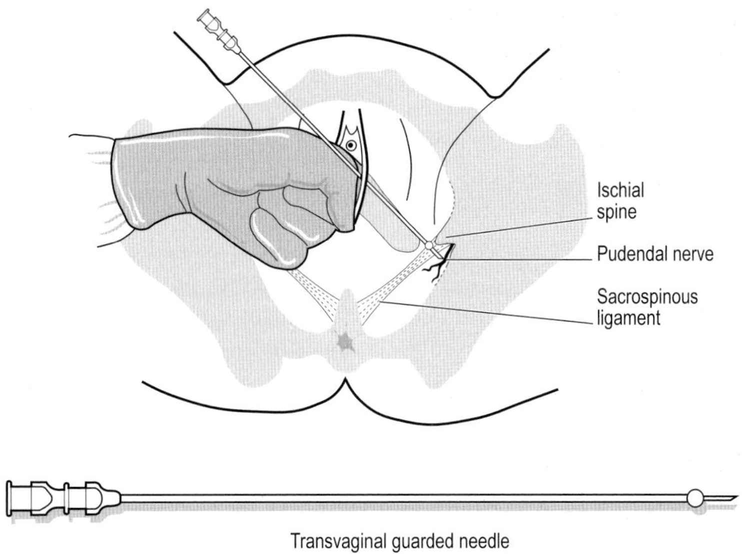

Figure 25.2 Transvaginal pudendal block.

if the point is firmly shielded between the fingers – this requires great care to avoid personal injury when making the final manipulation of the needle point through the sacrospinous ligament. After aspiration 5–8 ml of local anaesthetic is injected around the pudendal nerve.

- *Transperineal* – this method is much more painful and less accurate than the transvaginal route and is only used if the presenting part is so low as to preclude the transvaginal technique. The skin is infiltrated with local anaesthetic half way between the anus and the ischial tuberosity. With one index finger in the vagina the ischial spine is palpated and a 10 cm spinal needle is advanced through the infiltrated skin and guided towards the ischial spine and sacrospinous ligament. Aspiration and infiltration around the pudendal nerve follows.

It has to be admitted that on many occasions pudendal blocks are incomplete. It is therefore a good idea to use the remaining local anaesthetic, starting at the fourchette and fanning out with local infiltration to the perineum, site of the episiotomy, and lower aspect of the labia. Supplemental inhalation analgesia may also be useful.

Paracervical block

This is a very simple and effective method of pain relief in the first stage of labour when other conservative methods fail and epidural analgesia is not available. Unfortunately potential fetal side-effects preclude its use with a viable fetus. Fetal bradycardia can occur following paracervical block and there have been several cases of intrauterine death. The rapid absorption of local anaesthetic from the very vascular paracervical tissues may lead to high fetal levels and cause myocardial and central nervous system depression. If modified techniques with less toxic local anaesthetics are developed it may become safer in the future, but at present its use in labour with a viable fetus cannot be recommended. It may, however, be useful in cases of labour with a dead or non-viable fetus and it can also be useful in cases requiring intrauterine manipulation following delivery, such as manual removal of retained placenta and acute uterine inversion if epidural, spinal or general anaesthesia is not available.

The technique is simple, using a specially designed needle and guard, such that the needle protrudes only 3–5 mm from the guard. Between 3 and 4 o'clock and 8 and 9 o'clock 5–10 ml of local anaesthetic is injected into each lateral fornix where the cervix reflects off from the vagina (Fig 25.3). Frequent aspiration is essential as the paracervical space is extremely vascular.

Local anaesthesia for caesarean section

Depending upon available facilities and personnel, or lack thereof, there may be occasions when caesarean section needs to be performed under local anaesthesia. Inhalation analgesia with nitrous oxide may be used to augment the local anaesthetic.

Make up 100 ml 0.5% lidocaine to which 0.5 ml of 1 in 200 000 epinephrine (adrenaline) has been added. Using a 20 ml syringe the principle is to 'inject as you go':

- 15–20 ml along the line of the proposed skin incision
- 10–15 ml under the rectus sheath and adjacent rectus muscle
- 10–15 ml in the extraperitoneal tissue and transversalis fascia
- The peritoneum is then opened
- 10 ml in the utero-vesical peritoneal fold – this fold is then incised and the uterine muscle exposed

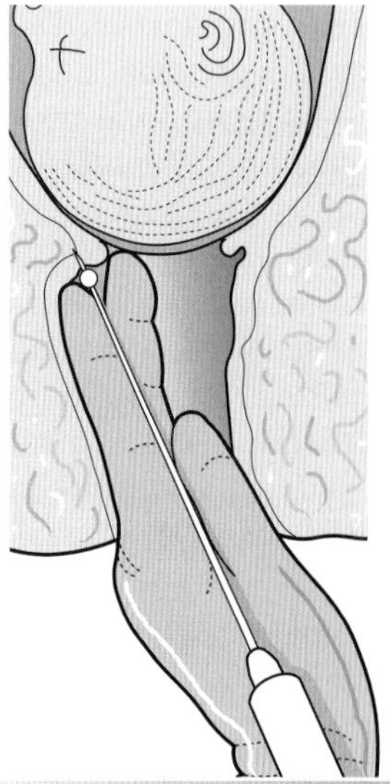

Figure 25.3 Paracervical block.

- The uterine muscle is relatively insensitive to incision but the muscle may be infiltrated with 10–15 ml before incision
- Once the infant has been delivered the mother should be given intravenous morphine.

The above methods of pain relief can be administered or guided by an obstetrician. Administration of epidural, spinal or general anaesthesia is beyond the scope of this book.

References

1. American College of Obstetricians and Gynecologists. Committee Opinion, No. 295. Pain relief during labor. Obstet Gynecol 2004; 104:213.
2. Horowitz ER, Yogev Y, Ben-Haroush A, Kaplan B. Women's attitude toward analgesia during labour – a comparison between 1995 and 2001. Eur J Obstet Gynecol Reprod Biol 2004; 117:30–32.

Bibliography

Baskett TF. Edinburgh connections in a painful world. J R Coll Surg Edin Irel 2005; 3:99–107.

Bricker L, Lavender T. Parental opiods for labour pain relief: a systematic review. Am J Obstet Gynecol 2002; 186S:94–109.

Campbell DC. Parenteral opioids for labor analgesia. Clin Obstet Gynecol 2003; 46:616–622.

D'Angelo R. New techniques of labor analgesia: PCEA and CSE. Clin Obstet Gynecol 2003; 46:623–632.

Hawkins JL. Anesthesia-related maternal mortality. Clin Obstet Gynecol 2003; 46:679–687.

Hodnett ED, Lowe NK, Hannah ME, et al. Effectiveness of nurses as providers of birth labor support in North American hospitals. A randomized controlled trial. JAMA 2002; 288:1373–1381.

Hodnett ED. Pain in women's satisfaction with the experience of childbirth: a systematic review. Am J Obstet Gynecol 2002; 186S:160–172.

Kuezkowski KM. Neurologic complications of labor analgesia: facts and fiction. Obstet Gynecol Surv 2003; 59:47–51.

Leighton BL, Halpernin SH. The effects of epidural analgesia on labour, maternal, and neonatal outcomes: a systematic review. Am J Obstet Gynecol 2002; 186:S69–77.

McInnes RJ, Hillan E, Clark D, Gilmour H. Diamorphine for pain relief in labour: a randomised controlled trial comparing intramuscular injection and patient-controlled analgesia. Br J Obstet Gynaecol 2004; 111:1081–1089.

Rosen MA. Paracervical block for labor analgesia: a brief historic review. Am J Obstet Gynecol 2002; 186S:127–130.

Rosen MA. Nitrous oxide for relief of labour pain: a systematic review. Am J Obstet Gynecol 2002; 186S:110–126.

Simkin PP, O'Hara MA. Non-pharmacologic relief of pain during labor: a systematic review of five methods. Am J Obstet Gynecol 2002; 186S:131–159.

Waldenström U, Hildingsson I, Ryding EL. Antenatal fear of childbirth and its association with subsequent caesarean section and experience of childbirth. Br J Obstet Gynaecol 2006; 1132:638–646.

26

Procedures and techniques

Acute tocolysis

In certain obstetric complications, rapid uterine relaxation is required for their successful resolution. Until recently acute uterine tocolysis required the institution of general anaesthesia with halogenated agents and involved rapid sequence induction and tracheal intubation with its associated maternal risks. The recent application of β-adrenergic drugs, oxytocin antagonists and nitroglycerine to achieve rapid uterine relaxation has obviated the need for general anaesthesia in these circumstances.

First use of uterine tocolysis

'I found it impossible to get my hand into the uterus to deliver the placenta. Bearing in mind the remarkable power which nitrite of amyl possesses in relaxing tension in the blood-vessels, I determined to test its action on the uterine spasms. The patient had three drops of the nitrite of amyl given her on a handkerchief to inhale. During the inhalation, the ring of muscular fibres around the os interna, which had been so rigid as to be absolutely undilatable, steadily yielded, until I could pass the whole hand into the uterus ...'

Fancourt Barnes
Hour-glass contraction of the uterus treated with nitrate of amyl. BMJ 1882; 1:377

Nitroglycerine

Nitroglycerine is an ester of nitric acid and exerts its relaxant effect on smooth muscle by the formation of nitric oxide. The drug is rapidly metabolized by the liver so that the half life is only 2 minutes. It has a low molecular weight of 227 and therefore crosses the placenta, but no adverse fetal or neonatal effects have been described in either animal studies or humans. In addition to uterine tocolysis the smooth muscle relaxation effect causes peripheral vasodilatation and reduced venous tone. Provided there is no hypovolaemia this causes only a mild and clinically insignificant hypotension. However, if there is associated hypovolaemia, rapid infusion of intravenous crystalloid is necessary to avoid acute and severe maternal hypotension. The peripheral vasodilation responds to epinephrine (adrenaline) and the uterine relaxation responds to oxytocin.[1]

Beta-adrenergic drugs

The biggest experience with this group of drugs has been with ritodrine, terbutaline and hexoprenaline. These selective β-2 receptor agonists have the main effect of relaxing arteriolar and uterine smooth muscle. They may cause mild hypotension and tachycardia and there have been isolated reports of atrial fibrillation. These agents cross the placenta and may cause a mild transient fetal tachycardia. They abolish uterine activity for 15–30 minutes.[2]

Atosiban

Atosiban is a synthetic analogue of oxytocin which acts as an oxytocin antagonist by binding to myometrial cell oxytocin receptors. The half life is about 12 minutes and it crosses the placenta, but umbilical vein levels are only 10% of those in the maternal uterine vein.[3] The advantage of atosiban is that it has fewer cardiovascular side-effects compared with the β-adrenergic agents. Atosiban has been used mainly in attempts to suppress preterm labour but it may also have an application for acute tocolysis in intrapartum fetal distress.[4]

Indications

Rapid uterine relaxation may be necessary in the following clinical situations.

Uterine hypertonus

This can occur in spontaneous labour but is more common in response to oxytocic drugs, either oxytocin or, more likely, the longer acting prostaglandins used for cervical ripening and induction of labour.[2,5,6]

Breech delivery

Unless the uterus is relaxed there may be difficulty with delivery of extended arms and/or the after-coming head of the preterm breech. This can occur with both vaginal and caesarean delivery but is more likely with the latter. The fetal breech, trunk and legs may be easily delivered through the uterine incision but the unrelaxed uterine muscle may clamp down around the fetal head, leading to delay, asphyxia and potential trauma. This is particularly likely in the preterm breech, but can also occur with the term fetus.[7,8]

Intrapartum version of fetal malpresentations

Uterine relaxation is usually necessary to safely and effectively carry out both external cephalic and internal podalic version at both vaginal and caesarean delivery of the second twin (see Chapter 15). With regional anaesthesia uterine relaxation is often inadequate and additional tocolysis is necessary.

Shoulder dystocia

In rare cases of shoulder dystocia that cannot be resolved with the traditional manoeuvres, cephalic replacement may be considered (see Chapter 10). In this situation, replacement of the head is facilitated by uterine relaxation, which may also help restore the utero-placental circulation and fetal oxygenation.

Retained placenta

Acute tocolysis may aid relaxation of a contraction ring and allow spontaneous delivery of the separated but retained placenta.[9] On other occasions, tocolysis may be necessary to facilitate the manual removal of a non-separated placenta, in which a contraction ring prevents manual access.

Acute uterine inversion

Manual replacement of acute uterine inversion may be possible using acute tocolysis, obviating the need for general anaesthesia.[10]

In many of the above situations, regional anaesthesia in the form of epidural or spinal analgesia may be in effect. However, these regional techniques, while providing excellent analgesia, do not provide uterine relaxation, so that additional tocolysis may be necessary.

Administration of tocolytics

Nitroglycerine

This can be given by the sublingual or intravenous routes. Sublingual administration is via an aerosol spray in doses of 400 μg. However, the mucosal absorption is not as predictable or precise as the intravenous route and the latter is usually chosen for acute tocolysis.

Nitroglycerine comes in an ampoule containing 5 mg in 1 ml solution. If this is added to a 100 ml bag of normal saline it produces a solution of 50 μg per ml. Draw up 20 ml into a syringe – this allows the precise titration of 50 μg per ml administered. Nitroglycerine is rapidly degraded and its effect is usually obvious within 90 seconds and lasts for a further 1–2 minutes. At the time of its administration intravenous crystalloid should be running rapidly, particularly if there is any question of hypovolaemia. The dose is titrated depending on the initial response and the clinical situation.[11,12] For cases of fetal entrapment a rapid response is necessary and one usually starts with a dose of 200 μg, repeating this at about 2-minute intervals until appropriate uterine relaxation is achieved.[13] In cases with retained placenta or acute uterine inversion, hypovolaemia should be corrected and smaller initial doses (100 μg) may be given.

In all cases in which oxytocin or prostaglandins has been previously administered, higher doses of nitroglycerine may be required.

Terbutaline

It is most commonly given as 250 μg subcutaneously, but can be given intravenously in 5 ml saline, slowly over 5 minutes.[14] The antagonist to terbutaline is propranolol 1–2 mg IV.

Ritodrine

This is given as 6 mg mixed in 10 ml normal saline and administered intravenously over 3 minutes.

Hexoprenaline

Give 5 μg in 10 ml normal saline intravenously over 5 minutes.

Atosiban

Mix 6.75 mg of atosiban in 5 ml normal saline and give intravenously over 1 minute.[4]

For rapid short-lived tocolysis necessary to deal with malpresentations and third stage complications, nitroglycerine is the drug of choice. For more sustained uterine relaxation needed with uterine hypertonus, atosiban, terbutaline or ritodrine are more appropriate.

References

1. Lau IC, Adaikau PC, Arulkumaran S, Ng SC. Oxytocics reverse the tocolytic effect of glyceryl trinitrate on the human uterus. Br J Obstet Gynaecol 2001; 108:164–168.
2. Ingemarsson I, Arulkumaran S, Ratnam SS. Single injection of terbutaline in term labor. I Effect on fetal pH in cases with prolonged

bradycardia. II Effect on uterine activity. Am J Obstet Gynecol 1985; 153:859–869.

3. Lamont RF. The development and introduction of anti-oxytocic tocolytics. Br J Obstet Gynaecol 2003; 110:108–112.
4. Afschar P, Schöll W, Bader A, Bauer M, Winter R. A prospective randomised trial of atosiban versus hexoprenaline for acute tocolysis and intrauterine resuscitation. Br J Obstet Gynaecol 2004; 111:316–318.
5. Palomaki O, Jansson M, Huhtala H, Kirkinen P. Severe cardiotocographic pathology at labor: effect of acute intravenous tocolysis. Am J Perinatol 2004; 21:347–353.
6. Shekarloo A, Mendez-Bauer C, Cook V, Freese V. Terbutaline (intravenous bolus) for the treatment of acute intrapartum fetal distress. Am J Obstet Gynecol 1989; 160:615–618.
7. Ezra Y, Wade C, Robin SH, Farine D. Uterine tocolysis at caesarean breech delivery with epidural anesthesia. J Reprod Med 2002; 47:555–558.
8. Craig S, Dalton R, Tuck M, Brew F. Sublingual glyceryl trinitrate for uterine relaxation at caesarean section – a prospective trial. Aust NZ J Obstet Gynaecol 1998; 38:34–39.
9. DeSimone CA, Norris MC, Leighton DL. Intravenous nitroglycerine aids manual extraction of a retained placenta. Anesthesiology 1990; 73:787–789.
10. Altabef KM, Spencer JT, Zinberg S. Intravenous nitroglycerin for uterine relaxation of an inverted uterus. Am J Obstet Gynecol 1992; 166:1237–1238.
11. Axemo P, Fu X, Lindberg B, Ulmstan U, Wessen A. Intravenous nitroglycerine for rapid uterine relaxation. Acta Obstet Gynecol Scand 1998; 77:50–53.
12. O'Grady JP, Parker RK, Patel SS. Nitroglycerin for rapid tocolysis: development of a protocol and a literature review. J Perinatol 2001; 20:27–33.
13. Dufour P, Vinatier S, Pouch F. The use of intravenous nitroglycerin for cervico-uterine relaxation: a review of the literature. Arch Gynecol Obstet 1997; 261:1–7.
14. Chandraharan E, Arulkumaran S. Acute tocolysis. Curr Opin Obstet Gynecol 2005; 17:151–156.

Version

Version refers to the procedure that changes the presenting part of the fetus. This may be carried out by *external* manipulation of the fetus, *internal* manipulation, or *combined (bipolar)* internal and external manoeuvres. Bipolar version is discussed in the chapter on antepartum haemorrhage.

External cephalic version

External cephalic version (ECV) is used to alter the presentation of the fetus in the later weeks of pregnancy. Breech presentation, transverse or oblique lie may be converted to cephalic presentation. This may also be achieved in early labour in some women, particularly the multiparous. Following delivery of the first twin, external cephalic version may be undertaken for breech or oblique lie of the second twin.

EXTERNAL CEPHALIC VERSION

'In all cases, where, after eight months of gestation the head occupies either the iliac fossa or the superior uterine segment, we should perform cephalic version by external manoeuvres … The first stage of the operation consists in rendering the foetus moveable … To facilitate this displacement of the breech, we may at the same time exert slight pressure in an opposite direction over the cephalic extremity. The two fetal extremities being moveable and accessible, and the hands being applied over them, we should make slow and continued pressure in such a manner as to cause the breech to ascend and the head to descend by the shortest route.

Adolpe Pinard
A Treatise on Abdominal Palpation, as Applied to Obstetrics, and Version by External Manipulations. English Edition. New York: J. H. Vail & Co, 1885, p75–78

Assessment

- Potential associations with malpresentations such as placenta praevia should be considered and excluded.
- For antepartum cases it is usual to delay version until 36 weeks gestation. Version before this gestation increases the chance that the fetus will revert to its original malpresentation by the onset of labour. From 37 weeks only 5–10% will revert to breech presentation after successful version. In addition, rare complications of version may necessitate immediate delivery which is more acceptable if the fetus is mature.
- A detailed ultrasound examination is undertaken to confirm gestational age, exclude fetal anomalies, identify the type of breech presentation, locate the placenta and assess the amount of amniotic fluid.
- If the woman has a single previous transverse lower segment caesarean scar, and is planning labour and vaginal delivery, it is permissible to attempt gentle external cephalic version in selected cases.

Technique

- Some obstetricians feel that these patients should be fasting because of the rare cases that require immediate delivery due to complications of the version. It is unpleasant for pregnant women to fast and, in addition, the fetus is often very quiet with maternal fasting. As it is helpful to have fetal movement to assist the version (see below) a reasonable compromise is to offer the woman a light snack 1–2 hours before the planned version.
- Ideally, a 20 minute pre-version cardiotocograph should show a reactive fetal heart rate.

- Perform an ultrasound scan to confirm the malpresentation, localize the placenta and determine the amount of amniotic fluid.
- The woman should be reasonably comfortable with slight elevation of the head of the bed and a minor left lateral tilt. After the ultrasound, remove the gel from the woman's abdomen and substitute talcum powder. This allows one's hands to move easily and smoothly over the abdomen and to avoid the use of excess force. It also facilitates the changing positions of the hands during the version. Others may use extra gel for the same purpose.
- It is usual to turn the fetus by promoting flexion, so that the fetus is moved in the direction it is 'looking'. This principle should be explained to the woman. Tell her she will feel pressure from your hands and that this will be sustained but she should not feel pain.
- The essential first step, upon which success depends, is the displacement and elevation of the breech from the pelvis. This can require sustained, albeit gentle pressure from both hands (Fig 26.1). Once this has been achieved the right hand continues to elevate the breech while the left hand is moved behind the fetal head (Fig 26.2). With the hands working in unison, intermittent pressure is applied to both fetal poles. It is at this point that fetal movement may help propel the fetus in the right direction. Throughout the procedure, gentleness is the guiding rule. Discretion is the better part of valour and the procedure is either going to be achieved gently and without pain, or it should be abandoned. If these principles are followed it is extremely rare for there to be any maternal or fetal complications.
- Once the fetus has been turned ultrasound is again used to confirm the new presentation and assess the fetal heart rate. It is not uncommon for there to be transient bradycardia due to the manipulations. Some will use the ultrasound or doptone over the fetal thorax to monitor the fetal heart rate during version. After version the fetal heart rate should be monitored for about 30 minutes and, provided this is normal and the woman is clinically well and without abdominal pain or vaginal bleeding, she can be discharged.

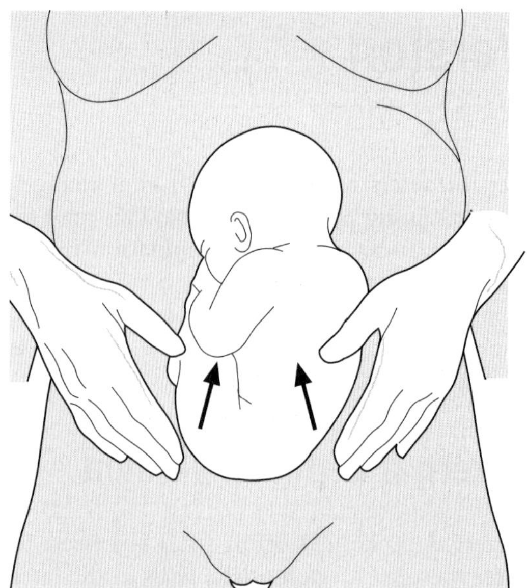

Figure 26.1 External cephalic version: elevation of the breech from the pelvis.

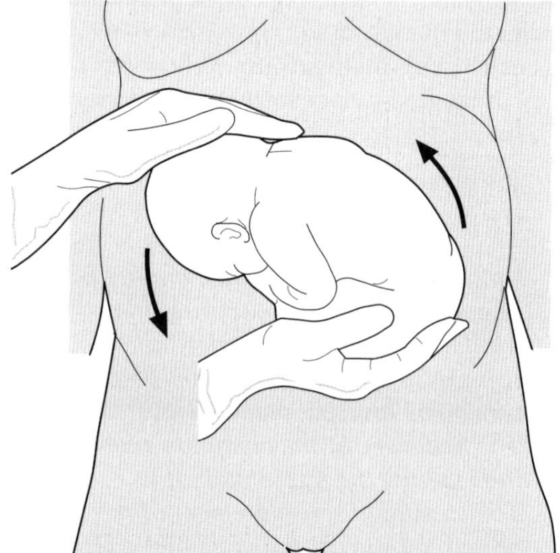

Figure 26.2 External cephalic version: one hand elevates the breech and the other provides pressure behind the fetal head, neck and back.

- If the woman is Rh negative, blood should be drawn for Kleihauer testing and an appropriate dose of Rh immune globulin given.

- Although there are some studies that support the use of uterine tocolysis to aid ECV the results are mixed and most will not use routine tocolysis. However, if attempted version without tocolysis fails, and the failure is thought to be due to good uterine tone, it is rational to consider tocolysis. The options include intravenous ritodine, subcutaneous terbutaline and sublingual or intravenous nitroglycerine, as outlined in the section on acute tocolysis in Chapter 26. The longer acting agents ritodrine and terbutaline are preferable.
- On rare occasions, if the need to achieve external cephalic version is felt to be compelling, epidural or spinal anaesthesia may increase the chance of success. Obviously the risks of the regional anaesthetic have to be balanced against the ultimate goal. In addition, with the removal of maternal pain sensation the obstetrician has to be very careful to avoid using excessive force in these circumstances.
- A reasonable compromise in cases of failed ECV for breech presentation is to assess the cervix on the morning of the booked elective caesarean section. If the cervix is favourable the epidural is established and ECV performed. If the fetus is converted to a cephalic presentation, oxytocin and amniotomy induction of labour can be in instituted and caesarean delivery potentially avoided.

Predictive factors

There are a number of factors which increase or diminish the chance of successful version:

- *Parity* is the most important and success rates are much higher in multiparous women, probably due to diminished abdominal and uterine muscle tone.
- *Gestational age:* the closer to term the lower the success rate. This is particularly evident when version is attempted at 40 weeks gestation or later, as the relative fetus to amniotic fluid volume ratio works against successful version.
- *Anterior placenta* may reduce the chances of success but this is not a major factor.
- *Obesity* reduces the chances of success.
- *Frank breech presentation* with the legs splinting the fetal body is less amenable to version compared with complete or footling breech.

Complications

- Abruptio placentae.
- Feto-maternal bleed which may initiate or worsen isoimmunization.
- Umbilical cord entanglement which may cause abnormal fetal heart rate patterns with variable deceleration, prolonged deceleration or fetal bradycardia. If sustained this may lead to fetal asphyxia. If this occurs one may have to turn the fetus back to the previous malpresentation in an attempt to alleviate the cord entanglement. On rare occasions this is the complication that leads to immediate delivery.

Internal podalic version

Internal podalic version involves the obstetrician placing one hand inside the uterus to turn the fetus from transverse or oblique lie to breech presentation. Probably the only justifiable indication for internal podalic version and breech extraction in modern obstetrics,

INTERNAL PODALIC VERSION

'And then let him put his hands gently into the mouth of the womb, having first made it gentle and slippery with much oil; and when his hand is in let him find out the form and situation of the child ... and so turn him that his feet may come forwards ... and when he hath them both out, let him join them both together, and so by little and little let him draw the whole body from the womb.'

Ambroise Paré
The Works of Ambroise Paré (1549). Translated by T. H. Johnson. London: Clark, 1678

when caesarean section is an available alternative, is in delivery of the second twin. The risk of uterine rupture and fetal trauma with internal version associated with singleton pregnancy and neglected transverse lie or shoulder presentation in advanced labour is no longer acceptable.

A sine qua non for the performance of internal version is adequate analgesia and uterine relaxation. Epidural or spinal anaesthesia will provide good analgesia but no uterine relaxation. Thus, this procedure should either be carried out under general anaesthesia with halogenated agents for uterine relaxation or under regional anaesthesia with uterine tocolysis, usually in the form of intravenous nitroglycerine (see acute tocolysis, p 287). The importance of good uterine relaxation for the safe performance of internal podalic version and breech extraction cannot be over-emphasized. The ease of this procedure and the lack of trauma to the fetus and the uterus depend entirely upon adequate uterine relaxation.

Recognition of fetal landmarks

Practice is required to become familiar with palpation of fetal anatomical landmarks to delineate the correct position and lie of the fetus. This familiarity can be gained by practicing palpation of the newly delivered infant with one's eyes closed. The main landmarks and potential pitfalls are as follows:

- *Foot and hand:* The toes of the foot are roughly equal in length and the separation between the big toe and the others is less distinct. The fingers of the hand are not equal and the separation between the thumb and the remaining fingers is obvious. The heel of the foot is more prominent than the heel of the hand. It is possible to tell whether the hand is right or left by 'shaking hands with the fetus' (Fig 26.3). To a degree the same can be said for 'shaking hands with the foot'.
- *The shoulder* can be recognized by the confluence of the humerus, scapula and clavicle. If in doubt the adjacent ribs can often be palpated.
- *Knee and elbow:* The flexed elbow has a prominent olecranon process, whereas the flexed knee has a dimple between the patella and tibia (Fig 26.4).
- *Mouth and anus:* Usually these can be easily distinguished but in an oedematous face presentation the mouth may be mistaken for the anus. The anus is smaller with greater tone and the adjacent ridges of the spines of the sacrum can usually be felt. In the case of the mouth the softer lips and adjacent gums and tongue should help make the distinction.

Technique

- With a long glove and the hand and forearm well lubricated the operator introduces the hand gently into the vagina and uterus. The external hand rests on the abdomen. Provided adequate uterine relaxation has been achieved the membranes should not be tense and one

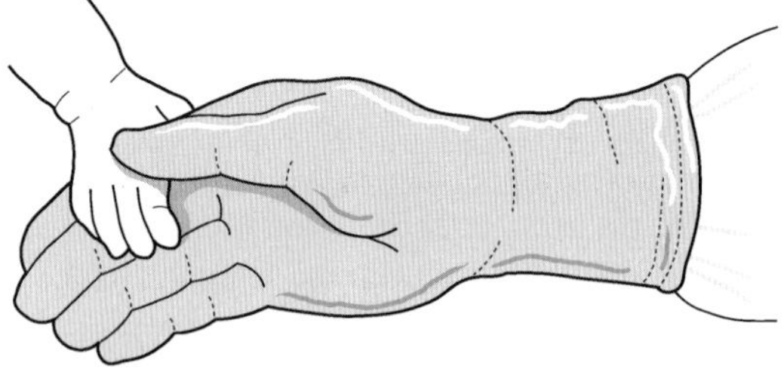

Figure 26.3 Internal podalic version: distinguishing the particular hand by 'shaking hands with the fetus'.

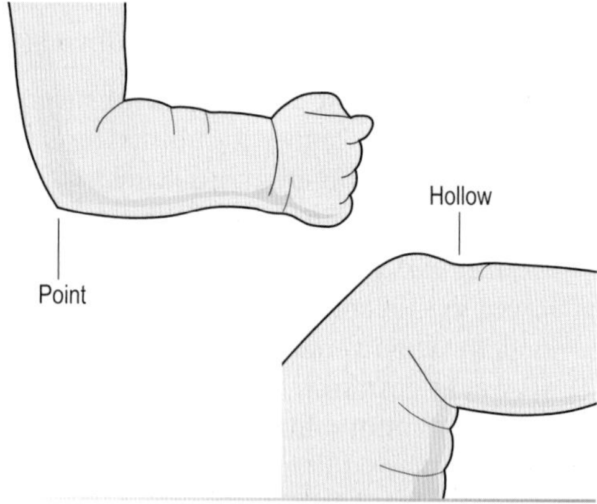

Figure 26.4 Internal podalic version: distinguishing features between the elbow and the knee.

should be able to establish the lie and position of the fetus, with particular reference to the anatomical landmarks noted above.

- The anterior fetal foot should be identified, grasped and steady but gentle downward traction applied. The external hand helps by manipulating the fetal trunk and head to the vertical position (Fig 26.5). If it is possible to grasp both feet this is most desirable (Fig 26.6).
- At some point during this downward traction the membranes will rupture. However, by this time the fetus has been converted to a longitudinal lie and the breech will already be entering the pelvis. If it has only been possible to grasp the posterior leg, then during the downward traction there should be 180° rotation, such that the posterior leg becomes anterior. This prevents the anterior buttock from becoming impacted above the symphysis (Fig 26.7). The remainder of the delivery is accomplished by breech extraction as outlined in Chapter 14.
- At times the membranes rupture during the manipulations and the fetal hand and arm will prolapse. It is difficult and often

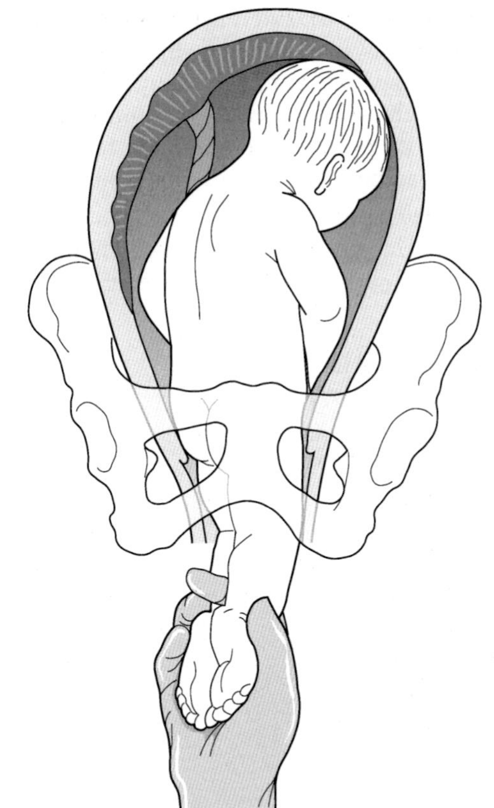

Figure 26.6 Internal podalic version: ideally both feet are grasped and with steady downward traction the fetus is converted to a longitudinal lie.

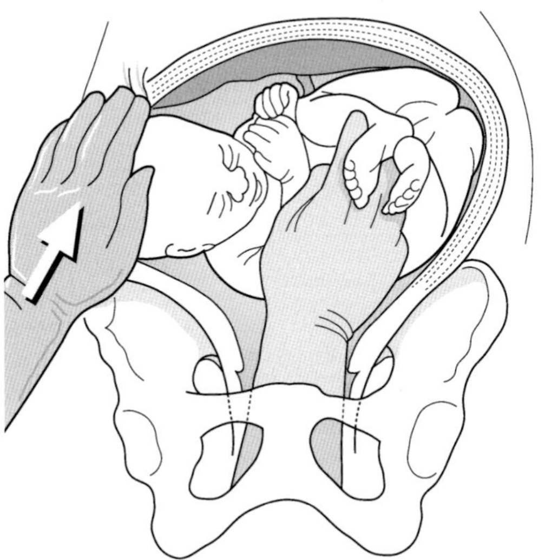

Figure 26.5 Internal podalic version: the external hand manipulates the fetal head and trunk to the vertical position and the internal hand seeks the anterior fetal foot.

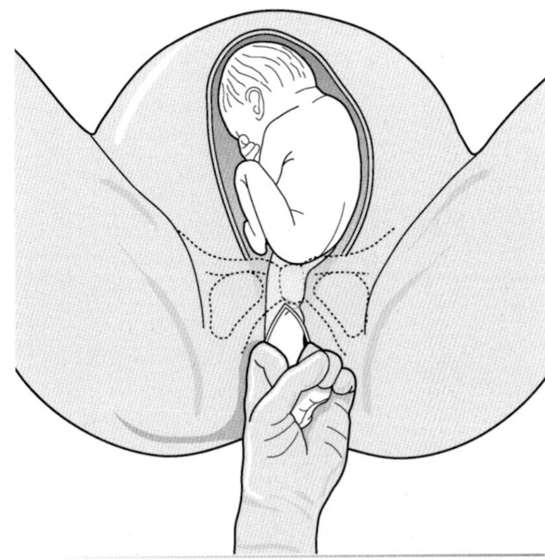

Figure 26.7 Internal podalic version: if only the posterior leg is delivered the anterior buttock may straddle the symphysis and become obstructed.

traumatic to try and replace the hand and arm. Thus, one should just proceed and grasp the foot, or feet, and pull them down through the introitus. As the fetal body turns the arm will automatically follow and can be delivered with the shoulders.

- Following delivery of the infant the uterus, cervix and upper vagina should be carefully explored for any lacerations.

Bibliography

American College of Obstetricians and Gynecologists. Practice Bulletin No. 13. External cephalic version. Washington, DC: ACOG, 2000.

Boggess KA, Chisholm CA. Delivery of the non-vertex second twin: a review of the literature. Obstet Gynecol Surv 1997; 52:728–735.

Dufour P, Vinatier D, Vanderstichele S, Ducloy AS, Monnier JC. Intravenous nitroglycerin for internal podalic version of the second twin in transverse lie. Obstet Gynecol 1998; 92:416–419.

Rabinovic IJ, Barkai G, Richman B, Serr DM, Mashiach S. Internal podalic version with unruptured membranes for the second twin in transverse lie. Obstet Gynecol 1988; 71:428–429.

Uterine tamponade

When oxytocic agents fail to control postpartum haemorrhage, examination under anaesthesia is warranted. These cases may end in laparotomy and, if conservative surgical methods fail, hysterectomy is commonly required. A survey in the UK found that hysterectomy was the most common surgical procedure in women who did not respond to combinations of uterotonics, and that methods to reduce the need for hysterectomy were urgently needed.[1]

Uterine tamponade is a less invasive procedure which is simple, does not require major surgery, can be done within minutes, and will often immediately reduce or stop the bleeding. It can be tried as soon as uterotonics are found to be ineffective. If it stops the bleeding this will be apparent within minutes and the need for definitive surgery either averted or confirmed promptly. Thus, it may avoid the need for laparotomy and hysterectomy as well as reducing the need for blood transfusion with its inherent risks. It is ideal for postpartum haemorrhage due to non-traumatic causes and for those without any retained tissue in utero.

Rationale

A principle of first aid to stop bleeding is to apply pressure to the bleeding site sufficient to compress the blood vessels. The pressure created on the blood vessels can be end-on or side-on compression that is greater than the pressure of blood flow in that vessel. Once the applied pressure stops the bleeding, the blood can clot and form a permanent seal. Blood flows into the uterus with a mean arterial pressure of about 90 mmHg, although the spiral arteriolar arrangement in the uterus probably lowers the arterial pressure as the blood flows through the uterine muscle. After placental separation the venous sinuses and spiral arterioles are exposed, which results in bleeding from the placental bed if the uterus does not contract and retract efficiently.

If, despite the appropriate use of oxytocic drugs, uterine atony continues, bimanual compression is undertaken after excluding any obvious lower genital tract trauma. If this does not stop the bleeding the uterus should be explored under anaesthesia to exclude retained products within the uterus and any uterine or lower genital tract trauma. If the bleeding is due to uterine atony a 'tamponade test' is useful to decide whether uterine tamponade itself would be therapeutic or whether laparotomy is needed to arrest the bleeding.[2]

Techniques

Uterine packing

In the past, uterine tamponade could only be achieved by packing the uterus with cotton gauze. While this can be life-saving, there are a number of disadvantages: general, spinal or epidural anaesthesia is needed, the packing is done blindly, and it is hard to be sure that the entire uterine cavity is tightly packed. Incomplete and ineffectual packing can occur due to the fear of perforation (Fig 26.8). Packing the uterus in this manner requires several metres of 10 cm gauze tightly packed into the uterine cavity manually and with ring forceps. The vagina is also firmly packed and a Foley catheter placed in the bladder.[3] The gauze packing is removed in 12–24 hours.

Whether packing has been effective is not known for several minutes as the blood has to first soak through the pack before revealing itself at the cervix. To overcome some of these difficulties a sterile plastic bag may be introduced into the uterus first and the bag then packed with gauze. This facilitates more complete packing of the uterine cavity and makes for easier removal of the gauze. However, gauze packing can be cumbersome to place and remove, takes time, and is not always effective.[4] The use of balloon tamponade may overcome some of these drawbacks.

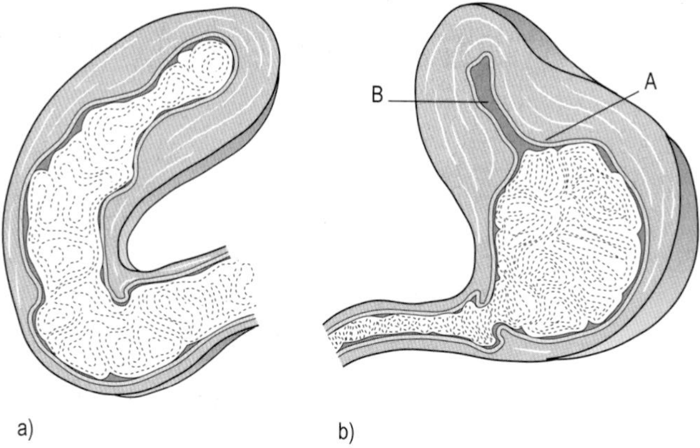

Figure 26.8 Correct and incorrect method of uterine packing: (a) uterus carefully packed with gauze, (b) uterus with only the lower uterine segment packed. A = retraction ring, B = upper cavity of uterus unpacked.

Balloon tamponade

There are several reports in the literature describing success using hydrostatic balloon tamponade either alone or in combination with additional surgical methods. Different types of balloons have been used, including the Sengstaken–Blakemore tube[5–7] (Fig 26.9), Rüsch urological balloon[8] and the Bakri balloon[9] (Fig 26.10) filled with sterile water or saline at room or higher temperature.[10] Most experience is with the Sengstaken–Blakemore tube, used by surgeons for many decades to arrest bleeding from oesophageal varices. When uterotonics and uterine massage do not stop the bleeding, causes of local trauma or retained tissue in the uterus should be excluded. Under adequate analgesia a Sengstaken–Blakemore tube (pre-sterilized by gas or by soaking in 2% glutaraldehyde for 20 minutes) is inserted into the uterine cavity. The tube distal to the stomach balloon is cut off to facilitate easy insertion and retention of the balloon in the uterine cavity. Insertion may be achieved by performing a vaginal examination, identifying the cervix and manually passing the stomach balloon into the uterine cavity without need for complex anaesthesia. Alternatively, under direct vision a vaginal speculum is passed and the anterior lip of the cervix is secured with sponge forceps. The stomach balloon of the Sengstaken–Blakemore tube is held with another sponge forceps and is inserted into the uterine cavity. The stomach balloon is filled with about 200–500 ml of warm saline or sterile water. Care must be taken not to overfill the balloon which may cause it to bulge out through the cervix and to be expelled.

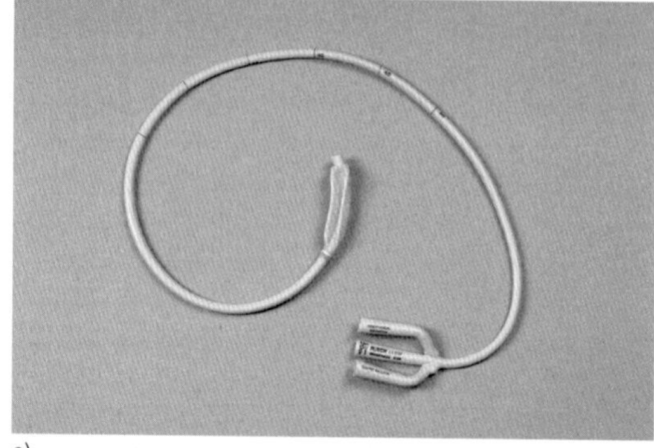

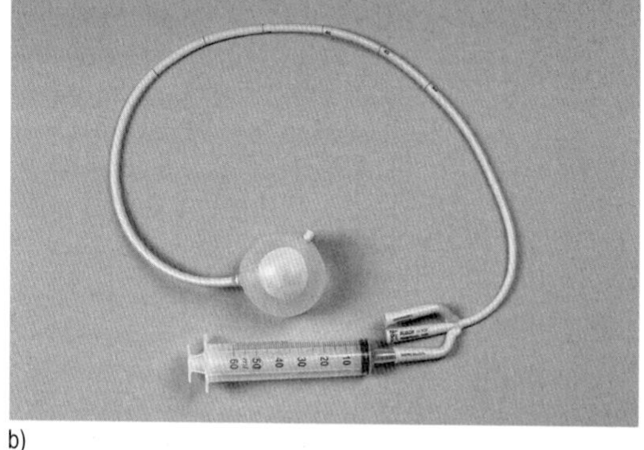

Figure 26.9 Sengstaken–Blakemore tube: (a) uninflated, (b) inflated.

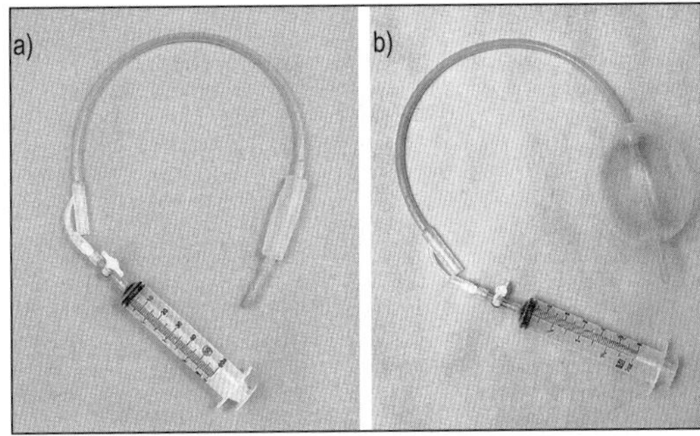

Figure 26.10 Bakri balloon: (a) uninflated, (b) inflated.

If the Sengstaken–Blakemore tube, Rüsch urological balloon or Bakri balloon are not available a simplified version can be fashioned as follows. Tie the cuff of a surgical glove to a straight plastic urinary catheter with any suture material. Place the glove and attached catheter into the uterus and fill the glove via the catheter with a large syringe, using the same principles outlined above.[11] Others have improvised by using a condom to provide balloon tamponade.[12]

In the case reports available in the literature the volume used has been arbitrary (200–500 ml) and the practice has been to fill the balloon until part of it is visible via the cervix. At this stage if there is no bleeding through the cervix and none through the drainage channel of the catheter the test of tamponade is pronounced successful and no further fluid is added.[2] If bleeding continues the test is a failure and further surgical treatment is needed. Further research is in progress to allow measurement of the pressure within the balloon. When the intra-balloon pressure exceeds the arterial pressure of the patient no additional fluid need be added. At this stage the bleeding should stop. If not, it indicates the need for surgery in the form of laparotomy provided one is sure the bleeding is not from the lower genital tract.

Whether tamponade is going to be successful or not is known within minutes. Once found to be successful the uterine fundus is palpated abdominally and a mark is made with a pen to provide a reference line from which any enlargement or distension of the uterus would be judged during the period of observation.

Care after tamponade

The woman should be kept fasting and under close surveillance after insertion of the balloon. Her pulse, blood pressure, uterine fundal height and signs of any vaginal bleeding or bleeding via the lumen of the catheter should be monitored. Her temperature should be recorded every 2 hours and urinary output measured hourly via an indwelling Foley catheter. The woman should receive broad-spectrum antibiotics from the time of insertion for up to 3 days. A low dose infusion of oxytocin, 40 units in 1 L of normal saline, is continued to keep the uterus contracted over the balloon. After 6 hours, if the uterine fundus remains at the same level and there is no active bleeding around the balloon via the cervix or via the central lumen of the catheter, it is safe to remove the catheter provided the woman is stable and adequate blood replacement has been given if required.

First the balloon is deflated but is not removed for 30 minutes. Provided there is no bleeding the oxytocin infusion is stopped for another 30 minutes and if there is still no bleeding the catheter is removed. These precautions are taken in case the woman starts bleeding when the balloon is deflated or the oxytocin is stopped, in which case the balloon can be re-inflated. In our experience there has not been an instance when the balloon needed to be refilled.[2] Six hours is usually sufficient for the placental bed to clot and stop bleeding. Few immediate problems such as bleeding or sepsis, or long-term complications such as menstrual problems or infertility have been reported.

In one series, 16 consecutive cases were described in which balloon tamponade was used as a last measure before embarking on laparotomy and it was successful in all but two cases.[2] This case series and others illustrate that balloon tamponade and its associated 'tamponade test' can be used in cases of primary and secondary postpartum haemorrhage, and for cases of bleeding after second trimester miscarriage.[13,14] It may also be considered after caesarean section in cases without discrete bleeding points or retained tissue:

for example, to provide tamponade of the poorly contracting lower uterine segment in placenta praevia.

About 80–90% of cases of primary postpartum haemorrhage are due to uterine atony. In those cases unresponsive to the usual oxytocic drugs, laparotomy and surgical measures, such as uterine compression sutures, major vessel ligation and hysterectomy may be required. Another alternative is interventional radiological embolisation of the internal iliac arteries. These procedures are covered elsewhere in this chapter but all require sophisticated facilities. If these facilities are not available, balloon tamponade and uterine packing can be used as an alternative or as a stop-gap measure until the woman can be transferred to an appropriate hospital or the personnel brought to her.

References

1. Mousa HA, Alfirevic Z. Major postpartum haemorrhage: survey of maternity units in the United Kingdom. Acta Obstet Gynecol Scand 2002; 81:727–730.
2. Condous GS, Arulkumaran S, Symonds I, Chapman R, Sinha A, Razvi K. The 'Tamponade Test' in the management of massive postpartum hemorrhage. Obstet Gynecol 2003; 101:767–772.
3. Maier RC. Control of postpartum hemorrhage with uterine packing. Am J Obstet Gynecol 1993; 169:17–23.
4. Drucker M, Wallach RC. Uterine packing: a re-appraisal. Mount Sinai J Med 1979; 46:191–194.
5. Katesmark M, Brown R, Raju KS. Successful use of a Sengstaken–Blakemore tube to control massive postpartum hemorrhage. Br J Obstet Gynaecol 1994; 101:259–260.
6. Condie RG, Buxton EJ, Payne ES. Successful use of a Sengstaken–Blakemore tube to control massive hemorrhage. Br J Obstet Gynaecol 1994; 101:1023-1024.
7. Chan C, Razvi K, Tham KF, Arulkumaran S. The use of a Sengstaken–Blakemore tube to control postpartum hemorrhage. Int J Gynaecol Obstet 1997; 58:251–252.
8. Johanson R, Kumar M, Obhrai M, Young P. Management of massive postpartum hemorrhage: use of a hydrostatic balloon catheter to avoid laparotomy. Br J Obstet Gynaecol 2001; 108:420–422.
9. Bakri YN, Amri A, Abdul Jabbar F. Tamponade-balloon for obstetrical bleeding. Int J Gynaecol Obstet 2001; 74:139–142.
10. Turner GD. Uterine haemorrhage controlled by an intrauterine balloon insufflated with hot water. Hosp Med 2002; 63:438.
11. Baskett TF. Surgical management of severe obstetric haemorrhage: experience with an obstetric haemorrhage equipment tray. J Obstet Gynaecol Can 2004; 26:805–808.
12. Akhter S, Begum MR, Kabir Z, Rashid M, Laila TR, Zabeau F. Use of a condom to control massive postpartum haemorrhage. Med Gen Med 2003; 5:38.
13. Danso D, Reginald P. Combined B-Lynch suture with intrauterine balloon catheter triumphs over massive postpartum haemorrhage. Br J Obstet Gynaecol 2002; 109:963.
14. Marcovici I, Scoccia B. Postpartum hemorrhage and intrauterine balloon tamponade: a report of three cases. J Reprod Med 1999; 44:122–126.

Uterine compression sutures

Uterine compression sutures of an improvised type have been used for decades: for example, figure-of-eight sutures in the lower uterine segment in cases of placenta praevia. In recent years more specific techniques for the application of compression sutures have been developed. In most cases these haemostatic sutures are used at the time of caesarean section; although they are occasionally used when all other methods of haemostasis have failed following vaginal delivery, and laparotomy is undertaken with a view to definitive arrest of haemorrhage by hysterectomy. In such cases major vessel ligation and/or uterine compression sutures may be used as a last-ditch attempt before resorting to hysterectomy. As with uterine tamponade, major vessel ligation and other rarely performed procedures it is wise for each labour unit to have the equipment and instruments readily available in an identifiable pack so that it can be made rapidly available when needed.[1,2] Diagrams of the various techniques of compression sutures can be added to the obstetric haemorrhage pack.[2]

Strong suture material is required for compression sutures, such as No. 1 polyglactin 910 (Vicryl), polyglycolic acid (Dexon) or *poliglecaprone* (Monocryl). If available, No. 2 chromic catgut is also suitable. For most compression sutures a curved needle of at least 70–80 mm and sometimes larger is required; straight needles should be 8–10 cm long. In many of the standard packaged suture materials the needles are not of adequate dimension. It may therefore be advisable to have larger-eyed needles available in the haemorrhage equipment pack.

With all of the techniques for uterine compression sutures it is important to assess the efficacy of the technique. To this end the patient should be placed in the Lloyd Davies (frog-legged) position and so that an assistant can remove any clots from the vagina. With both hands providing compression of the uterus it can be seen whether or not this will stop the bleeding. If it does the compression suture is applied and, upon its completion, a careful appraisal will confirm whether the bleeding has been controlled – the 'test of tamponade'.[3]

B-Lynch suture

The first of the uterine compression sutures was described and named by B-Lynch and colleagues in 1997.[4] This type of suture is performed following low transverse caesarean section and is usually done for uterine atony unresponsive to oxytocic agents. With the uterus out of the abdominal incision and using a large (≥ 70 mm) round bodied, preferably blunt needle the first suture is placed from outside in to the uterine cavity approximately 3 cm below the lateral margin of the lower transverse caesarean incision and guided through the uterine cavity and out 3 cm above the caesarean incision. The suture material is then looped over the fundus of the uterus down to the posterior wall of the uterus opposite the caesarean incision. The suture is carried through the posterior wall into the uterine cavity and out on the other side roughly opposite the lateral margins of the caesarean incision. This suture is then looped over the posterior wall of the uterus down the anterior wall and placed through the uterus 3 cm above the other lateral margin of the caesarean incision and out 3 cm below (Fig 26.11a). Each of the suture insertion points is placed about 4 cm from the lateral border of the uterus. The two ends of the suture are then progressively tightened with an assistant applying continuous anteroposterior compression to the uterus with both hands. The loops of the sutures over the fundus of the uterus are placed approximately 4 cm from each lateral border of the uterus. It is very important that there be progressive compression and tightening of the suture which may take 1–2 minutes to be completely effective. Once it is achieved the two ends of the suture are

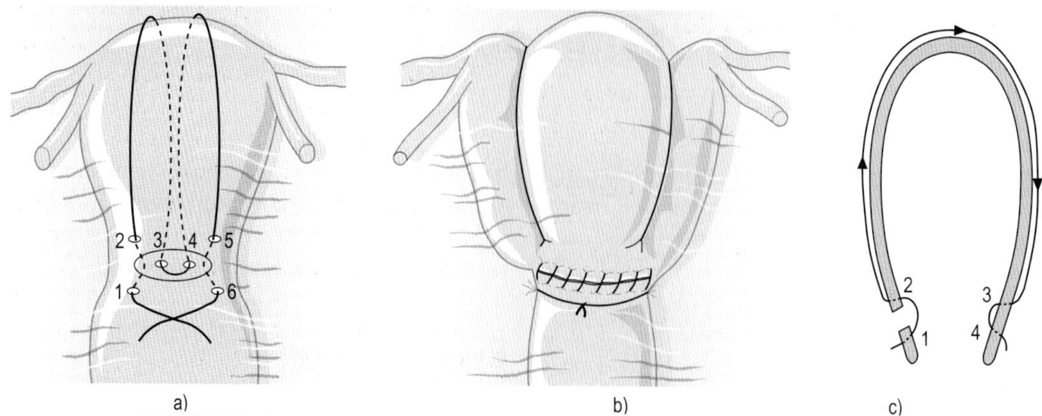

Figure 26.11 B-Lynch compression suture.

tied across the midline below the transverse caesarean incision (Fig 26.11b). At this point the assistant carefully checks the blood loss from the vagina to ensure that the suture has passed the 'tamponade test'. If so, the low transverse incision is closed in the routine fashion followed by closure of the abdomen. The placement of the suture is further illustrated in Figure 26.11c.

Modified B-Lynch suture

A simplified adaptation of the B-Lynch suture has been proposed by Bhal et al.[5] This retains the same principles but uses two separate sutures, one for each side. Figure 26.12a shows the entry and exit points of both sutures. As in the B-Lynch technique, progressive manual compression and tying down of the suture is vital. As shown in Figure 26.12b each of the sutures is tied across in the midline. The advantages of this technique are that it is a little easier to remember and by using one suture on each side the standard length (70 cm) of a polyglactin 910 suture is adequate on each side. With the B-Lynch technique one may have to tie two suture lengths together to achieve the entire suture placement.

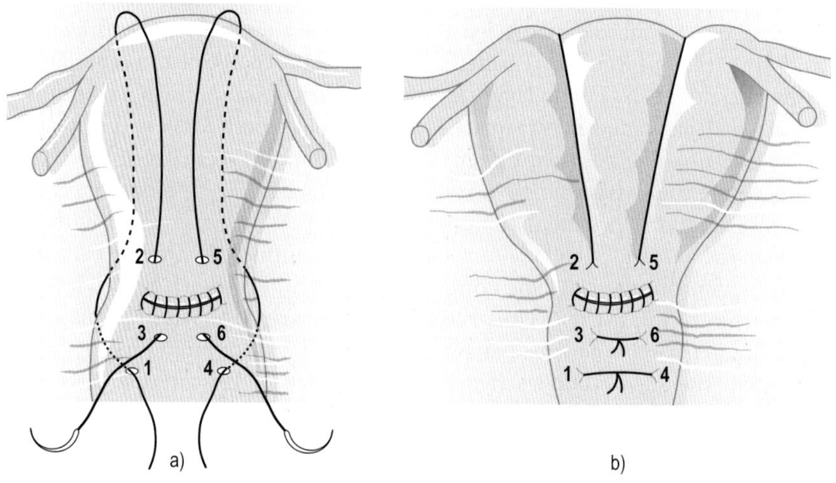

Figure 26.12 Modification of B-Lynch compression suture (After Bhal et al[5]).

Vertical uterine suture

This is an even simpler modification proposed by Hayman et al.[6] Using a straight needle and ensuring that the bladder is well reflected the individual vertical sutures are passed from anterior to posterior approximately 3 cm below the site of a transverse caesarean incision. Depending on the width of the uterus anywhere from 2 to 5 of these sutures may be placed. The usual manual compression is carried out and the sutures are tied at the fundus (Fig 26.13). The advantages of this technique are its simplicity, the fact that it can be done with or without a caesarean incision and the variable number of sutures which can be placed depending upon the width of the uterine fundus.

Square compression sutures

In this technique the anterior and posterior walls of the uterus are compressed together using a straight needle passing from front to back through the entire uterine wall and, moving laterally approximately 3 cm coming back through the uterine wall from back to front. From this exit point the needle is placed 3 cm below from front to back and then laterally 3 cm to a final pass of the needle from back to front to complete the square (Fig 26.14). The anterior and posterior anterior walls are then compressed together and the suture snugly tied down.[7] This technique can be repeated at a number of sites, if necessary to cover the entire uterine cavity.

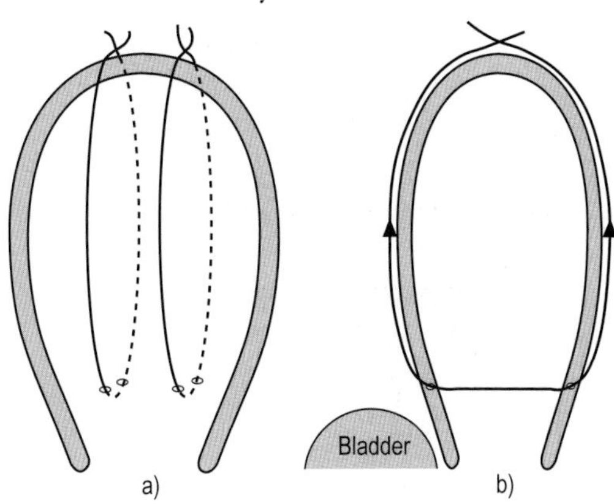

Figure 26.13 Vertical compression sutures.

In cases of bleeding from the lower uterine segment in placenta praevia, with or without partial accreta, this technique may be used in the lower segment alone, assuming the upper uterine segment is well contracted.

In many cases the application of an individual compression suture technique will be adequate. In others more than one type of suture may be necessary. For example, the B-Lynch technique may leave 'shoulders' of a very broad uterine fundus that appear not to be compressed. In such cases additional square sutures may be useful.

In all of the techniques it is important to ensure that the lower uterine segment is not completely obliterated and that there is egress for blood and lochia. This is particularly so with the use of square compression sutures in the lower segment associated with placenta praevia.

Complications of compression sutures are relatively few. With all techniques it is important to ensure that the bladder is reflected inferiorly to avoid inclusion in the suture. Theoretically, as the uterus involutes, long-lasting suture material may remain as loops and bowel could potentially become

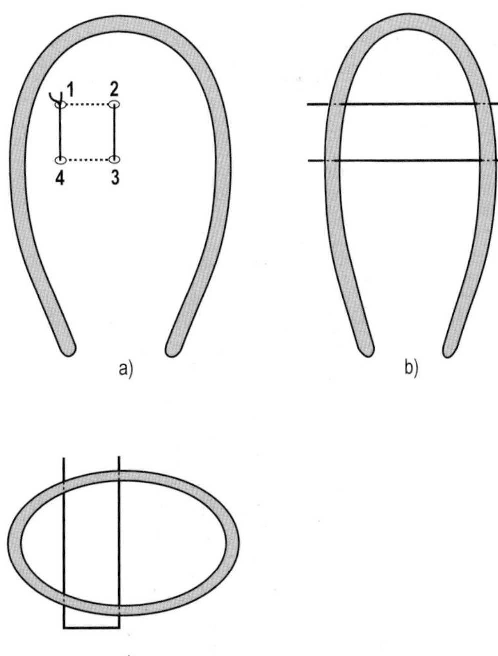

Figure 26.14 Square compression sutures.

entangled and obstructed. No cases of this have been described. For this reason, at least on theoretical grounds, long-acting sutures such as PDS should be avoided. Isolated cases of pyometra have been described. In most cases, however, follow-up hysterosalpingogram and hysteroscopy have shown a normal uterine cavity and, where it has been desired, subsequent fertility has been achieved. In some cases at caesarean section in a subsequent pregnancy a slight grooving of the uterine muscle from the vertical suture can be seen, so presumably a degree of ischaemic necrosis occurs in some cases.

Thus, by and large, it seems that the complications of these techniques are limited and these must be put in the context of a procedure that is usually being done as a last resort before moving to hysterectomy. In most, but not all cases reported, uterine compression sutures have been successful in arresting haemorrhage and avoiding hysterectomy and it is with this perspective that subsequent effects on fertility should be judged.

References

1. Anderson ER, Black R, Brocklehurst P. Acute obstetric emergency drill in England and Wales: a survey of practice. Br J Obstet Gynaecol 2005; 112:372–375.
2. Baskett TF. Surgical management of severe obstetric haemorrhage: experience with an obstetric equipment tray. J Obstet Gynaecol Can 2004; 26:805–808.
3. Condous GS, Arulkumaran S, Symonds I, Chapman R, Sinha A, Razvi K. The 'tamponade test' in the management of massive postpartum hemorrhage. Obstet Gynecol 2003; 101:767–772.
4. B-Lynch C, Cocker A, Lowell AH, Abu J, Cowan MJ. The B-Lynch surgical technique for control of massive postpartum haemorrhage: an alternative to hysterectomy? Five cases reported. Br J Obstet Gynaecol 1997; 104:372–375.
5. Bhal K, Bhal N, Mullik V, Shankar L. The uterine compression suture – a valuable approach to control major haemorrhage with lower segment caesarean section. J Obstet Gynaecol 2005; 25:10–14.
6. Hayman RC, Arulkumaran S, Steer PJ. Uterine compression sutures: surgical management of postpartum hemorrhage. Obstet Gynecol 2002; 99:502–506.
7. Cho JH, Jun SH, Lee CN. Hemostatic suturing technique for uterine bleeding during cesarean delivery. Obstet Gynecol 2000; 96:129–131.

Bibliography

Allahdin S, Aird C, Danielian P. B-Lynch sutures for major primary postpartum haemorrhage at caesarean section. J Obstet Gynaecol 2006; 26:638–642.

Dacus AV, Busowski MT, Busowski JD. Surgical treatment of uterine atony employing the B-Lynch technique. J Matern Fetal Med 2000; 9:194–196.

El-Hamamy E, B-Lynch C. A worldwide review of the uses of uterine compression suture techniques as alternative to hysterectomy in the management of severe postpartum hemorrhage. J Obstet Gynaecol 2005; 25:143–149.

Ferguson JE, Bourgeiois FJ, Underwood PB. B-Lynch suture for postpartum hemorrhage. Obstet Gynecol 2000; 95:1020–1022.

Mousa HA, Walkinshaw W. Major postpartum haemorrhage. Curr Opin Obstet Gynecol 2001; 13:595–603.

Price N, B-Lynch C. Technical subscription of the B-Lynch brace suture for treatment of massive postpartum hemorrhage and review of published cases. Int J Fertil 2005; 50:148–163.

Smith KL, Baskett TF. Uterine compression sutures as an alternative to hysterectomy for severe postpartum haemorrhage. J Obstet Gynaecol Can 2003; 25:197–200.

Tamizian O, Arulkumaran S. Surgical management of postpartum haemorrhage. Curr Opin Obstet Gynecol 2001; 13:127–131.

Wohlmuth CT, Gumbs J, Quebral-Ivie J. B-Lynch suture: A case series. Int J Fertil 2005; 50:164–173.

Pelvic vessel ligation and embolisation

In other parts of this book, measures to deal with life-threatening obstetric haemorrhage have been outlined including: the use of oxytocic agents, uterine tamponade, uterine compression sutures and hysterectomy. In this section we are concerned with the role of major pelvic vessel ligation or embolisation when other methods to control bleeding have failed. The main indications for pelvic vessel ligation or embolisation are bleeding of uterine origin in which preservation of the uterus is sought, and in vaginal and paravaginal trauma when local measures fail to achieve haemostasis. These indications may include haemorrhage from placentae praevia, placenta accreta, abruptio placentae with Couvelaire uterus, uterine atony unresponsive to oxytocics, extension of lower segment caesarean incision into the broad ligament or vagina, uterine rupture, paravaginal haematoma, and extensive cervical and/or vaginal lacerations.

For cases of haemorrhage occurring at the time of caesarean section, or at laparotomy for uterine rupture, recourse to major vessel ligation at an early stage in an attempt to preserve the uterus is logical. For cases delivered vaginally other efforts to control haemorrhage without moving to laparotomy and pelvic vessel ligation should be tried. If these are unsuccessful one has the option of either resorting to laparotomy and pelvic vessel ligation or, if facilities are available, interventional radiology and pelvic vessel embolisation.

Anatomy and haemodynamics

The common iliac artery bifurcates at the level of lumbo-sacral junction in front of the sacro-iliac joint. The external iliac artery runs lateral and superior, while the internal iliac (hypogastric) artery descends medially and inferiorly toward the sacral hollow. The ureter runs antero-laterally to the internal iliac artery just below the bifurcation. Posterior to the internal iliac artery lies the internal iliac vein, which is very close and vulnerable to trauma during attempts to ligate the artery. The internal iliac artery runs for 3–4 cm before dividing into anterior and posterior divisions. The posterior division divides into three branches: the ilio-lumbar, lateral sacral and the superior gluteal arteries – the latter leaves the pelvis through the greater sciatic foramen to supply the gluteal muscles. The anterior division usually has eight branches: the superior and inferior vesical, obturator, middle haemorrhoidal, uterine, vaginal and the terminal internal pudendal and inferior gluteal arteries (Fig 26.15). There are, however, variations and the internal pudendal and obturator arteries can arise from the posterior division.

There are a number of collateral anastomoses, the three main ones being:[1]

- the lumbar artery arises from aorta and anastomoses with the ilio-lumbar artery from the internal iliac artery
- the middle sacral artery from the aorta anastomoses with the lateral sacral artery of the internal iliac artery
- the superior haemorrhoidal artery, which is the terminal branch of the inferior mesenteric artery from the aorta, joins the middle haemorrhoidal artery of the internal iliac artery (Fig 26.16).

Other collaterals that may link the aorta with branches of the internal iliac artery include: the ovarian artery and the uterine artery; the femoral artery with the internal pudendal artery via the profunda femoris and femoral circumflex vessels; and the circumflex iliac arteries from the common iliac with the superior gluteal artery of the internal iliac artery.

The haemodynamics of pelvic blood flow after internal artery ligation were demonstrated by Burchell in the 1960s.[2] He showed that unilateral ligation reduced the pulse

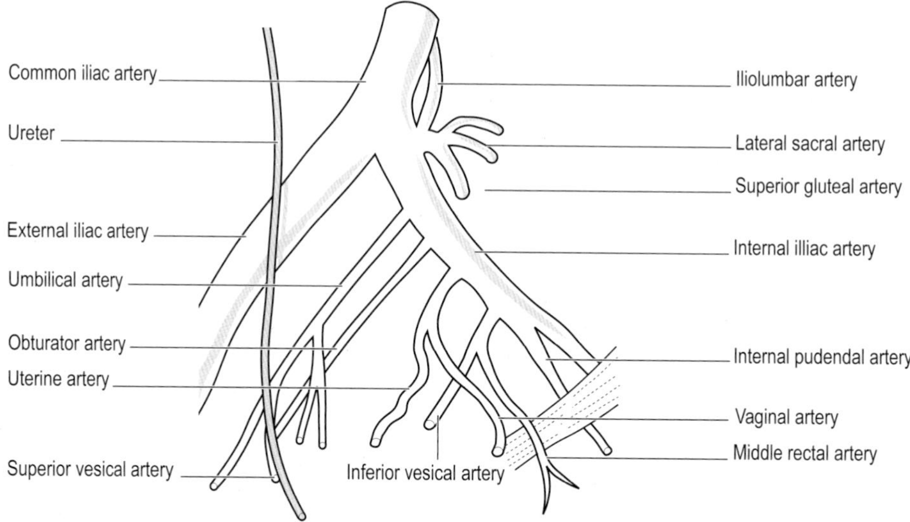

Figure 26.15 Branches of the internal iliac artery.

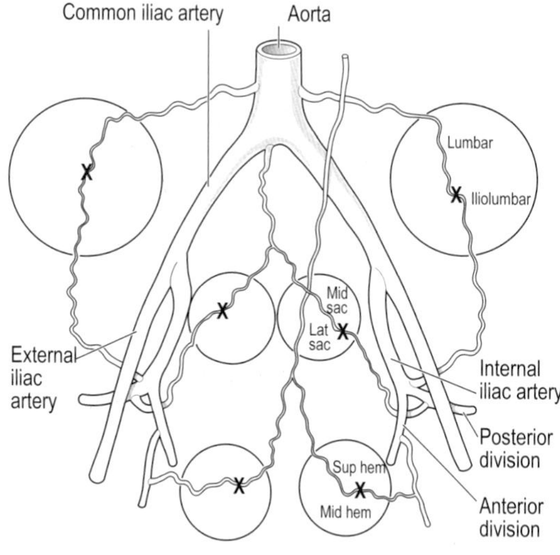

Figure 26.16 The three main anastomoses between branches of the internal iliac artery and the aorta.

pressure by about 75% on that side, and with bilateral ligation the reduction was 85%. The mean arterial pressure was reduced by 25% but the blood flow by almost 50%. Thus, bilateral internal iliac artery ligation almost reduces the pulse pressure to that of a venous system and allows clotting to occur. Blood flow does not stop completely due to the presence of the previously outlined collateral anastomoses. These collateral channels open immediately after ligation of the internal iliac artery and flow is reversed so that all branches of the iliac artery are again filled with flowing blood, but at the reduced pressures noted above. This collateral system opens immediately and is so efficient that even bilateral internal iliac artery ligation does not result in tissue necrosis or interfere with subsequent menstrual or reproductive function.[3]

The uterine artery carries the majority of the blood supply to the body of the uterus. The ovarian artery arises directly from the aorta just below the renal arteries and passes down to the pelvis in the infundibulo-pelvic ligament to the mesovarium and mesosalpinx. It passes superior to the ovary, provides branches to the ovary and tube, and ends by anastomosing with the ascending uterine artery about the level of the utero-ovarian ligament. It thus contributes to the blood supply of the uterine fundus.

Uterine artery ligation

Uterine artery ligation is the simplest major vessel ligation and may be effective for uterine haemorrhage.[4] It is usually carried out in association with the equally simple ovarian artery ligation. It is only likely to be effective for haemorrhage from the body of the uterus as the technique described involves ligation of the ascending branch of the uterine artery. Haemorrhage from the lower uterine segment, cervix and paracolpos will not be effectively treated by this technique.

The uterus should be elevated out of the abdominal incision and the fundus tilted away from the side to be ligated. Using a large curved tapered needle with No. 0 or 1 absorbable suture the needle is passed through the myometrium from anterior to posterior, about 2 cm medial to the lateral edge of the uterus (Fig 26.17). The suture is then brought back through an avascular space in the broad ligament and tied. Including a good 'cushion' of myometrium ensures inclusion of all branches of the uterine vessels and helps stabilize the ligature (Fig 26.18). The level at which one places the suture is approximately 2–3 cm below a low transverse caesarean incision.

It is important to ensure that the bladder is well away from the placement of the suture to avoid ureteric or bladder injury. The procedure is repeated on the other side. Uterine artery ligation has been reported to have 80–95% success rate in dealing with postpartum haemorrhage unresponsive to oxytocics at the time of caesarean section.[4–6] Not all of us have this high level of success, but uterine artery ligation is very simple, safe, can be rapidly performed and has no detrimental effect on subsequent menstrual and reproductive function.

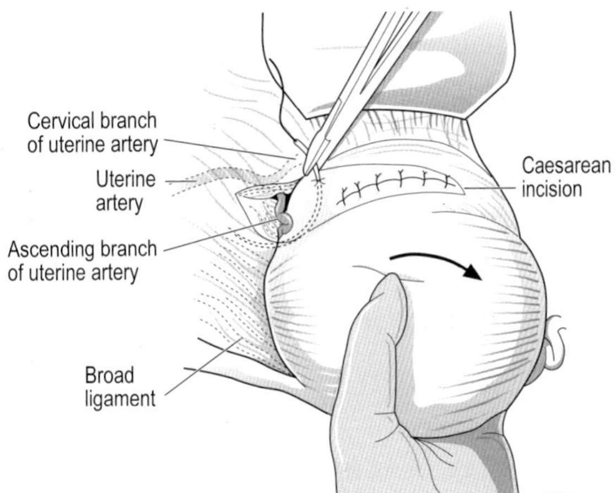

Figure 26.17 Uterine artery ligation: tilt fundus of uterus to opposite side; place suture 2–3 cm below the caesarean incision and include 2–3 cm of the lateral myometrium.

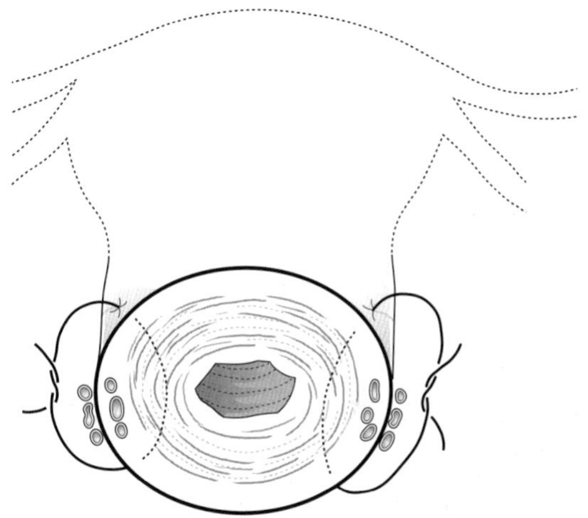

Figure 26.18 Uterine artery ligation: coronal view of lower uterine segment and placement of suture to include adjacent myometrium and all branches of the uterine vessels.

Ovarian artery ligation

Because of the previously mentioned anastomosis of the ovarian artery with the ascending branch of the uterine artery it is logical to include ovarian artery ligation when performing ligation of the uterine artery. The technique is identical to ligation of the uterine artery except that the suture is placed just below the utero-ovarian ligament. Ligation at this point does not interfere with the blood supply to the tube or ovary (Fig 26.19).

Internal iliac artery ligation

Uterine and ovarian ligation can only reduce or stop bleeding from the body of the uterus.

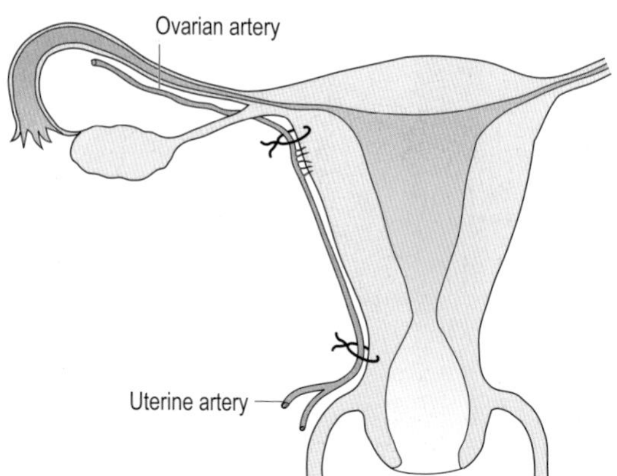

Figure 26.19 Uterine and ovarian artery ligation sites.

Bleeding from the lower uterine segment, cervix, broad ligament and vaginal and paravaginal areas may require internal iliac artery ligation. This is a more intimidating procedure for the general obstetrician and gynaecologist, but the principles are straightforward. The key is to familiarize oneself with the anatomy of the retroperitoneal space, which is best done when performing elective abdominal hysterectomy in gynaecology.

The uterus is elevated out of the abdominal incision and the fundus tilted away from the side to be ligated. The mid portion of the round ligament is clamped and divided between two forceps. This permits entry to the retroperitoneal space and the avascular posterior leaf of the broad ligament is further opened with sharp dissection. Using a moistened gauze on a sponge forceps the retroperitoneal space is opened with gentle blunt dissection. If not immediately visible the common iliac artery and its bifurcation can be located by palpation. At this point the ureter should be identified and retracted medially with the attached peritoneum. Either using a gentle suction cannula or a moistened 'peanut' sponge identify the bifurcation of the common iliac and clear the areola tissue around the internal branch. It is also wise to identify the external iliac artery and be in a position to palpate the femoral pulse. The main hazard is trauma to the adjacent external iliac veins or to the internal iliac vein which lies just beneath the internal iliac artery.

There is a theoretical advantage to ligation of only the anterior division of the internal iliac artery. By ligating the artery distal to the posterior division its terminal superior gluteal artery is preserved and the risk of subsequent ischaemic buttock pain is avoided – although the latter is rare. However, it is not always easy to identify the anterior and posterior divisions and attempts to do so may risk damage to adjacent veins. Thus, it is best to ligate the internal iliac artery about 3 cm from the bifurcation which should avoid the posterior division. It may be helpful to elevate the artery gently with a Babcock clamp and pass a double strand of No. 1 absorbable suture behind the artery with a right angle forceps. Pass the forceps from lateral to medial to reduce the risk of trauma to adjacent veins. The artery is then doubly ligated but not divided (Fig 26.20). The same procedure is carried out on the other side. Success rates with internal iliac ligation are variable, between 40 and 90%.[7–12]

Pelvic vessel embolisation

In the past 25 years numerous reports have confirmed the value of angiographic embolisation of pelvic vessels in the control of obstetric haemorrhage.[13–19] Success rates are in the 95% range. The main limitation is the immediate availability of interventional radiologists and the relatively sophisticated equipment required. This technique is particularly

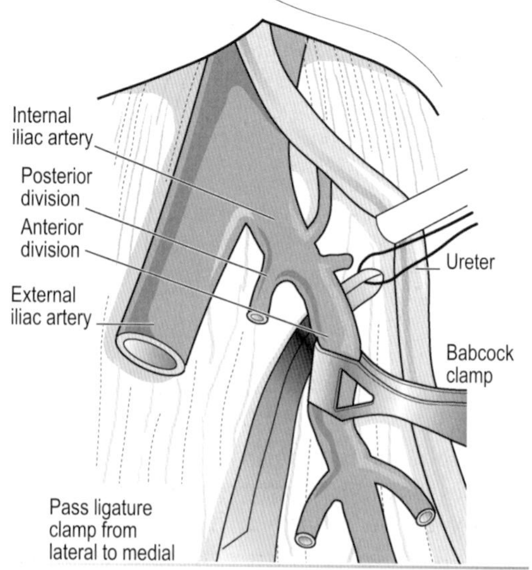

Figure 26.20 Internal iliac artery ligation.

valuable in women who have delivered vaginally but have intractable postpartum haemorrhage from uterine atony, cervical and vaginal lacerations, or paravaginal haematoma. Sometimes temporary measures such as uterine and/or vaginal tamponade will allow one to transfer the patient to a hospital with facilities for angiographic embolisation.

The procedure is done under local anaesthesia and, via a femoral artery puncture, under angiographic control a vascular catheter is guided to the aortic bifurcation and an aortogram performed to define the vascular anatomy and locate extravasation of contrast material from bleeding vessels. Angiography will detect flow rates of 1–2 ml per minute, which is usually present in cases of severe postpartum haemorrhage. However, in some cases of uterine atony there may be no discrete extravasation of contrast but just a general picture of uterine hypervascularization. If discrete bleeding points are seen the cannula is advanced to that vessel which is embolised using either gelatin sponge pieces (Gelfoam) or polyvinyl alcohol particles (PVA). It is usual to embolise the contralateral vessel, even if no collateral circulation is identified. If no discrete bleeding points are found the anterior division of both internal iliac arteries are usually embolised.[18,19]

As with vessel ligation, subsequent menstrual and reproductive functions are usually unaffected, although uterine necrosis can occur on rare occasions.[20]

Both surgical ligation and embolisation of pelvic vessels have a role in the management of severe postpartum haemorrhage. Each technique aims to stop bleeding and preserve the uterus. For women who deliver vaginally with extensive cervical and/or vaginal lacerations, and/or vulvovaginal haematomas unresponsive to local treatment, vascular embolisation saves the woman laparotomy and is usually more effective in dealing with the bleeding vessels than internal iliac artery ligation. Similarly, in cases of uterine atony that are unresponsive to uterine tamponade, embolisation, provided the woman can be sustained until the procedure is undertaken, is advisable. In women delivered by caesarean section with uterine haemorrhage there is much to recommend the simple and safe combination of uterine and ovarian artery ligation. If the bleeding is from the lower uterine segment and paracolpos bilateral internal iliac artery ligation may be successful. The problem with this is that it may not be within the general obstetrician's competence and, if it is performed and fails to control the haemorrhage, subsequent vascular embolisation is rendered more difficult and in some cases impossible, with no access for the vascular catheter to the internal iliac artery.[18,19]

References

1. Burchell RC, Olsen G. Internal iliac ligation: aortograms. Am J Obstet Gynecol 1966; 94:117–124.
2. Burchell RC. Physiology of internal iliac artery ligation. J Obstet Gynaecol Br Commonw 1968; 75:642–651.
3. Likeman RK. The boldest procedure possible for checking the bleeding – a new look at an old operation, and a series of 13 cases from an Australian hospital. Aust NZ J Obstet Gynaecol 1992; 32:256–262.
4. O'Leary JL, O'Leary JA. Uterine artery ligation for control of postcesarean hemorrhage. Obstet Gynecol 1974; 43:849–852.
5. Fahmy K. Uterine artery ligation to control postpartum hemorrhage. Int J Gynaecol Obstet 1987; 25:363–367.
6. O'Leary JA. Uterine artery ligation in the control of post-cesarean hemorrhage. J Reprod Med 1995; 40:189–193.
7. Clark SL, Phelan JP, Bruce SR, Paul RH. Hypogastric artery ligation for obstetric hemorrhage. Obstet Gynecol 1985; 66:353–356.
8. Evans S, McShane P. The efficacy of internal iliac ligation. Surg Gynecol Obstet 1985; 160:250–253.
9. Chattopadhyay SK, Deb RB, Edress YB. Surgical control of obstetric hemorrhage; hypogastric artery ligation or hysterectomy. Int J Gynaecol Obstet 1990; 32:345–351.
10. Fehrman H. Surgical management of life-threatening obstetric and gynecologic hemorrhage. Acta Obstet Gynecol Scan 1988; 67:125–128.

11. Nandanwar YS, Jhalam L, Mayadeo N, Guttal DR. Ligation of internal iliac arteries for control of pelvic haemorrhage. J Postgrad Med 1993; 39:194–195.

12. Thavarasah AS, Sivolingam N, Almohdzar SA. Internal iliac and ovarian artery ligation in the control of pelvic haemorrhage. Aust NZ J Obstet Gynaecol 1989; 29:22–25.

13. Corr P. Arterial embolisation for haemorrhage in the obstetric patient. Best Pract Res Clin Obstet Gynaecol 2001; 15:557–561.

14. Hansch E, Chitkara V, McAlpine J. Pelvic arterial embolisation for control of obstetric haemorrhage: a five-year experience. Am J Obstet Gynecol 1999; 180:1454–1460.

15. Mitty HA, Sterling KM, Alvarez M. Obstetric hemorrhage: prophylactic and emergency arterial catheterization and embolotherapy. Radiology 1993; 188:183–187.

16. Stanacato-Pasik A, Mitty HA, Richard HA, Eskhar N. Obstetric embolotherapy; effect on menses and pregnancy. Radiology 1997; 204:791–793.

17. Vedantham S, Goodwin SC, McLucas B. Uterine artery embolisation: an underused method of controlling pelvic hemorrhage. Am J Obstet Gynecol 1997; 176:938–948.

18. Boulleret C, Chahid T, Gallot D, et al. Hypogastric arterial selective and superselective embolisation for severe postpartum haemorrhage: a retrospective review of 36 cases. Cardiovasc Intervent Radiol 2004; 27:344–348.

19. Hong TM, Tseng HS, Lee RC, Wang JH, Chang CY. Uterine artery embolisation: an effective treatment for intractable obstetrical haemorrhage. Clin Radiol 2004; 59:96–101.

20. Cottier JP, Fignon A, Tranquart F, Herbreteau D. Uterine necrosis after arterial embolisation for postpartum hemorrhage. Obstet Gynecol 2002; 100:1074–1077.

Obstetric hysterectomy

Elective caesarean hysterectomy may be carried out for conditions such as cervical cancer, ovarian cancer and uterine fibroids – but these indications are rare. We are concerned here with emergency hysterectomy carried out following caesarean section or vaginal delivery. The incidence varies from about 1 in 350[1] to 1 in 7000[2] deliveries and the associated maternal death rates range from 0% to 30%. The higher incidence and mortality rates tend to occur in regions and hospitals with limited resources.[3] In developed countries the incidence of emergency obstetric hysterectomy is about 1 in 2000 to 1 in 4000 deliveries.[4–6] Compared with vaginal delivery there is a strong association between caesarean section and emergency hysterectomy.[5,7] Multiple pregnancy has been shown to have a 2–8-fold increased risk of hysterectomy, compared with singletons.[8,9] Because of the increasing rates of both caesarean delivery and assisted reproductive technology induced multiple pregnancy, the incidence of emergency obstetric hysterectomy is likely to rise worldwide. In Canada, between 1991 and 2003, the rate of obstetric hysterectomy rose significantly from 0.26 per 1000 deliveries to 0.46 per 1000 deliveries.[10]

The need for blood transfusion, intensive care and the associated risks of trauma to the bladder and ureter make this one of the markers of severe maternal morbidity and potential 'near-miss' mortality in both developed and developing countries.[5,6,10]

Indications

Emergency obstetric hysterectomy is usually required for complications of delivery associated with haemorrhage. In most cases it is a last resort life-saving procedure, undertaken when other more conservative measures to control haemorrhage have failed. There is a fine balance between premature recourse to hysterectomy and excessive delay associated with repeated ineffectual application of conservative measures. Included in this equation will be the woman's age, parity and desire for future child-bearing. The main reasons for emergency hysterectomy are as follows.[11–16]

Abnormal placentation

With the rising caesarean section rate the number of pregnant women with a previous caesarean delivery has increased. These women have a higher incidence of placenta praevia and/or placenta praevia accreta in subsequent pregnancies. In developed countries these two conditions are now the commonest reason for emergency obstetric hysterectomy. In cases of placenta praevia with accreta over an old caesarean scar, removal of the placenta can cause torrential haemorrhage obscuring the field of surgery and acutely compromising the mother. In these cases it is best to proceed to total hysterectomy with the placenta in situ.

Under exceptional circumstances abruptio placentae may be so severe as to cause extensive extravasation of blood into the myometrium (Couvelaire uterus). Usually the myometrium will still respond to oxytocics but on occasion atony may prevail and hysterectomy is necessary.

Uterine atony

The range of modern oxytocic drugs has improved the management of uterine atony (see Chapter 18). However, on rare occasions the uterus may be refractory to all of the available oxytocic agents. This is most commonly found in prolonged labour with chorioamnionitis – the exhausted and infected uterus may not respond to oxytocic drugs. Other structural abnormalities of the uterus, such as congenital anomalies and uterine fibroids, are slightly more prone to uterine atony.

Uterine rupture

This is most commonly associated with a previous uterine scar – the majority of these are caesarean section scars (see Chapter 13). In multiparous women, the intact uterus may rupture in response to inappropriate use of oxytocic drugs during the first or second stage of labour. Traumatic uterine rupture can be caused by obstetric manipulation, such as internal version and breech extraction in obstructed labour, or instrumental manipulation such as the classical application of the anterior blade of Kielland's forceps or uterine exploration for postpartum haemorrhage, either manually or with a curette. External trauma, such as a fall, domestic violence, or motor vehicle accident, may rarely cause uterine rupture.

Sepsis

This is an uncommon indication for obstetric hysterectomy but can occur when postpartum intrauterine sepsis does not respond to appropriate antibiotic treatment. This is more common with clostridial infections in which there may be myometrial abscesses refractory to antibiotic treatment. Another septic cause is that related to uterine scar infection, necrosis and dehiscence, usually manifest 1–3 weeks after caesarean delivery ('rotting scar').[17] Some cases of secondary postpartum haemorrhage, with or without overt infection, may not respond to curettage or other supportive treatment and require hysterectomy for a combination of bleeding and infection. Another rare cause of intractable, delayed postpartum haemorrhage is arteriovenous fistula formation secondary to uterine trauma and/or infection.[18]

Chronic recurrent uterine inversion

In most instances acute uterine inversion responds to replacement and does not recur (see Chapter 20). Rarely, however, uterine inversion, despite successful manual replacement may recur in the days immediately following delivery. In these cases hysterectomy may be necessary.

Ectopic pregnancy

There are a number of rare varieties of ectopic pregnancy, including cornual and cervical pregnancies that may require hysterectomy to control haemorrhage.

Surgical considerations

While many of the surgical principles of emergency obstetric hysterectomy are similar to hysterectomy in the gynaecological patient there are a number of anatomical and physiological changes in the pregnant uterus and pelvis that create potential difficulties.[19] The uterus is greatly enlarged and all the adjacent pelvic tissues are oedematous and friable. The uterine and collateral vessels are enlarged (up to five times normal calibre), engorged and tortuous.

The choice of abdominal incision will depend upon the circumstances. If the hysterectomy is being done following caesarean section then the incision is likely to have been of the Pfannenstiel variety. If laparotomy is being performed with a view to hysterectomy following vaginal delivery a lower midline incision is preferable due to speed and greater pelvic access. With either type of incision it is advisable to manually eventrate the uterus and, if there was a caesarean section, this can be easily achieved by hooking the fingers in the uterine incision.

The choice between total and subtotal hysterectomy will depend upon the indications for the procedure. If the trauma and/or bleeding is confined to the upper uterine segment there is much to recommend subtotal hysterectomy – which can be performed more rapidly and with less risk of trauma to the ureters and bladder – since it may be difficult to define the limits of the softened cervix. If the cervix and paracolpos are involved then total hysterectomy will be needed to achieve haemostasis. Be careful in women with prolonged labour and dystocia at full cervical dilatation that are delivered by caesarean section. In these cases, in addition to bleeding from the upper uterine segment associated with the uterine atony, there may be cervical trauma from the prolonged pressure and distension of the cervix – so that bleeding may continue from this area after the body of the uterus has been removed. Thus, in cases of subtotal hysterectomy it is advisable to clean out the vagina and check for continued blood loss before closing the abdomen.

In cases of haemorrhagic urgency, initial steps will have to be taken to reduce or stop the bleeding before definitive hysterectomy is performed. In cases of uterine trauma this will involve the use of Green–Armytage clamps and/or sponge forceps to the bleeding edges of uterine muscle. On each side, adjacent to the uterus, a large straight clamp is applied to include all adnexal structures: round ligament, utero-ovarian ligament and fallopian tube. This will control the collateral flow from the ovarian vessels. The uterus is elevated and the broad ligament transilluminated on each side to find an avascular space opposite the level of a lower uterine segment caesarean incision. Through these two spaces in the broad ligament a catheter, penrose drain, or intravenous tubing can be passed and tightly twisted around the lower segment, just above the cervix, to occlude the uterine arteries. The twisted catheter, drain or tubing can be held tightly in place with a straight clamp. These measures should stem the flow of blood so that hysterectomy can then be systematically performed.

The main vascular pedicles are often thick and oedematous. These should be double clamped. The proximal clamp is removed first and replaced by a free tie. The distal clamp is then replaced by a transfixing suture (Fig 26.21). In this way haematoma formation in the pedicle is prevented. Avoid taking too much tissue in the clamp – the proximal one-third of a pedicle within a clamp is not secure. Thus, substantial pedicles should only be grasped to fill the distal two-thirds of the clamp to ensure security. Pedicles should be held in the normal anatomical plane whilst clamping and tying. Untwisting of the pedicle, especially if it had too much tissue, is one reason for suture slippage and subsequent haemorrhage.

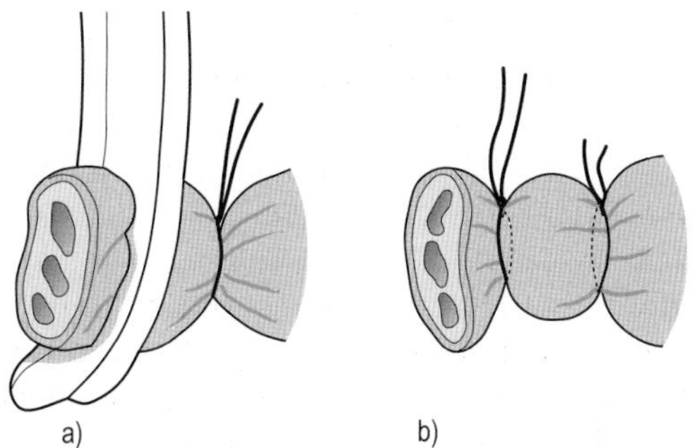

Figure 26.21 Double clamp technique: (a) the proximal clamp is replaced by a free tie, (b) the distal clamp is replaced with a transfixing suture.

Surgical technique

The uterus is lifted out through the incision and the adnexal structures placed on tension by the assistant. On each side a long straight clamp is applied close to the uterine body and across the adnexal structures – round ligament, utero-ovarian ligament and fallopian tube. The round ligament is grasped with a short straight clamp about 3 cm from its attachment to the uterus and is incised just medial to this clamp, allowing access to the broad ligament between the two leaves of peritoneum. The areolar tissue within the broad ligament is gently separated using the index finger. The anterior leaf of the broad ligament is now incised infero-medially. If a lower segment caesarean section has been performed this incision of the anterior leaf joins up with the lateral aspect of the incision of the utero-vesical peritoneum. When ligating the round ligament it is important to ensure that the small artery (Sampson's artery) that consistently runs beneath the round ligament is included.

The posterior leaf of the broad ligament is now transilluminated and incised either with scissors or a finger. The now-exposed pedicle containing the utero-ovarian ligament and fallopian tube is isolated medial to the ovary and secured with a curved clamp. The posterior leaf of the broad ligament can now be transilluminated and incised down to the level of the utero-sacral ligaments. Further dissection of the areolar tissue in the base of the broad ligament with the index finger and, if necessary, by gentle sharp dissection should allow exposure of the uterine vessels. The above technique is used on each side.

It is important to identify and dissect the bladder free of the operative field. With a previous caesarean section it is common for the posterior wall of the bladder to be adherent to the lower uterine segment. Precise sharp dissection is required to free this adherence. Blunt dissection with gauze is not recommended as this may cause more bleeding, tearing, and perforation of the friable adherent posterior bladder wall. When dissecting the bladder down limit the lateral dissection to avoid the vascular bladder pillars. At this stage, dissection of the bladder is only required sufficient to safely place curved clamps across the uterine vessels. This vascular bundle is doubly clamped and ligated. The level of placement of the uterine clamps is at the junction of the cervix with the isthmus of the uterus. This can be hard or impossible to appreciate at full cervical dilation, but is usually about 2 cm below the transverse incision of a caesarean section. From now on all clamps are placed medially to the uterine clamps to avoid ureteric damage. The ureter runs about 2 cm below the uterine artery – 'water flows under the bridge'.

Large curved clamps can now be placed across the lower uterine segment at the junction of the cervix on each side, allowing excision of the body of the uterus. If the bleeding is due to uterine atony or trauma in the upper uterine segment, the haemorrhage should now be controlled. If there is no bleeding from the cervix then this subtotal hysterectomy should suffice. If the bleeding involves the cervix this will now be more readily accessible – although it can be very hard to distinguish the level of the cervix if the hysterectomy was performed at full cervical dilatation. At this point a finger placed through the uterine incision should allow one to identify the rim of the cervix (Fig 26.22). The clamps holding the angle of the cervix are ligated with a transfixing suture and held. The rim of cervix is carefully identified to ensure that the entire body of the uterus has been excised – if not, the edges can be trimmed to achieve this. In the case of the cervix that is fully dilated the area to be stitched is quite broad. This is achieved with figure-of-eight haemostatic

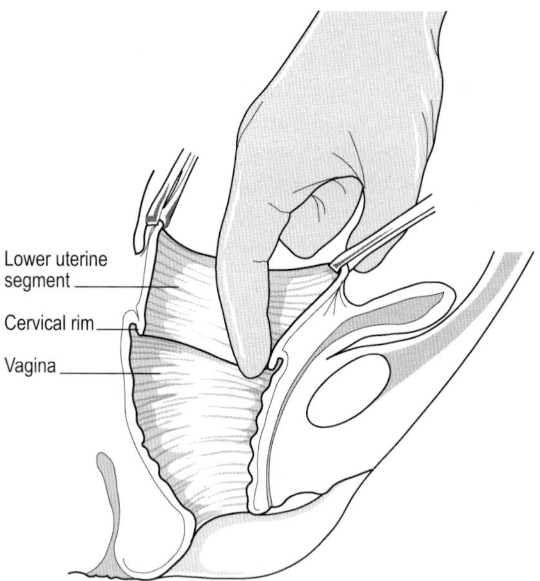

Figure 26.22 The body of the uterus has been excised and the finger can more readily identify the rim of the cervix.

sutures or a continuous locking suture in one or two layers as required.

If removal of the cervix is deemed necessary the bladder will have to be further dissected from the anterior part of the cervix. Here again careful identification of the rim of cervix is necessary. The utero-sacral and cardinal ligaments are taken with curved clamps and the angle of the vagina is incorporated into the cardinal ligament suture ligation. Depending upon whether drainage is deemed necessary the vaginal cuff can either be closed with a continuous locking suture, or interrupted figure-of-eight sutures. Alternatively, drainage can be encouraged by a continuous locking suture of the edges of both the anterior and posterior walls of the vagina.

In 1–4% of cases the bladder is inadvertently entered. This is less likely if care is taken with sharp dissection of the bladder from the cervix. However, even with good technique, bladder injuries may occur. The important thing is to recognize the injury and repair it at the time, otherwise there is a risk of vesico-vaginal fistula. It is therefore essential to test the integrity of the bladder in all cases once the hysterectomy has been achieved. This may be done by manipulating the bulb of the Foley catheter through the bladder wall, so that a hole in the bladder becomes obvious if the bulb of the catheter is seen. Alternatively, and more accurately, the bladder can be filled with a marking medium such as methylene blue or sterile milk taken from the nursery. In many ways milk is preferable as it does not cause permanent staining of the tissues – so that after repair, or in dealing with continued haemorrhage, further use of milk installation in the bladder can be seen more easily than the permanently methylene blue-stained tissues.

If there is a tear in the bladder it should be closed in two layers using continuous running sutures of 3/0 vicryl or its equivalent. Ensure that the ureteric orifices are not involved in the repair, which is especially likely in posterior tears of the bladder wall adherent to a previous caesarean scar.

Identification of the ureter is advisable and it is particularly vulnerable at three sites. If bleeding has necessitated removal of the ovary and tube on one side, the ureter may be caught when clamping the infundibulopelvic ligament lateral to the tube and ovary. During clamping of the uterine vessels the ureter is very close as it runs beneath the vessels. It is best to identify the ureter at the pelvic brim on the medial leaf of the broad ligament and follow its course down beneath the uterine vessels. Provided all subsequent clamps are placed medially to the uterine vessel clamps, and the bladder is dissected from the front of the cervix, the ureter as it enters the bladder (the third vulnerable site) should be avoided. From a medicolegal point of view it is wise to include a description of the identification of the bladder and ureters in the operation record. If there is any doubt about the integrity of the ureters, cystoscopy should be performed postoperatively, preferably having given intravenous indigo carmine 10–15 minutes before to highlight the efflux of dye-stained urine from the ureters. If no cystoscope is available a diagnostic laparoscope or hysteroscope can be used. Provided the condition of the patient allows it, and the resources are available, it is preferable to identify and treat ureteric obstruction or damage at the time of the initial operation.

Once the operation is complete the pelvis can be filled with water or saline to check that all pedicles are intact and that there are no additional bleeding sites. It is not necessary to reperitonize the pelvis.

Perioperative antibiotic prophylaxis should be given and, depending on the duration of labour or potential chorioamniotitis, this may be continued for 24–48 hours. Thromboprophylaxis should also be instituted once haemostasis is secure.

In hospital reviews of obstetric hysterectomy up to 25% may be in primiparous women with its potentially devastating fertility-ending implications.[5]

Described elsewhere in this book are a number of alternative techniques and procedures that can be undertaken for the control of haemorrhage, which is the main reason for obstetric hysterectomy. These include the appropriate use of oxytocic drugs; uterine tamponade; uterine compression sutures; and major vessel ligation and embolisation. The obstetrician should be familiar with these alternatives and be prepared to perform them as both a life-saving and uterus-preserving alternative to hysterectomy.

Once the woman's initial postoperative recovery is secure the whole sequence of events should be reviewed and discussed with her by an experienced obstetrician and appropriate follow-up arranged.

References

1. Korejo R, Jafarey SN. Obstetric hysterectomy – five years experience at Jinnah Postgraduate Medical Centre, Karachi. J Pakistan Med Assoc 1995; 45:86–88.
2. Yamamoto H, Sagae S, Nishik WA, Skuto R. Emergency postpartum hysterectomy in obstetric practice. J Obstet Gynaecol Res 2000; 26:341–345.
3. Ezechi OC, Kalu BK, Njokanma FO, Nwokoro CA, Okeke GC. Emergency peripartum hysterectomy in a Nigerian hospital: a 20-year review. J Obstet Gynaecol 2004; 24:372–373.
4. Englesen IB, Albrechtsen S, Iverson OE. Peripartum hysterectomy – incidence and

maternal morbidity. Acta Obstet Gynecol Scand 2001; 80:409–412.

5. Baskett TF. Emergency obstetric hysterectomy. J Obstet Gynaecol 2003; 23:353–355.
6. Baskett TF, O'Connell CM. Severe obstetric maternal morbidity: a 15-year population-based study. J Obstet Gynaecol 2005; 25:7–9.
7. Kacmar J, Bhinmai L, Boyd M, Shah-Hosseini R, Piepert J. Route of delivery as a risk factor for emergency peripartum hysterectomy: a case-controlled study. Obstet Gynecol 2003; 102:141–145.
8. Walker MC, Murphy KE, Pan S, Yang Q, Wen SW. Adverse maternal outcomes in multifetal pregnancies. Br J Obstet Gynaecol 2004; 111:1294–1296.
9. Francois K, Ortiz J, Harris C, Foley MR, Elliott JP. Is peripartum hysterectomy more common in multiple gestations? Obstet Gynecol 2005; 105:1369–1372.
10. Wen SW, Huang L, Liston RM, Heaman M, Baskett TF, Rusen ID. Severe maternal morbidity in Canada, 1991–2001. Can Med Assoc J 2005; 173:759–763.
11. Chew S, Biswas A. Caesarean and postpartum hysterectomy. Singapore Med J 1998; 39:9–13.
12. Bakshi S, Meyer BA. Indications for and outcomes of emergency peripartum hysterectomy: a five-year review. J Reprod Med 2000; 45:733–737.
13. Abu-Heija AT, Jallad FF. Emergency peripartum hysterectomy at the Princess Badeea Teaching Hospital in North Jordan. J Obstet Gynaecol Res 1999; 25:193–195.
14. Sebitalone MH, Moodley J. Emergency peripartum hysterectomy. East African Med J 2001; 78:70–74.
15. Bai SW, Lee HJ, Cho JS, Park YW, Kim SK, Park KH. Peripartum hysterectomy and associated factors. J Reprod Med 2003; 48:148–152.
16. Sheiner E, Levy A, Katz M, Major M. Identifying risk factors for peripartum cesarean hysterectomy: a population-based study. J Reprod Med 2003; 48:622–626.
17. Rivlin ME, Carroll CS, Morrison JC. Conservative surgery for uterine incisional necrosis complicating cesarean delivery. Obstet Gynecol 2004; 103:1105–1108.
18. Aziz N, Lenzi TA, Jeffrey RB, Lyell DJ. Postpartum uterine arteriovenous fistula. Obstet Gynecol 2004; 103:1076–1078.
19. Baskett TF. Peripartum hysterectomy. In: B-Lynch C, Keith LG, Lalonde AB, Karoshi M (eds). A textbook of postpartum haemorrhage. Duncow: Sapiens Publishing 2006. pp 312–315.

Symphysiotomy

'I believe the operation fills a most useful place in practice, and that is the opinion of many others, and if everyone would deliberately struggle against taking up an extensive extreme position with regard to the operation, that place could be more exactly determined'.

Munro Kerr, 1908

The operation of symphysiotomy has had a rather chequered history. It was originally performed upon the dead as an alternative to postmortem caesarean section by Claude Dela Courveé in 1665. It was performed on the living by Jean René Sigault in 1777. The patient was a rachitic dwarf, said to have an obstetric conjugate of 6.5 cm. She had four previous stillborn infants and Sigault performed a symphysiotomy and produced a live child: although the patient developed a vesico-vaginal fistula and was unable to walk for 2 months. Symphysiotomy enjoyed some popularity on the continent but this was short-lived due to the postoperative urological and orthopaedic morbidity. It enjoyed a resurgence on the continent, in Ireland and in South America in the late 19th and early 20th centuries.

In modern obstetrics the use of symphysiotomy is almost completely confined to the developing world; although a plea has been made for its occasional use in specific rare situations in countries with well developed health services.[1,2]

Symphysiotomy is the surgical division of the fibrocartilaginous symphysis pubis. A 2–3 cm separation of the pubic symphysis increases the area of the pelvic brim by 15–20% and increases all the pelvic transverse diameters by about 1 cm. This increase is permanent and carries over into subsequent pregnancies. About 85% of women with cephalopelvic disproportion treated by symphysiotomy will deliver vaginally in a subsequent pregnancy.[3,4] The main role for symphysiotomy, therefore, is in those countries where clinical and cultural factors mitigate against caesarean section for cases of mild-to-moderate cephalopelvic disproportion. This is especially so in some African communities in which caesarean section may be seen as a 'failure' of maternal achievement. Furthermore, in a subsequent pregnancy the woman previously delivered by caesarean section may avoid hospital confinement and rupture her uterus in a remote community. If contraceptive services are not available or unacceptable to the woman she may have to endure the risks of multiple repeat caesarean sections. This was one of the reasons for the popularity of symphysiotomy in predominately Catholic countries in the late 19th and early 20th centuries.

Indications

Cephalopelvic disproportion

As discussed above, women with obstructed labour and mild-to-moderate cephalopelvic disproportion may, for clinical and cultural reasons, be managed with symphysiotomy. It is not appropriate to expect symphysiotomy to safely overcome severe disproportion. Thus, only two-fifths or less of the fetal head should be palpable above the maternal pelvic brim and the degree of moulding of the fetal head should not show an irreducible overlap of the cranial bones.[5]

Breech presentation

A rare but dreaded complication of vaginal breech delivery is entrapment of the after-coming head due to disproportion. This should be rare in a properly conducted labour for vaginal breech delivery. However, it can occur and one option for dealing with this is rapid symphysiotomy. A number of case series have shown that this will save about 80% of such infants.[6,7]

Shoulder dystocia

Symphysiotomy has been put forward as a solution to severe cases of shoulder dystocia that do not resolve with the usual manoeuvres (see Chapter 10). Although this treatment has been suggested, and in theory may have some logic if symphysiotomy can be rapidly performed, there are very few cases reported and some of those show poor outcome for both mother and infant.[8,9]

Technique

The main advantages of the procedure are that it can be done under local anaesthesia by a doctor or a nurse trained to do symphysiotomy but who may not have the training or the facilities to perform caesarean section. In some settings it may be performed more rapidly than caesarean section and may thus be life-saving in some cases of obstructed labour with fetal distress or with entrapment of the after-coming head in vaginal breech delivery. The operative principles of symphysiotomy are as follows:[5,10–13]

- The operator should be familiar with the anatomy of the symphysis pubis (Fig 26.23).
- The woman is placed in the lithotomy position with her legs supported by two assistants. The angle between the legs should not exceed 80° (Fig 26.24). This restricted degree of abduction is necessary to avoid excessive separation of the symphysis with damage to the underlying urethra and bladder neck and to avoid excessive traction on the sacro-iliac joints.
- Local anaesthesia in the form of 1% lidocaine is infiltrated into the skin over the symphysis pubis and into the subcutaneous tissues as well as into the joint space. The local anaesthetic needle may be helpful to identify the space and can be left in place as a guide to the subsequent incision site. In addition, local anaesthetic should be infiltrated into the site of the proposed episiotomy.
- A number 14 Foley catheter is inserted into the bladder and the bulb inflated with 5 ml saline or sterile water. If the fetal head is firmly lodged in the pelvis a

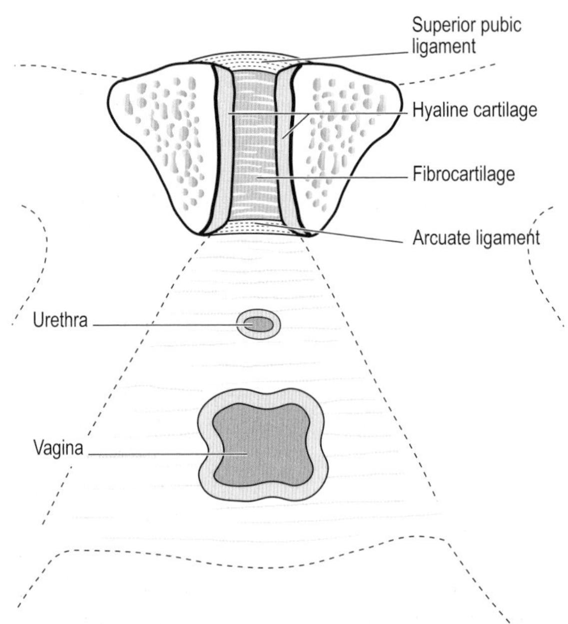

Figure 26.23 Anatomy of the symphysis pubis.

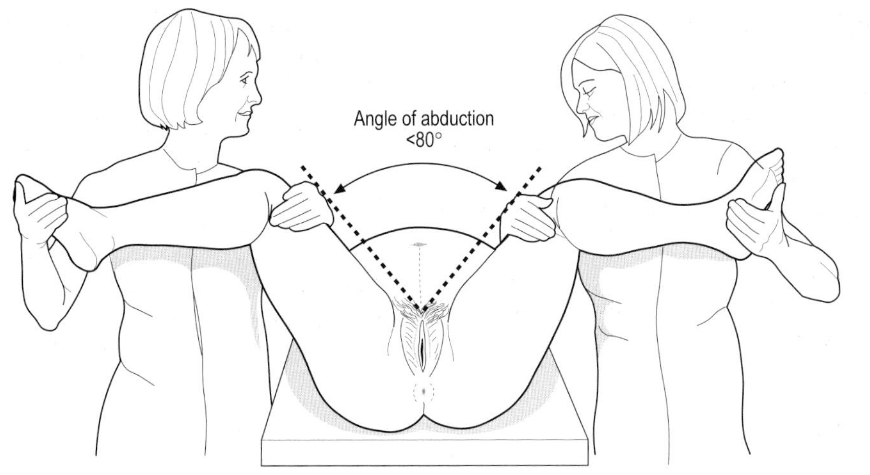

Figure 26.24 Assistants support the legs.

firmer silastic catheter may be necessary. It is essential to ensure that the bladder is completely drained. The index and middle fingers of the left hand are inserted vaginally and placed alongside the catheter in the urethra. These fingers push the catheter and the urethra to the side so that the middle finger lies underneath the symphysis pubis joint space – a firmer catheter may facilitate this lateral movement (Fig 26.25).

- Incision of the symphysis pubis is best done with a solid-bladed scalpel if available. A small incision is made through the overlying skin, just enough to allow the scalpel to gain access to the deeper tissues. The symphysis pubis joint should be incised in the midline starting at the junction of the upper and middle thirds. Using the left middle finger as a guide the scalpel blade is pushed through the joint until the tip is felt and, using a levering action, incises the lower two thirds of the symphysis. The scalpel blade is then withdrawn from the joint, rotated 180°, re-inserted and used to incise the upper third of the symphysis (Fig 26.26). During this time constant vigilance is kept by means of the vaginal finger lest there should be any intrusion of the blade into the tissues underneath the symphysis. The thumb of the left hand held in front of the symphysis will detect the onset of separation. This separation should not exceed the width of the thumb, approximately 2.5 cm (Fig 26.26).

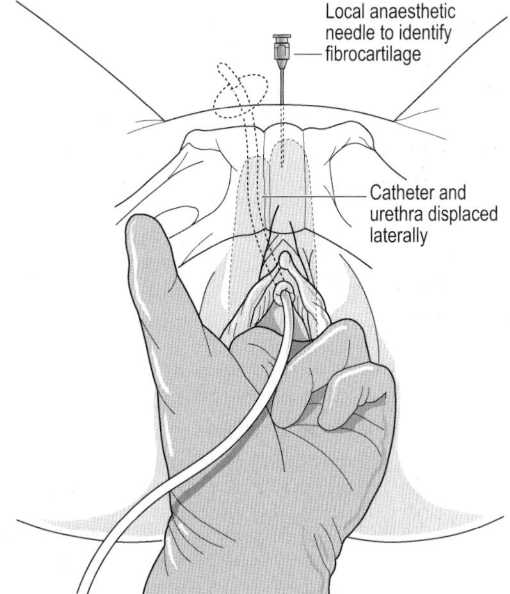

Figure 26.25 Catheter and urethra pushed to one side by the index and middle fingers of the operator's hand.

- At this point the anterior vaginal wall and underlying urethra and bladder neck are unsupported and vulnerable, so it is essential that the assistants maintain the support of the legs and do not allow separation beyond 80°.
- At the time of delivery a generous medio-lateral episiotomy is performed to reduce the tension and pressure on the anterior

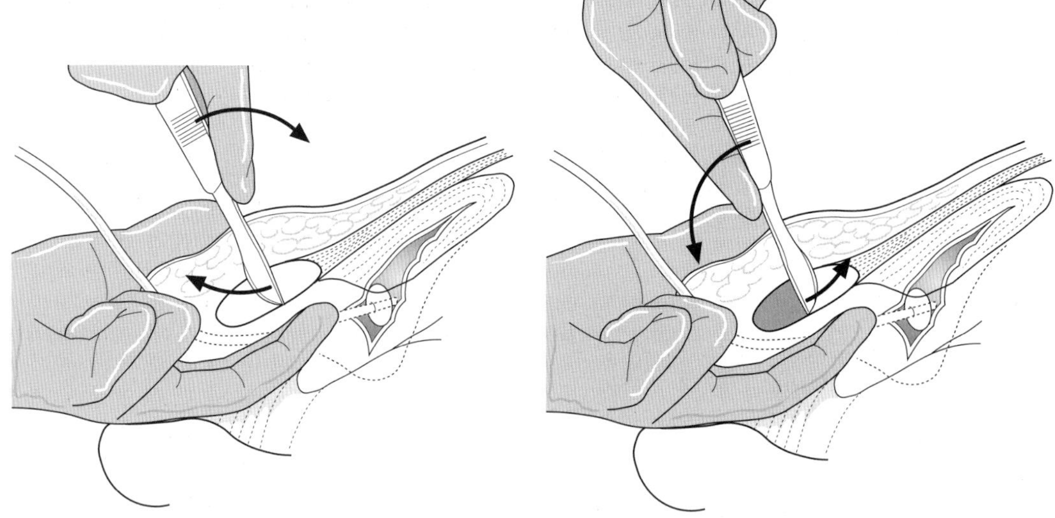

Figure 26.26 With the underlying middle finger as a guide, the symphysis is divided in two steps using a levering action of the scalpel.

vaginal wall. Often delivery of the head will be spontaneous, but if assistance is required the vacuum is preferred over forceps. To further reduce trauma to the tissues under the symphysis pubis the assistants are instructed to adduct the legs at the point of delivery of the fetal head.

- After delivery of the infant and the placenta, the symphysis and underlying soft tissues are compressed between the thumb above and the index and middle fingers below for 3–5 minutes. This should reduce the risk of bleeding from the very vascular inferior vesical plexus of veins around the upper urethra and bladder neck. The episiotomy and any vaginal lacerations should be sutured in addition to the stab wound over the symphysis.

Post-delivery care

- Bladder drainage should be continued for 4–7 days. If there is haematuria then drainage should be continued until the urine has been clear for at least 3 days.
- A broad-spectrum antibiotic is given for 1 week to reduce the risk of urinary tract infection and infection of the tissues of the symphysis.
- Depending on other risk factors thromboprophylaxis may be given.
- The patient should be nursed mostly on her side with her knees strapped loosely together to avoid inadvertent and excessive abduction. She should remain mostly at rest in this position for the first 3 days. Thereafter ambulation should be encouraged and, if necessary, assisted by walking-aids.
- The patient is discharged once she is confident with her walking but is advised against excessive physical activity for 3 months until the fibrous healing of the joint has occurred. Although the benefits of symphysiotomy will extend to her next pregnancy and likely result in uncomplicated vaginal delivery she is advised that subsequent deliveries should be in hospital.

Complications

Haemorrhage

Initial bleeding from the symphysis pubis can be brisk. However, this is usually venous in origin and responds to the pressure applied by the thumb and vaginal fingers outlined previously. The bleeding is likely to be more if the incision has been made away from the midline or too deep. Careful identification of the middle of the symphysis with the local anaesthetic needle and the guidance of the underlying finger should reduce this risk. A retropubic haematoma can occur postoperatively but is usually self-limiting.

Urinary complications

Infection of the urinary tract is common but reduced by prophylactic antibiotics. Inadvertent incision of the bladder can occur and if identified and small it should heal with 10–14 days of continuous bladder drainage. If a vesico-vaginal fistula is suspected this should be confirmed as soon as possible with urethrocystoscopy as it will often respond to 6 weeks of continuous bladder drainage without the need for subsequent surgery. The incidence of stress incontinence is likely to be increased but there are no good studies to confirm or deny this.

Orthopaedic

Osteitis pubis can occur but this complication is reported in less than 1% of cases. Instability of the sacro-iliac joints and pubic symphysis can cause significant ambulatory difficulties but the reported incidence is 1–2%. Overall in large series of symphysiotomy conducted by appropriately trained personnel the incidence of serious long-term orthopaedic and urinary complications is around 2%.[5]

Symphysiotomy has little or no role in countries with well-developed, hospital-based obstetric services. It does, however, have a significant and potentially life-saving role for both mother and infant in regions with less developed medical services. The conclusions of Myerscough in the 10th edition of this book 25 years ago remain relevant:

> *'Discussion will doubtedly continue for many years, but the question should be reviewed dispassionately. No reasonable person doubts the merit of a well-executed caesarean section even if it be performed in late labour, despite its immediate and remote hazards; but to condemn without thought the alternative procedure – which incidentally does not require elaborate technique for its performance – betokens intolerance of mind rather than exercise of reason. The morbidity and mortality following caesarean section are significantly greater, especially in the neglected, infected case. Besides, symphysiotomy spares the patient the risk of scar rupture in each and every subsequent labour. It is the experience of those workers who perform symphysiotomy that one of its chief virtues is the ease and safety with which subsequent spontaneous delivery takes place, for the pelvis readily expands on each occasion. To sum up, symphysiotomy may be reasonably considered in cases where descent of the head is obstructed as in moderate cephalopelvic disproportion, including cases of malposition of the head. It has a special place in some communities in order to avoid a caesarean section scar in cases of moderate pelvic contraction where the patient may not come under observation in a subsequent pregnancy and labour and where successful vaginal delivery has a strong cultural importance.'*

References

1. Wykes CB, Johnston TA, Paterson-Brown S, Johansen RB. Symphysiotomy: a life saving procedure. Br J Obstet Gynaecol 2003; 110:219–221.
2. Johanson R, Wykes CB. Symphysiotomy. In: Johanson R, Cox C, Grady K, Howell C, eds. Managing obstetric emergencies and trauma – the MOET course manual. London: RCOG Press, 2003:237–239.
3. VanRoosmalen J. Symphysiotomy as an alternative to caesarean section. Int J Gynaecol Obstet 1987; 25:451–458.
4. VanRoosmalen J. Safe motherhood: cesarean section or symphysiotomy? Am J Obstet Gynecol 1990; 163:1–4.

5. Bjorklund K. Minimally invasive surgery for obstructed labour: a review of symphysiotomy during the twentieth century (including 5000 cases). Br J Obstet Gynaecol 2002; 109:236–238.

6. Spencer JA. Symphysiotomy for vaginal breech delivery: two case reports. Br J Obstet Gynaecol 1987; 94:16–18.

7. Menticoglu SM. Symphysiotomy for the trapped aftercoming parts of the breech: a review of the literature and a plea for its use. Aust NZ J Obstet Gynaecol 1990; 30:1–9.

8. Goodwin TM, Banks E, Millar L, Phelan J. Catastrophic shoulder dystocia and emergency symphysiotomy. Am J Obstet Gynecol 1997; 177:463–464.

9. Hofmyer GJ. Obstructed labor: using better technologies to reduce mortality. Int J Gynecol Obstet 2004; 85(Supp 1):S62–S72.

10. Hartfield VJ. Subcutaneous symphysiotomy: time for a reappraisal? Aust NZ J Obstet Gynaecol 1973; 13:147–152.

11. Seedat EK, Crichton D. Symphysiotomy: technique, indications and limitations. Lancet 1962; 1:154–158.

12. Crichton D, Seedat EK. The technique of symphysiotomy. South Afr Med J 1963; 37:227–231.

13. Gebbie D. Symphysiotomy. Clin Obstet Gynaecol 1982; 9:663–683.

Destructive operations on the fetus

When caesarean section was still a lethal operation and serious degrees of pelvic contraction were commonplace throughout the world, obstructed labour frequently dragged on until the infant died. When it proved impossible to deliver the infant the man-midwife was called in to perform a destructive operation on the fetus to reduce its size and allow vaginal delivery in the hope that the mother's life could be saved.

The procedures to be considered here have for their objective the diminution of the bulk of the fetus, in order to permit of its more easy passage through the birth canal. Such procedures are only performed on the fetus with a lethal anomaly or in the fetus already dead. Other than the special case of drainage of the hydrocephalic fetal head these procedures have no place in modern obstetrics in regions with developed health services. However, similar to the arguments in favour of symphysiotomy there are occasions, for cultural and clinical reasons, in regions with poorly developed health services, when destructive operations on the fetus may be necessary to save the life of the mother. When training and facilities for caesarean section are absent or unsafe these procedures may allow safe delivery of the mother, in addition to avoiding a uterine scar that may rupture if she is unable or unwilling to find suitable hospital-based obstetric care in a future pregnancy.

Even in developing countries the incidence of destructive operations is decreasing and is usually well under 1%.[1–3] In about 80% of cases the indication is obstructed labour with a dead fetus.[4] When hospital facilities are limited, caesarean section for obstructed labour, particularly with a shoulder presentation in an over-distended and infected uterus, may carry higher maternal mortality than a fetal destructive procedure. In addition the caesarean incision may have to be of the classical type with the implications for uterine rupture in subsequent pregnancy.

The role of these operations will depend upon the clinical circumstances and the level of obstetric services available – particularly safe caesarean section. In cases of obstructed labour with mild-to-moderate cephalopelvic disproportion and a live fetus, symphysiotomy may be chosen. If there is gross disproportion and the fetus is alive then caesarean section should be performed. Similarly if obstructed labour is due to a transverse lie, shoulder or compound presentation and the fetus is alive, caesarean section will be less risky to both mother and infant than internal version and breech extraction – which are fraught with the risk of uterine rupture and a potentially fatal outcome for both infant and mother. However, when the fetus is dead and facilities for safe caesarean section are absent or marginal, craniotomy may be necessary for cases of cephalopelvic disproportion and decapitation may be indicated for transverse lie.[5] In addition, the social and cultural context in which the women lives may lead her to refuse caesarean delivery under all circumstances.

General principles

In the majority of cases with obstructed labour the woman has been through a prolonged, painful and harrowing experience. She is likely to be exhausted, demoralized, dehydrated, septic and in pain.

- Initial first aid management should involve resuscitation with intravenous crystalloids and placement of a Foley catheter to monitor and guide fluid management.
- Blood should be taken for full blood count, cross-match and coagulation screen if possible. Many of these women are already anaemic and, with prolonged obstructed labour, atonic postpartum haemorrhage is more likely. In addition, trauma to

the genital tract during the destructive procedure may increase blood loss.

- Infection is likely and, indeed, may be assumed so that intravenous broad-spectrum antibiotics should be administered.
- In addition to her physical condition the woman may be so exhausted and demoralized as to be barely able to comprehend her situation. She may not even know yet that the fetus is dead. After the initial resuscitation manoeuvres have been undertaken and analgesia provided the woman and her husband and, if appropriate, a senior relative should be involved in the discussion and plan for delivery. Fully informed consent in these situations is difficult but every effort must be made to obtain this to the extent feasible under the circumstances.
- The choice of anaesthesia will depend on what is available and the patient's condition. General anaesthesia has some advantages for both the patient and operator under these trying circumstances. However, spinal anaesthesia combined with sedation may be a safer option. If these are not available local anaesthesia with pudendal block, paracervical block and intravenous sedation may be adequate.
- Ideally the cervix should be fully dilated for the performance of these procedures, although an experienced operator may be able to work within a cervix of 7 cm or more dilatation. The true conjugate of the pelvic brim should be at least 8 cm.
- In all cases of neglected obstructed labour the possibility of uterine rupture should be considered before embarking upon the procedure.

Operative procedures

Craniotomy

This is the most commonly performed destructive operation and is used for a neglected obstructed labour with a dead fetus in cephalic presentation. The ease and safety of this procedure depends upon the degree of pelvic contraction, the size of the fetal head and the experience of the operator. In general, if the fetal head is palpable more than three-fifths above the pelvic brim or is mobile at the pelvic brim then the procedure is difficult, dangerous, and can be impossible. In such cases, even with a dead fetus, caesarean section is usually less hazardous for the mother.

In addition to adequate anaesthesia it is essential to confirm that the Foley catheter is properly placed and that the bladder is empty. The ideal instrument for perforation of the fetal head is Simpson's perforator (Fig 26.27). The depth of the two cutting blades is limited by the instrument's shoulders beneath them. The handles are held together by a hinged-crossbar and are wide apart when the cutting blades are in apposition. By pressing the handles together the cutting blades are separated. The head of the infant is steadied by the assistant using suprapubic pressure. The fingers of one hand are used to protect the maternal tissues and guide the points of the perforator to the anterior or posterior fontanelle, whichever is more accessible. The perforator should be at right angles to the surface of the skull as the instrument is pushed into the head up to the shoulders of the blades and opened as widely as possible to make a longitudinal incision on the scalp and the bone below, usually by separation of the sutures. This is followed by closing the blades and turning the perforator through 90° and repeating the procedure to produce a cruciate incision in the skull (Fig 26.28).

Keeping the perforator inside the cranium it should be opened and closed, and the points of the instrument pushed into the skull and the brain broken up in all directions. Provided the perforator is kept in the skull up to the instrument's shoulders, and this is monitored by the fingers of the other hand, there

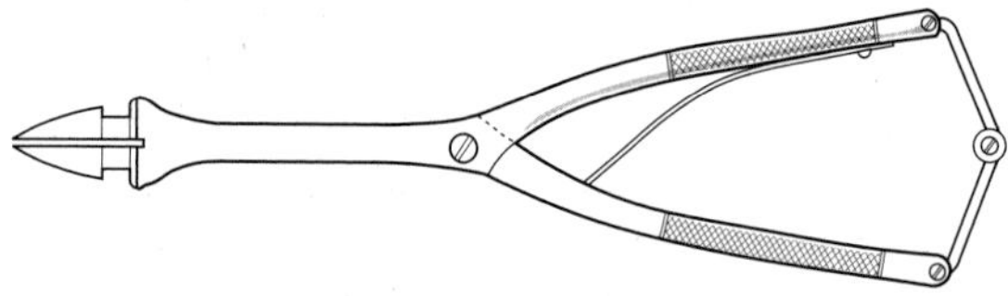

Figure 26.27 Simpson's perforator.

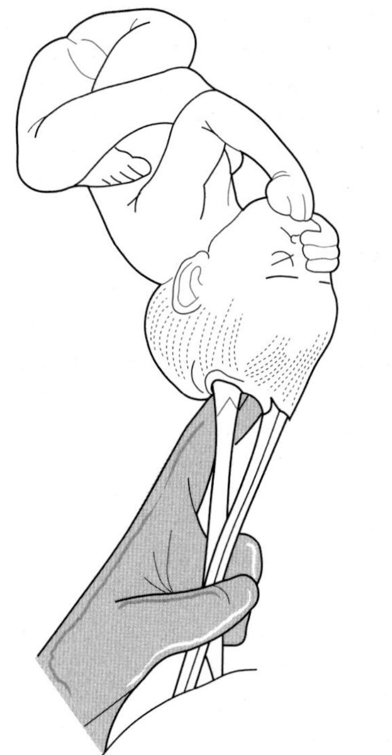

Figure 26.28 Perforation of the skull. The perforator is pushed into the skull in the neighbourhood of the anterior fontanelle, the ideal site for perforation. The blades are separated by pressing the handles together and the opening of the skull is enlarged.

should be no risk of trauma to the maternal soft tissues. The perforator is now withdrawn under protection of the other hand. Brain matter will usually ooze out of the incision and this evacuation can be assisted digitally.

If Simpson's perforator is not available, sharp Mayo's or similar scissors can be used to make a cruciate incision on the fetal scalp followed by introduction of the scissors into the fetal head via the most accessible fontanelle or suture line. The scissors are retained in the fetal skull and opened repeatedly in all directions to facilitate evacuation of the brain tissue.[6]

Once the head has been reduced in size delivery can be assisted by traction on the edges of the cranium by Kocher's forceps or vulsella. If the cervix is not yet fully dilated, a bandage can be tied through the handles of these forceps and a weight applied to the end to facilitate complete cervical dilatation and delivery of the head during subsequent uterine contractions. If the degree of pelvic contraction is slight and the decompressed head is low in the pelvic cavity then ordinary obstetric forceps such as Simpson's or Neville–Barnes may be used to effect delivery of the fetal head. In cases of face presentation the most convenient site for perforation is the palate.

Craniotomy of the after-coming head

This may be required for the dead fetus with the breech delivered and an obstructed after-coming head. Once the arms of the infant have been brought down the assistant ensures that the fetal back is anterior and applies traction to the legs in a direction that facilitates access of the operator to the occipital region. Protecting the maternal tissues with the fingers of one hand, Simpson's perforator is pushed through the skull in the neighbourhood of the posterior lateral fontanelle (Fig. 26.29). In some cases of contracted pelvis this may be difficult to reach, in which case the occipital bone is perforated in the midline. The manoeuvres to enlarge the incision and evacuate the contents of the skull are the same as with the forecoming head. Once the size of the head has been reduced it may be delivered by the Mauriceau–Smellie–Veit manoeuvre or forceps to the after-coming head.

Craniocentesis

Minor degrees of hydrocephalus that are diagnosed in the antenatal period by ultrasound and in which the infant is felt to have a reasonable chance of survival and good quality of life are likely to be delivered by caesarean section. We are concerned here with cases of severe hydrocephalus in which the infant is either dead or because of the degree of hydrocephalus, and perhaps other associated anomalies, the chance of infant survival after birth is remote. Of all the procedures under consideration in this chapter, craniocentesis – the drainage of the excess cerebrospinal fluid (CSF) is the easiest. The fetus almost invariably presents by the head or breech – transverse lie or shoulder presentation is extremely rare with severe hydrocephalus.

If the fetus presents by the head, the CSF can be drained transabdominally using a spinal needle, preferably under ultrasound guidance. As labour progresses it may be necessary to drain additional fluid transvaginally. Once the cervix has dilated, transvaginal drainage can be carried out using a spinal needle or pudendal block needle – the latter has the advantage of a guard which can be introduced through the vagina and cervix en route to the fetal head. If the fetus is already dead or severely malformed, the head may also be drained transvaginally using a Drew–Smythe catheter or Simpson's perforator or a pair of sharp scissors. These more comprehensive methods of drainage are more likely to result in the infant being stillborn.

If the fetus presents by the breech, labour can be allowed to progress until the body of the infant is delivered. If, as is not uncommon, there is an associated spina bifida, a catheter is passed through this opening up to the cranium and the CSF will drain effectively. If there is no spina bifida it is possible to transect the thoracic spine (spondylotomy) and pass a catheter up the canal into the head to drain the CSF. Alternatively, the base of the fetal skull can be entered with Simpson's perforator as for craniotomy of the after-coming head (Fig 26.29). With all these methods of drainage the delivery of the head is usually spontaneous or easily assisted.

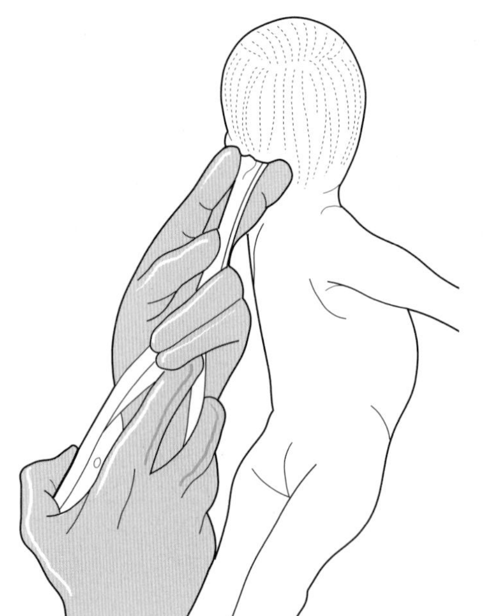

Figure 26.29 Perforating the after-coming head through the posterolateral fontanelle.

Decapitation

Of all the procedures outlined in this chapter decapitation is the most distressing for all involved. It is indicated in cases of neglected labour with a dead fetus in transverse lie with a prolapsed arm or shoulder presentation. In this situation the alternative of internal version or breech extraction carries such a high risk of uterine rupture that it is contraindicated. The safest and most simple technique is to use a Blond–Hiedler saw (Fig 26.30). The operator mounts the thimble on one thumb and attaches the wire to the slot in the thimble. If there is a prolapsed arm, counter traction is put on this to make the fetal neck accessible. The thumb with the thimble is passed in front of the fetal neck and the fingers behind.

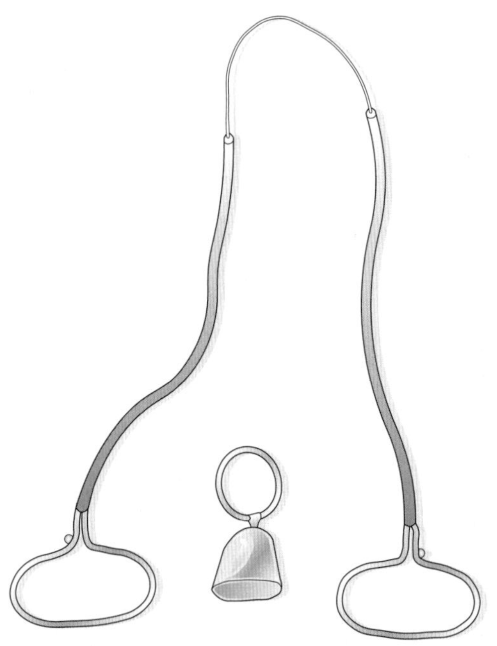

Figure 26.30 The Blond–Heidler and thimble decapitating wire. The ends of the wire (saw) are protected with rubber tubing. The traction handles are detachable.

The middle finger feels for the metal loop that projects from the thimble and, having secured it, pulls the thimble with the attached wire off the thumb and round the fetal neck (Fig 26.31).

The ends of the wire are now mounted on the handles shown in Figure 26.30 and by a to-and-fro motion the neck is severed. This technique is much safer, simpler and less traumatic to the maternal tissues than the previously used decapitation hooks. After the head is completely severed the trunk is removed by traction on the arm (Fig 26.32). The head is steadied by applying suprapubic pressure and can usually be delivered by finger traction

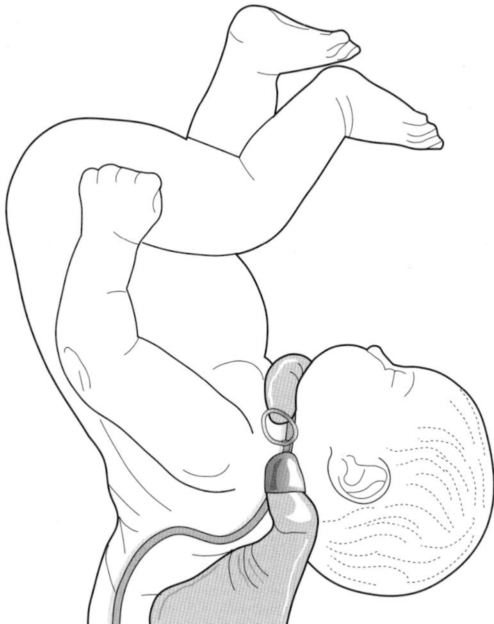

Figure 26.31 Method of passing the decapitating wire around the fetal neck using the Blond–Heidler thimble.

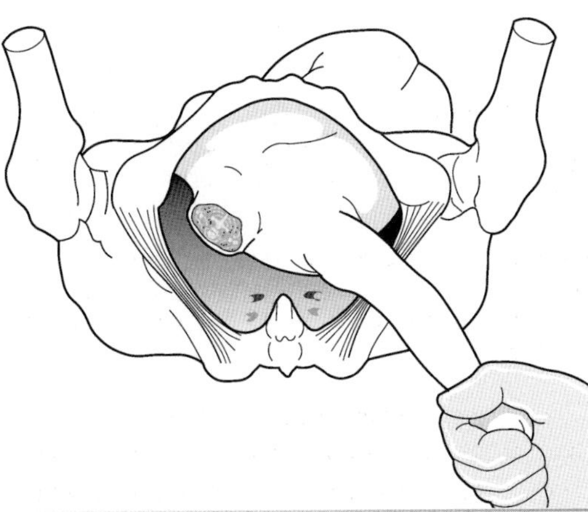

Figure 26.32 Extraction of the trunk by traction on the fetal arm.

through the baby's mouth, or by the application of forceps, or by using vulsellum or other toothed forceps on the fetal scalp. Care must be taken during delivery of the head that sharp bony protrusions of the cervical spine do not injure the maternal tissues.

Evisceration

The operation of evisceration consists in the removal of the abdominal and/or thorax contents, with the object of diminishing the bulk of the child so it can be extracted vaginally. Obviously this is only considered in the case of a dead fetus. It is occasionally necessary in the fetus with a distended abdomen or thorax due to a fluid or a tumour. Using a perforator or embryotomy scissors the abdomen or thorax, whichever is accessible, is opened. The organs are removed manually or by traction with sponge forceps. Entry from the thorax to the abdomen and vice versa can be gained via the diaphragm.

Paracentesis

If there is fetal hydrops of a degree that obstructs labour, and if the fetus is dead or not viable, this can be drained by passing a spinal needle through the maternal abdomen and into the fetal peritoneal cavity. If the fetus is in breech presentation and the legs and breech are delivered with the distended fetal abdomen causing obstruction, this can be drained by a spinal or pudendal block needle guided vaginally. If necessary, scissors, a perforator, or a Drew–Smythe catheter can be used to enter the abdomen and drain the fluid.

Cleidotomy

This is considered in cases where the head is delivered, large shoulders are obstructing delivery and the fetus is dead. If delivery of the shoulders cannot be achieved by the usual manoeuvres used to overcome shoulder dystocia (see Chapter 10) the operation of cleidotomy – division of one or both clavicles to reduce the bulk of the shoulder girdle – is performed. One hand is placed vaginally along the ventral aspect of the fetus and under this protection strong straight embryotomy scissors are introduced to cut the clavicle. It is best to cut the skin over the clavicle first and push the scissors round the bone. Considerable strength is often required to break the bone at about its mid-point.

Post-delivery care

- Active management of the third stage of labour should be carried out and an oxytocin infusion continued for 6–8 hours as the risk of atonic postpartum haemorrhage following prolonged obstructed labour is high.
- The genital tract should be carefully inspected for any signs of trauma, including uterine exploration to rule out rupture. Lacerations of the cervix and vagina should be carefully repaired.
- The bladder in many cases has been distended for a prolonged period of time and an indwelling catheter should be left for 5–7 days to allow bladder tone to be regained.
- Broad-spectrum antibiotics should be continued for several days.
- Thromboprophylaxis should be instituted.
- As much as possible the infant should be restored anatomically with suturing. This, along with careful and tasteful placement of blankets should help reduce the trauma to the parents when they view their newborn dead infant.
- In addition to attention to the physical welfare of the mother her psychological wellbeing and that of her husband/partner and close family members should be considered. The most knowledgeable and senior member of the staff involved should review all of the events with the woman and the implications and plans for subsequent pregnancy care.

It bears re-emphasis that in all cases when destructive operations are considered the operator should consider the alternative of delivery by caesarean section, even if the fetus is dead. This decision will be guided by the availability of safe caesarean section, the operator's experience in destructive operations, and other clinical, social, and cultural aspects, which may include the woman's refusal to have a caesarean delivery and the implications of a caesarean section scar in future pregnancies should she agree to caesarean delivery.

References

1. Giva-Osagie OF, Azzam BB. Destructive operations. Progress in Obstetrics and Gynaecology 1987; 6:211–221.
2. Amoh-Mensah S, Elkins T, Ghosh T, Greenway F, Waite V. Obstetric destructive procedures. Int J Gynaecol Obstet 1996; 54:167–168.
3. Biswas A, Chakraborty PS, Das HS, Bose A, Kalsar PK. Role of destructive operations in modern day obstetrics. J Indian Med Assoc 2001; 99:248,250–251.
4. Arora M, Rajaram P, Oumachigui A, Parveena P. Destructive operations in modern obstetrics in a developing country at a tertiary level. Br J Obstet Gynaecol 1993; 100:967–968.
5. Lawson J. Delivery of the dead or malformed fetus. Clin Obstet Gynaecol 1982; 9:745–755.
6. St. George J. A simple and safe method of vaginal delivery of cases of prolonged obstructed labour with head presentation. West Afr Med J 1975; 23:34–40.

Index

Note: Page numbers in **bold** refer to figures or tables.

A

B

C

D

E

F

G

H

I

K

L

M

R

S

V

W

Y

Z